Occupational Therapy:
Principles & Practice

Alice J. Punwar, M.S., OTR, FAOTA

PROFESSOR, OCCUPATIONAL THERAPY PROGRAM
SCHOOL OF ALLIED HEALTH PROFESSIONS
UNIVERSITY OF WISCONSIN-MADISON
MADISON, WISCONSIN

Occupational Therapy: Principles & Practice

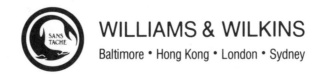

WILLIAMS & WILKINS
Baltimore • Hong Kong • London • Sydney

Editor: John Butler
Associate Editor: Victoria M. Vaughn
Copy Editor: Elizabeth Cowley
Text Design: Alice Sellers/Johnson
Production: Raymond E. Reter
Cover Design: Bets, Ltd

Copyright © 1988
Williams & Wilkins
428 East Preston Street
Baltimore, MD 21202, U.S.A.

Printed in the United States of America

Library of Congress Cataloging in Publication Data

Punwar, Alice J.
  Occupational therapy.

  Includes bibliographies and index.
  1. Occupational therapy—Vocational guidance.
2. Occupational therapy—United States.   3. Occupational
therapy—History.   I. Title. [DNLM: 1. Occupational
Therapy. WB 555 P9840]
RM735.4.P86   1988   615'.8'515   87-10438
ISBN 0-683-06974-8

90 91 92

10 9 8 7 6 5 4

Much have I learned from my teachers,
more from my colleagues, but
most from my students.

Talmud, Ta'anith, 7b

Preface

This book was written to introduce beginning students to the field of occupational therapy and the career opportunities it offers. It is directed at students in both technical and professional occupational therapy programs, since the author believes that beginning students have similar needs for basic information about the field. Throughout the book the contributions of both levels of personnel are discussed, and the author hopes that students will recognize the complementary roles of the registered occupational therapist and the certified occupational therapy assistant and will learn how each supports the other in clinical practice. Nontechnical language has been used as much as possible, and where technical terms appear they have been defined in a glossary that appears at the end of the book.

The text is divided into three major sections. Part I provides background information about the origins of the field, its basic concepts and philosophy, its educational patterns, and the basic practice functions of registered occupational therapists and certified occupational therapy assistants. Part II looks at patterns of health care in the United States and how they developed, discusses team concepts in health care, and gives an overview of the process of service delivery in occupational therapy. The remaining chapters in this section look at practice within a number of specialty areas in the field as well as private practice and indirect service careers. Part III discusses occupational therapy organizations, international occupational therapy, and current trends and future projections for the field. The text is intended to provide basic information for students who are considering a career in occupational therapy. It does not discuss advanced theoretical concepts or practice techniques. There are excellent texts available for such content and the author had no intention of duplicating these efforts.

Many topics of current interest in occupational therapy are discussed only briefly in the text. For this the author apologizes to her colleagues and suggests that the lists of references be used if more in-depth study of specific topics is desired. Although strenuous attempts were made to ensure the accuracy of information presented, there may be errors or omissions that the author hopes students and colleagues will call to her attention. Because publication of a book is a lengthy process, some information may be outdated by the time the book appears in print. This is regretable but unavoidable, and it is suggested that instructors using the text add updated information from current periodicals where necessary. The discussion questions were intended to stimulate students to think about some of the issues raised in each chapter and to engage in discussion of the topics presented.

Each occupational therapist and therapy assistant is likely to have his or her own view of the field and the issues that confront it. This book represents a personal view. Readers should recognize that there are differences of opinion on many of the topics presented. The perspectives given here represent the author's point of view and are not intended to represent the official views of the American Occupational Therapy Association or any other professional organization.

Acknowledgments

This book could not have been completed without the help of many academic and clinical colleagues who provided material, read drafts of chapters, gave both positive and negative feedback, and offered frequent encouragement throughout the writing process. I am most grateful for their help and support.

I would like to acknowledge Dean G. Alan Stull of the School of Allied Health Professions and the Board of Regents of the University of Wisconsin System who approved a two-semester sabbatical leave that enabled me to work on the text uninterrupted by other duties. The patience and perseverence of the Occupational Therapy Program's clerical staff who handled the word processing of the manuscript is gratefully acknowledged.

Special thanks are due to those who made direct contributions of chapters or case material. Martha Stavros and Daraleen Sitka at the University of Michigan Hospitals contributed the chapter on the health care team.

Many clinicians contributed case studies to illustrate aspects of occupational therapy practice. Although all of them could not be included in the text, I am most grateful to the practitioners who responded to my request for case material. The following clinicians provided the case studies that were included in the text and reviewed the chapter in which it appeared for accuracy and currency of information.

Amy Letourneau, OTR, and Pamela Pichette, OTR St. Vincent's Hospital, Green Bay, WI
Joan Loeffelholz, OTR St. Mary's Medical Center, Madison, WI

Chris T. Sparrow, OTR, and staff Sacred Heart Rehabilitation Hospital, Milwaukee, WI
Linda Speer, OTR, and staff Mary Cariola Children's Center Inc. Rochester, NY
Bridget Connolly, OTR and Patti Mader Ebert, OTR Cooperative Educational Service Agency 8, Oshkosh, WI
Cindy Wegrzyn Jernegan, OTR Leader Nursing and Rehabilitation Center, Madison, WI
Margaret Montejano, COTA/L Mercy Hospital and Medical Center, Chicago, IL

Jo Barker, President of the World Federation of Occupational Therapists, served as a consultant for the chapter on international occupational therapy. The staff of the Instructional Media Development Center, who redrew the figures used in the body of the text, made the text visually much more interesting. Tom Diamond, LPT, assisted with the development of the index. I am also grateful to John P. Butler, Senior Editor at Williams & Wilkins, for his encouragement and support and to Victoria Vaughn, Associate Editor, for her direct assistance with the manuscript. My husband, whose unfailing encouragement helped me to complete this project, also deserves special recognition.

ALICE J. PUNWAR, M.S., OTR, FAOTA
University of Wisconsin-Madison
January 30, 1987

Contents

Overview of
Occupational Therapy

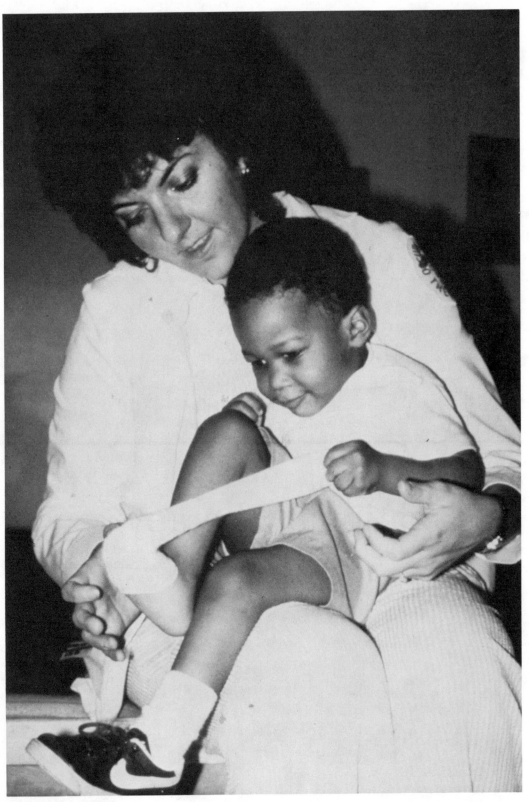

ONE

Defining Occupational Therapy

Passengers were boarding for a four-hour flight to San Francisco and a middle-aged businessman was searching for his seat. He found it and settled in beside an attractive young woman. As the plane took off, he noticed that she was reading a magazine, apparently a trade journal of some kind. When the seat belt sign had been turned off, he introduced himself. "Hello!" I'm Sam Hoffman. I'm a salesman for an industrial equipment firm, and I'm on my way to a trade show in San Francisco. Are you flying for business or pleasure?" The young woman smiled and lowered her magazine. "Both," she admitted. "My name is Gerry White, and I'm on my way to a national occupational therapy conference there. I'm an occupational therapist at Hillside Rehabilitation Center in Chicago." Sam looked puzzled. "What do occupational therapists do?" he asked. "Oh wait, I know. You find jobs for disabled people." "No, not quite," Gerry corrected gently. "We work with people who have been injured or ill to help them regain their maximum function so they can pick up their lives again." Now Sam looked even more puzzled. "I thought physical therapists did that," he said. Gerry sighed. Then she resumed her efforts to explain occu-

pational therapy in a way that would be meaningful to Sam.

Most occupational therapists have had this conversation countless times during their career. *Occupational therapy* is not a household term, although many people have had family members or friends who have received occupational therapy services. Because the field is a broad one and has undergone many changes since its beginnings, it is difficult to define simply and accurately. People often confuse occupational therapists with other health professionals, such as physical therapists, recreational therapists, workers in dance, music, or art therapy, craft instructors, and vocational rehabilitation personnel. Occupational therapy shares some interests with all of these fields, but its chief focus is different.

The term *occupation* has been defined by Kielhofner as "the dominant activity of human beings that includes serious, productive pursuits and playful, creative, festive behaviors" (1). Purposeful goal-directed activity is an essential part of any person's life. Occupational therapy is based on the belief that purposeful activity (occupation) may be used to prevent physical and psychosocial dysfunction and to restore function to more normal levels. *Occupations*, as used in this sense, are activities that are selected for their therapeutic value and that the occupational therapist uses to help the client regain abilities that have been lost or limited due to physical or psychological disturbances. Although an occupational therapist may utilize art, music, dance, or craft activities, the focus is always on the achievement of a therapeutic goal. Activities are not used as recreation or to fill in empty time or for self-expression, but rather as a means to a therapeutic end. It is this goal directedness that characterizes the occupational therapist's use of activities. Each activity has a specific purpose and is used for a reason.

In 1979 the American Occupational Therapy Association adopted a philosophical statement that describes the profession's beliefs about how human activity is related to health and well-being:

Man is an active being whose development is influenced by the use of purposeful activity. Using their capacity for intrinsic motivation, human beings are able to influence their physical and mental health and their social and physical environment through purposeful activity. Human life includes a process of continuous adaptation. Adaptation is a change in function that promotes survival and self-actualization. Biological, psychological, and environmental factors may interrupt the adaptation process at any time throughout the life cycle. Dysfunction may occur when adapation is impaired. Purposeful activity facilitates the adaptive process. Occupational therapy is based on the belief that purposeful activity (occupation), including its interpersonal and environmental components, may be used to prevent and mediate dysfunction and to elicit maximum adaptation. Activity as used by the occupational therapist includes both an intrinsic and a therapeutic purpose (2).

Definitions of occupational therapy have changed over the years. Early definitions emphasized the use of occupation as remedial activity to help restore the individual to an improved state of physical and mental health. It was viewed as a medically prescribed form of treatment and was usually conducted in a hospital, sanitorium, or community workshop. Arts and crafts activities were considered the primary tools of the occupational therapist during these formative years of the field, and the therapist was viewed as a specialist in the selection and application of planned programs of activity that were expected to directly improve the condition of the client. The goal of such programs was to help the individual resume as much of his or her normal pattern of living as possible. This included the work role as well as the daily home tasks of the client. Occupational therapy was regarded as a gradual preparation of the client to return to work responsibilities or, if that was impossible, to explore feasible vocational alternatives. The relationship of occupational therapy to the work roles of clients has made for some confusion of occupational therapists with vocational rehabilitation workers, who provide counseling and job training for individuals who are unable to return to their previous jobs.

As occupational therapy grew and expanded, it was used with clients who had many different kinds of limitations and who were being cared for in a variety of settings. Occupational therapists began to work in outpatient clinics, community mental health centers, public and private schools, nursing homes, home health care agencies, and private or group practices. Therapists were working with clients of all age levels and with a wide range of physical and psychosocial disorders. This diversity of practice made it difficult to define the field simply and yet comprehensively. The American Occupational

Therapy Association, however, has provided definitions to reflect the growing scope of the field. A recent statement was published in 1981 when some states were beginning to adopt state licensure for occupational therapists. The following definition describes current occupational therapy practice and is one of several in general use today.

Occupational therapy is the use of purposeful activity with individuals who are limited by physical injury or illness, psychosocial dysfunction, developmental or learning disabilities, poverty and cultural differences or the aging process in order to maximize independence, prevent disability, and maintain health. The practice encompasses evaluation, treatment, and consultation. Specific occupational therapy services include: teaching daily living skills; developing perceptual-motor skills and sensory integrative functioning; developing play skills and prevocational and leisure capacities; designing, fabricating, or applying selected orthotic and prosthetic devices or selective adaptive equipment; using specifically designed crafts and exercises to enhance functional performance; administering and interpreting tests such as manual muscle or range of motion tests; and adapting environments for the handicapped. These services are provided individually, in groups, or through social systems. (3)

This definition describes well the diverse practice and scope of occupational therapy today. There are several key phrases in the definition that are important to the understanding of occupational therapy. The concept of *purposeful activity* is a central one to the field. There is always a reason for the selection of a given client activity, and therapists draw on their scientific knowledge of their clients' condition and needs as well as their repertoire of potential activities in making that selection.

The 1981 definition also clearly defines the populations with which occupational therapists work. With all clients, the end goals of occupational therapy intervention are "to maximize independence, prevent disability, and to maintain health" (3). This goes farther than earlier definitions in its inclusion of prevention and health maintenance as valid outcomes of occupational therapy. The specific services of occupational therapists are spelled out by the definition, as well as patterns of service delivery. Because of the increasing need for containment of health care costs, occupational therapy clients are being seen more often in groups today, although individual treatment still occurs. Occupational therapists are also becoming more involved in the legislative process and are serving as advocates for their client populations when health and social welfare issues are under consideration by legislative bodies.

This definition of occupational therapy accurately reflects the broad scope of the field today. We may well see further changes in the definition of occupational therapy as health care and services change to meet the needs of society. But let's get back to our in-flight conversation. Gerry is just finishing her explanation of occupational therapy to Sam by saying, "Although I myself work with the physically handicapped, other therapists are working with learning-disabled children, the mentally retarded, people who have psychological problems, or older people who need help in adapting to the changes caused by aging. Even though we work with so many different kinds of people, our goal is basically the same: to help people live as normally and as fully as possible within their own environment." "I see," said Sam enthusiastically, "you help people learn to help themselves." "That's it!" agreed Gerry, beaming. "Now you've got it!" Both settled back in their seats for the flight ahead.

DISCUSSION QUESTIONS

1. What are some of the misconceptions you have heard about occupational therapy?

2. When people ask you what occupational therapy is, how do you define it?

3. How did you learn about occupational therapy as a potential career?

REFERENCES

1. Kielhofner G: *Willard and Spackman's Occupational Therapy*, ed. 6. Philadephia, JB Lippencott, 1983, p. 31.
2. The philosophical base of occupational therapy. Minutes of the 1979 AOTA Representative Assembly. *AJOT* 33:785, 1979.
3. Resolution Q: Definition of occupational therapy for licensure. Minutes of the 1981 AOTA Representative Assembly. *AJOT* 35:798–799, 1981.

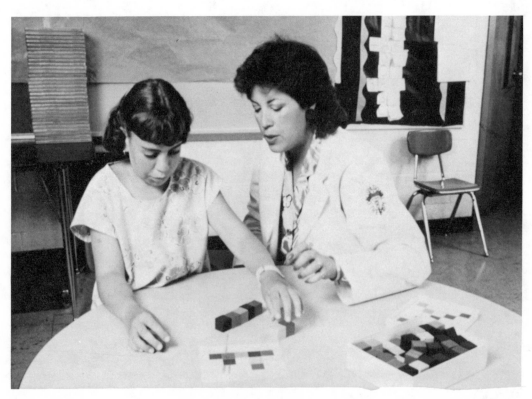

TWO

Use of Activity as a Therapeutic Tool

Occupational therapy uses purposeful activity as its medium to help clients accomplish their desired goals. Occupational therapists and therapy assistants are activity specialists; their primary role is to draw on their knowledge of activities and select and apply those that are most likely to meet the needs of their clients. This chapter discusses how occupational therapists and certified occupational therapy assistants use activities to promote and maintain health, prevent injury or disability, and help their clients develop or redevelop needed abilities and skills.

When occupational therapists discuss their field, they are careful to describe their methods as *purposeful activity*, a term that the American Occupational Therapy Association has defined.

Individuals engage in purposeful activity as part of their daily life routine. Purposeful activity, in this natural context, can be defined as tasks or experiences in which the individual actively participates. Engagement in purposeful activity requires and elicits coordination between one's physical, emotional, and cognitive systems. An individual who is involved in purposeful activity directs attention to the task itself, rather than to the internal processes required for achievement of the task. Activities may yield immediate results or may require sustained effort and multiple repetition. They may represent novel and singular responses or be part of complex, long-standing patterns of behavior. Purposeful activities, influenced by the individual's life roles, have unique meaning to each person (1).

When we look at healthy people, we see that activity is part of the normal pattern of life. We all engage in many different activities each day, and often complete them with little conscious thought or effort. The routine self-care tasks of getting up in the morning, bathing, dressing, combing our hair, shaving or putting on makeup, eating breakfast, and getting ourselves off to work or school do not take up much of our attention; yet they are essential parts of our daily life. It is only when some circumstance—an injury, an illness, or psychological stress—interferes with our ability to perform these tasks in the ordinary way that we begin to be concerned and realize how much we have taken for granted.

Each individual has his or her own

pattern of daily activities. The pattern may be influenced by the individual's environment, age or developmental level, socioeconomic status, life-style, family and friends, and culture. As individuals grow and develop, their activity pattern changes as their life roles and societal expectations change. Play forms an important part of the young child's pattern of daily activities. Through play the child learns how to interact with the environment, to master gross and fine motor skills, to communicate, and to relate to people. Rest or sleep is another large part of the child's daily activity schedule. Work activities are present only in the form of play, as new skills are practiced and refined. When the child begins school, learning activities become the "work." For the middle-aged person, work takes up a very large proportion of the daily activity pattern. Leisure hours may be few, since work may be taken home in the evening or thought about even though it was left at the workplace. The weekend is anticipated with pleasure, since it means a welcome break from the daily demands of a job. Sleep and rest take up a moderate amount of time, but often the amount of rest is considered insufficient. The daily activity pattern is dramatically different for these two individuals, but each is typical for the period of life represented. Cynkin (2) has written about how normal individuals use activity in their daily lives. "Health is manifested in the ability of an individual to participate in socioculturally delineated and prescribed activities with satisfaction and comfort." In other words, participation in the activities sanctioned by the culture is a mark of physical and psychological health.

When the ability to function in daily life is impaired because of injury, illness, psychological stress, changing developmental or environmental demands, or lack of skill, the individual becomes a candidate for occupational therapy services. The occupational therapist will evaluate the client's present performance abilities and, based on those findings, will develop a program of activities to help meet the client's needs. Activity experiences will be designed to offer the client opportunities to learn and practice needed skills so that much or all of the client's personal pattern of daily activities may be resumed. If the injury or disorder is complex, a remedial activity may be broken down into very small steps so that the client can work on each step sequentially. The end goal is accomplishment of the total task. In situations where the disability is permanent, the occupational therapist may decide to help the client adapt to the limitations by teaching different ways of performing needed tasks or by providing special pieces of equipment that will enable the client to function. In this way, the disability is compensated for and the client may continue to perform the desired activity.

Occupational therapy treatment activities must usually be individually planned for each client. Although two people may have similar disabilities, their attitudes, interests, goals, and life circumstances may be quite different. Occupational therapy attempts to meet these individual needs by designing activity programs that will provide the specific support and assistance needed by each client. Although occupational therapy does make use of group treatment approaches, individual client goals are never lost sight of. The group may be a vehicle for the achievement of some of those goals. Occupational therapy treatment activities cannot be routinely prescribed and applied. There are no "recipes" for the use of activity as a therapeutic tool.

OCCUPATIONAL PERFORMANCE AND PERFORMANCE COMPONENTS

One way to view the therapeutic use of activity is to look at the domain of occupational therapy. Mosey (3) has said that the domain of occupational therapy consists of "performance components within the context of age, occupational performance, and an individual's environment."

The term *occupational performance* refers to the individual's total life pattern, including activities of daily living, work, recreation or leisure, and the ability to organize one's time to meet one's roles and responsibilities (temporal adaptation). Occupational performance is the big picture of how the individual functions within the context of his or her environment. To function effectively, the individual must have a variety of subskills that contribute to total performance. These microabilities or performance components are the building blocks that support occupational performance and are necessary to normal functioning. Sensory integration refers to

one group of performance components that focus on the ability of the central nervous system to organize and use sensory stimuli for planned interaction with the external environment. Neuromuscular functions are another component of performance and refer to the ability to use one's body to move and respond effectively. Cognitive function is needed for performance and refers to the ability of the brain to learn, remember, understand, conceptualize, and solve problems. Psychological performance components include the ability to perceive oneself and others realistically and to express one's feelings and understand those of others. Social interaction components refer to the realm of human experience in which we learn to relate to others in meaningful ways and are able to function in group situations. As occupational performance describes the global

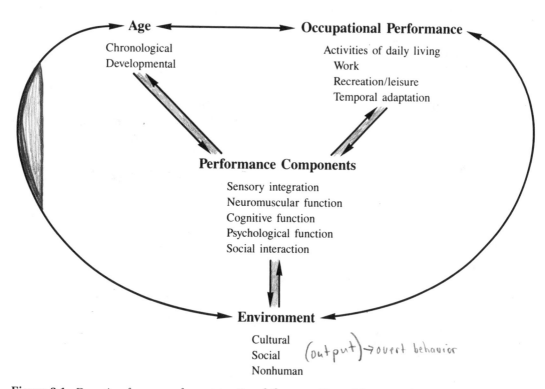

Figure 2.1. Domain of concern for occupational therapy. (From Mosey A: *Occupational Therapy: Configuration of a Profession*. New York, Raven Press, 1981, p. 75.

picture of the individual's ability to function in his or her environment, performance components describe the subskills that, when combined effectively, allow participation in a full range of daily activities. Figure 1 illustrates the relationships between occupational performance, performance components, and the environment.

Looking at the domain of occupational therapy in this way helps us to understand how activities are used as therapy in clinical occupational therapy programs. For individuals who show impairments in occupational performance, we need to look first at how those problems are being manifested. Is the individual unable to perform daily work tasks? Is the individual limited in carrying out daily self-care or having problems with the use of leisure time? Once the problem areas have been identified, we need to determine why the problems are occurring. Is a neuromuscular disorder interfering with the ability to move or coordinate movement? Is the client showing signs of depression and lack of self-esteem? Do perceptual disorders interfere with the client's ability to respond to sensory input? By evaluating the client's performance components, the occupational therapist attempts to identify the root causes of the limitations in occupational performance. Once these have been identified, the therapist will be able to set appropriate goals and design treatment activities intended to improve weak or damaged performance components or to compensate for them. Treatment goals are usually discussed with the client and mutually agreed upon. It is essential that the client's needs and wishes be taken into account when planning a therapeutic program, since the client's interest and active participation are critical to the achievement of a successful outcome. In planning a therapeutic program, the occupational therapist relies on his or her knowledge of effective activities used by other occupational therapists for this type of dysfunction, on the results of research, and on past experience working with this type of disorder.

CHANGING CONCEPTS OF THERAPEUTIC ACTIVITY

Activities are the tools of occupational therapy, but what kind of activities and how are they applied? In the early days of the field, arts and crafts activities were heavily used. They were considered a first step toward vocational training, and a strong work orientation was present in many of the early descriptions of therapeutic activities. Haas (4), writing in 1925, described a comprehensive occupational therapy program in the men's division of Bloomingdale Hospital, an institution for the mentally ill. Haas, an early occupational therapist, was a craftsman and a craft instructor. He utilized activities such as industrial brush making, chair caning, basketry, metal work, jewelry making, construction of concrete garden furniture, stringing tennis rackets, making tennis and basketball nets, and furniture making. The therapeutic uses of each activity were described, with case studies showing the benefits achieved by some of the residents of the institution. High-quality work was expected and good work habits were encouraged.

As times and conditions changed, occupational therapy media changed. Fidler (5), writing in 1948, suggested a method of analyzing potential treatment activities in terms of their psychological characteristics. She recommended that the mental as well as the physical processes demanded by an activity be considered and urged that therapists consider the opportunities an activity provided for creative expression, expression of feelings, assumption of social roles, and adaptability. Fields (6), writing in 1956, deplored the declining use of arts and crafts activities in occupational therapy and the increasing use of "industrial media." She urged the use of a broad range of activities as therapy, including the creative arts and music, to meet the diverse needs of clients.

TOOLS OF OCCUPATIONAL THERAPY

Mosey (3) in 1981 identified six "legitimate tools" of occupational therapy. We will look at these tools in detail and will describe how occupational therapists use them in programs of intervention.

THE NONHUMAN ENVIRONMENT

The physical surroundings are one tool that the occupational therapist can manipulate to help the client achieve security, mastery of environmental interactions, and a source of pleasure and relaxation. For example, the therapist or therapy assistant may suggest environmental modifications that will make an elderly client's home a safer and more convenient place to live.

THE CONSCIOUS USE OF SELF

Occupational therapists and therapy assistants learn to use their personalities as a therapeutic tool to alleviate client anxiety, provide reassurance or information, and assist the client in mobilizing and using inner resources. *Use of self* means that the therapist engages in planned interactions with clients to help them toward their therapeutic goals. Therapists must be well aware of their own feelings and reactions when engaged in such interactions and must be able to express their feelings as well as be sensitive and receptive to those of their clients. Effective use of self

depends heavily on the therapist's people skills and the ability to communicate clearly and directly.

THE TEACHING-LEARNING PROCESS

Each therapist-client interaction can be viewed as a teaching-learning situation in which the therapist helps clients to experience, learn, and practice new behaviors that will enable them to function more effectively in daily life. The therapist and therapy assistant are teachers, and study of learning theories and principles helps make the learning process easier and more effective for the client.

USE OF PURPOSEFUL ACTIVITIES

Purposeful activity involves interaction with both the human and nonhuman environments and is one of the ways in which people achieve mastery or competence. Activities may be realistic, symbolic, or a little of both. In occupational therapy, purposeful activities usually relate to the domains of work, leisure or self-care. They may be done in the natural environment or may be simulated. For example, handicapped homemakers may be taught adapted cooking methods in their own kitchens or in a simulated kitchen in a hospital occupational therapy clinic. To be effective, purposeful activities used as therapy must be relevant to the needs, interests, and capacities of the client. They must be sufficiently interesting that the client will be motivated to perform them, and they must lead to functions that the client wants to be able to perform in his or her daily environment. New activities are constantly being added to the occupational therapy repertoire. Many of the technologies now developing offer considerable promise as therapeutic activities. In 1983 Holm (7) suggested that videotape be utilized in occupational therapy clinical programs for a variety of therapeutic purposes. The sophisticated personal computers now available offer many possibilities for use in assessing client performance skills and training for needed abilities.

ACTIVITY GROUPS

Activity groups are made up of individuals who share common concerns or who need to work on similar problems or deficiencies. Because we all function in many kinds of group situations, we need to know how to relate to group members effectively, how to get our own needs met within groups, and how to recognize and help meet the needs of other group members. Mosey (3) describes activity groups as laboratories for learning, because they provide opportunities for individuals to try out and practice ways of dealing with others in a relatively safe environment. Activity groups involve a "doing" process. They differ from verbal therapy groups in that the group members work on purposeful activities as well as take part in group discussion. The activity helps to focus the group's attention on problems and issues in need of resolution and provides a structure and organization that many clients need. Many people find it easier to talk about themselves when they are engaged in an activity. Cooperative interaction is fostered, since the group must complete a common task. The occupational therapist or therapy assistant serves as a facilitator for the group and guides it toward positive interactions and resolution of conflicts. Therapists using group techniques must be familiar with group dynamics, communication, and group leadership methods.

In 1985 Duncombe and Howe (8) conducted a survey of occupational therapy practice to determine how occupational therapists used group techniques. They found that 60% of the therapists surveyed in all areas of practice were using group treatment approaches. Of these, 54% reported using activity groups, while 24% were using verbal groups. Specific types of groups being used included exercise groups, cooking groups, activities of daily living groups, self-expression groups, task groups, arts and crafts groups, feeling-oriented discussion groups, reality-oriented discussion groups, sensorimotor groups, and education groups.

ACTIVITY ANALYSIS AND SYNTHESIS

The occupational therapist and the therapy assistant must be skilled in the process of analyzing activities for their potential therapeautic value. Activity analysis is the process of examining the task or activity in terms of its smallest performance components. The task of selecting an appropriate treatment activity is essentially one of matching an activity to the specific needs of the client. If the match is a good one, the activity chosen will help the client to achieve his therapy goals.

Activity analysis may be general in nature or may be related to a specific theoretical frame of reference. A general activity analysis looks at the factors that have traditionally been accepted as part of the domain of occupational therapy. The sample activity analysis outline shown on page 18 is an example of this general approach (Schneider M, Cordero J, Decker J. Activity analysis form. Occupational Therapy Program. Univ. of Wisconsin at Madison. Unpublished.) The activity analysis outline shown on page 19–21 is one that has been derived from a theoretical frame of reference (9). The frame of reference is that of human occupation, as described by Kielhofner and his colleagues (9). In this approach a specific activity is analyzed in terms of the model of human occupation. The questions asked are different from those on the general activity analysis outline, because the model of human occupation looks at activities in their broadest sense, as a part of the whole spectrum of human occupation. To use this format to analyze an activity, one needs to be familiar with the concepts of human occupation and how these are applied in clinical occupational therapy programs. To effectively analyze any activity, one must be familiar with the activity, the materials used, the necessary tools, and the processes involved. The therapist or therapy assistant should have had direct experience with the activity. In educational programs that prepare registered occupational therapists and certified occupational therapy assistants, the study of activity analysis and the learning of a broad range of potentially therapeutic activities comprise an important part of the curriculum.

SELECTION OF THERAPEUTIC ACTIVITIES

Cynkin (2) offers some guidelines for the selection of appropriate therapeutic activities. She notes that treatment activities must be meaningful to the client and appropriate to the setting in which they are being used. They should be practical— easily administered and compatible with the amount of time available for treatment. They should be versatile and adaptable so that they can be graded and adjusted to different client needs. It should be possible to grade the activity in terms of difficulty, physical and psychological demands, cognitive requirements, and/or social characteristics. Therapeutic activities should lend themselves to a step-by-step progression and to a systematic, structured approach. One activity may build on another, so that each takes the client fur-

ther toward achievement of a treatment goal. The therapist must be alert to a client's changing needs and must be able to adjust the treatment activities accordingly. In planning the sequence of treatment, the therapist must anticipate events likely to occur during the treatment process and should be prepared to vary the program as needed (2).

EXAMPLES OF THERAPEUTIC ACTIVITY USE

Work

Let us now look briefly at some recent reports of how activity has been used as treatment in the three domains of work, use of leisure time, and self-care. In May of 1985 the *American Journal of Occupational Therapy* devoted an entire issue to work evaluation in occupational therapy. In a paper describing the historical involvement and interest of occupational therapy in work, Marshall (10) pointed out that in its earliest years, occupational therapy was developing work programs for the mentally ill. By the late 1930s, prevocational evaluation was becoming part of the practice of occupational therapy, and therapists were using crafts to develop skills that would be readily transferable to industry. The emphasis on work evaluation and training continued until the 1950s, when professionals in the field of vocational rehabilitation began to assume more of the responsibility for work evaluation and training programs. Occupational therapy largely neglected these areas until the 1970s, when there was a resurgence of interest in work roles and the contributions occupational therapy could make to preparing clients for work.

Therapists working with physical limitations have frequently been involved with work evaluation and training programs. Bettencourt and his colleagues (11) have described a comprehensive program of work simulation used with clients who had back injuries. The program was sponsored by an insurance company that provided rehabilitation services for policyholders who had been injured on the job. Treatment included client education, focusing on anatomy, body mechanics, and energy conservation so that clients would fully understand their treatment program. Activities were then begun to develop the physical abilities and skills needed for specific job performance. Elaborate equipment was developed for the program, including a balance monitor to determine distribution of weight by the client and a multiwork station that stimulated carpentry construction tasks, plumbing jobs, and electrical wiring jobs. A truck simulator was used to practice driving skills, and a pneumatic lift platform simulated lifting tasks. An upper extremity simulator provided graded practice with a variety of industrial tools. Much of the equipment was computerized and provided immediate feedback on the amount of muscular effort being exerted and other parameters of function. Such sophisticated programs provide close approximation of the work tasks that clients will be returning to and can directly prepare them to resume their jobs.

LEISURE

The use of leisure time is another area in which occupational therapy makes use of activity to contribute to the client's health and well-being. Occupational therapy has long been interested in the role of play in the growth and development of children. Gliner (12) has suggested that purposeful activity is an essential component to the learning of coordination and motor skills. He saw the therapist's role in motor development as one of structuring client-environmental interactions in a purposeful way to allow for the development or refinement of motor skills. Ayres (13) and her colleagues working with learning disabled and autistic children have used a variety of movement experiences and games to improve perceptual and motor planning skills. With adult clients, constructive use of leisure time is frequently a focus of occupational therapy intervention. Many people have difficulty finding satisfying ways of using their leisure time and may instead develop negative or destructive patterns of behavior. The occupational therapist or therapy assistant can serve as a guide to low-cost community activities that can provide social stimulation and personal satisfaction. With the middle-aged population, retirement planning may be a major concern. Broderick and Glazer (14) conducted a study of 60 retired men and found that those who had a high level of preretirement participation in leisure activities were the most likely to show a high degree of planning for their retirement. Those retired persons who were the most socially active also showed the most positive attitudes toward retirement. There is a definite role for occupational therapists and therapy assistants in helping the aging population find fulfilling leisure activities that can be carried into the retirement years.

Arnetz (15) reported the results of a study conducted in Sweden on the effects of a social activation program carried out in a senior citizen apartment building. She found that residents who participated in a six-month activity program showed a threefold increase in their activity level following the program. The people who benefited most were those who had been the most passive and isolated prior to the study. Arnetz concluded that occupational therapy programs play an important role in preventing social isolation in elderly persons who live in institional environments.

SELF-CARE

Self-care has been a traditional focus of occupational therapy services in the past and continues to be a necessary part of the treatment program of many clients. Traditionally, the phrase *activities of daily living* (frequently abbreviated ADL) has included feeding, dressing, personal hygiene, travel and transportation, and other abilities needed to function in daily life. In our society, independence in such tasks is highly valued and most of us are reluctant to accept help. Attention to the performance of daily living skills is essential to help many clients retain their sense of self-worth and competence.

With the advent of sophisticated electronic equipment, occupational therapists and therapy assistants have found new ways of making the performance of daily tasks easier for severely disabled clients. In a 1984 report, Seplowitz (16) described the case of a 39-year-old quadriplegic client who had suffered secondary neurologic complications. Seplowitz was able to adapt an inexpensive remote control unit, which enabled the client to operate his stereo, dictaphone, lights, television, telephone, CB radio, and tape recorder by himself. He was also able to operate his home computer with the use of hand splints. These adaptations allowed him to remain mentally active and productive and gave him some degree of control over his immediate environment. Seplowitz noted that advances in medical care and technology are enabling severely disabled clients to live longer. Such individuals are being discharged from medical facilities earlier than in the past and have very complex needs. Occupational therapy can play a major role in helping these people to be as productive and in control as they wish to be, even though seriously limited in their performance abilities.

Training and practice in self-care activities is also useful for clients with psychosocial disturbances or developmental disabilities. Many clients are unable to live independently in the community because they lack essential self-care skills. Learning to manage money, shop sensibly, perform household maintenance tasks, do laundry, or cook for themselves are skills that can be taught, either individually or in groups. With opportunities to learn and practice such skills, many disabled persons can live and function adequately in community settings.

Additional examples of the use of activity are found in the individual case studies in part II of this text. In writing about the occupational therapy heritage of activity, Kielhofner (17) summarized some of the most basic occupational therapy concepts. He noted that one of the premises of the field from its earliest times was that human beings have an occupational nature. When illness or disability interfered with the mental or physical activities of the individual, deterioration of both faculties could result. Because occupation was a natural method of maintaining the organization of both body and mind, it was logical to assume that it could be used as a means of restoring function. These fundamental beliefs about the nature and value of activity in human life continue to underly occupational therapy practice today and form the basis of all occupational therapy intervention.

DISCUSSION QUESTIONS

1. Activities can be used to maintain health and prevent problems as well as improve impaired functions. Can you think of some ways that you can utilize activities to maintain good physical and psychological health?

2. Think of a new skill that you have recently learned. What kind of cognitive abilities are required to perform this skill?

What kind of movements? What kind of social or psychological abilities?

3. Occupational therapy activities are constantly changing as new media are developed and as the needs of clients change. List some recently developed activities, materials, or pieces of equipment that might have application in occupational therapy.

4. Imagine that a group of people share a common need to be able to live in their homes or apartments without requiring constant help and support from their families or friends. How could an activity group be used to help them develop independent living skills?

5. Do the meanings of activities vary from one culture to another? Give an example of how an activity might be interpreted differently by people from different cultural backgrounds.

6. Constructive and satisfying use of leisure time may be a goal in some occupational therapy intervention programs. List several activities that might be useful in helping clients develop better social interactions with others through recreational opportunities.

7. Are some activities in our society gender related? Discuss some activities that might be considered primarily male or female oriented.

GENERAL ACTIVITY ANALYSIS FORMAT[a]

I. Information Identifying the Activity
   Equipment needed
   Materials needed
   Source of materials
   Time needed to complete
   Cost
   Precautions
   Appropriate age group
   Gender association
   Technical skill needed
II. Sensory Qualities of the Activity
   Tactile
   Auditory
   Gustatory
   Visual
   Olfactory
III. Physical Abilities Needed
   Position
   Range of motion
   Muscle strength
   Coordination
   Grasp and prehension pattern
   Movements
IV. Psychosocial Characteristics
   Amount of structure
   Amount of resistiveness
   Neatness/messiness
   Passive/aggressive
   Automatic/requires attention
   Reality oriented/symbolic
V. Cognitive Characteristics
   Amount of attention required
   Opportunity for decision making
   Opportunity for problem solving
   Memory requirements
VI. Interpersonal Characteristics of the Activity
   Individual
   Group
   Cooperative
   Competitive
VII. Perceptual Skills Required
   Visual figure-ground perception
   Form constancy
   Position in space
   Crossing the midline
   Motor planning
VIII. Adaptability
   How can the activity be adapted for varying physical, cognitive, or interpersonal abilities?

IX. Gradability

How can the activity be graded for varying physical, cognitive, or interpersonal abilities?

---

[a]Occupational Therapy Program, University of Wisconsin, Madison, Wisconsin.

OCCUPATIONAL ANALYSIS ACCORDING TO THE MODEL OF HUMAN OCCUPATION[a]

I. Environmental Analysis
  A. Objectives: What objects are used in this occupation, and what are their characteristics?
  B. Tasks: What action sequences must be carried out? What are important task characteristics?
  C. Social Groups/Organizations: What social groups or organizations use this activity?
  D. Culture: What is the cultural significance of this activity?

II. Volitional Analysis
  A. Personal Causation: Does this occupation provide experiences of personal effectiveness through use of skills relevant to everyday life? Does it provide experience in management of external and internal control? Are the outcomes of the occupation predictable?
  B. Values: What are the inherent performance standards? What awareness of time and of time use is developed in this occupation? What other values may be enacted?
  C. Interests: Does the occupation provide variety? Is it likely to be familiar to many people? Is it widely available?

III. Habituation Analysis
  A. Roles: Is this occupation important in the performance of the following roles? Worker, caregiver, home maintainer, family member, friend, student, volunteer, organization participant, religious participant, hobbyist/amateur, other? Explain briefly.
  B. Habits: Describe the primary habit systems that organize behavior in this occupation.

IV. Performance Analysis
  A. Perceptual-motor: How are perceptual-motor skills used in the performance of this occupation?
  B. Process: How are process skills used?
  C. Communication/Interaction: How are interpersonal skills used?

V. Output Analysis
  A. Work: How is this occupation used in work tasks?
  B. Play: How is this occupation used in play or leisure?
  C. Daily Living Tasks: How is this occupation used in daily living tasks?

---

[a]From Barris R (ed): *Workbook: Applying the Model of Human Occupation* in Kielhofner G: *A Model of Human Occupation*. Baltimore, Williams & Wilkins, 1985, pp. 426–435.

CLINICAL OCCUPATIONAL ANALYSIS

I. Exploratory Learning
  A. Skill Sequence: What graded behaviors need to be learned in order to perform this occupation?
  B. Occupational Environment: What arrangements of objects, tasks, social groups, or cultural contexts will encourage the learning of this occupation?

II. Competence Learning: How can the occupation be practiced as part of daily routines in
    A.   Daily living tasks
    B.   Leisure
    C.   Work

III. Achievement Learning: How can the occupation be used in role performance?
    A.   Standard of performance
    B.   Trials: identify a graded sequence of trials in using the occupation, including planning, implementation, and feedback.

OCCUPATIONAL RELEVANCE SCALE[a]

Evaluate the occupation on the following factors, placing check marks in the appropriate columns.

	High	Moderate	Low
Performance/output:			
Uses a variety of skills			
Important in work, play, and daily living tasks			
Behavioral organization:			
Used in many roles			
Generates practical habit patterns			
Motivation:			
Allows a wide range of choice			
Is highly valued in the dominant culture			
Environmental press:			
Can be easily practiced in ordinary settings			
Can generate various levels of arousal . .			

[a]From Barris R (ed): Workbook: Applying the Model of Human Occupation. In Kielhofner G: *A Model of Human Occupation*. Baltimore, Williams & Wilkins, 1985. pp. 426–435.

REFERENCES

1. Hinojosa J, Sabari J, Rosenfeld M: Purposeful activities. *AJOT* 37:805–806, 1983.
2. Cynkin S: *Occupational Therapy: Toward Health Through Activities*. Boston, Little, Brown & Co., 1979, pp. 33, 47–58.
3. Mosey A: *Occupational Therapy: Configuration of a Profession*. New York, Raven Press, 1981, pp. 74–79, 89–118.
4. Haas L: *Occupational Therapy*. Milwaukee, Bruce Publishing, 1925, pp. 38–50.
5. Fidler GS: Psychological evaluation of occupational therapy activities. *AJOT* II:284–287, 1948.
6. Fields B: *What is realism in occupational therapy? AJOT* X:9–10, 1956.
7. Holm MB: Video as a medium in occupational therapy. *AJOT* 37:531–534, 1983.
8. Duncombe LW, Howe MC: Group work in occupational therapy: a survey of practice. *AJOT* 39:163–170, 1985.
9. Barris R (ed): *Workbook: Applying the Model of Human Occupation*. In Kielhofner G: *A Model of Human Occupation*. Baltimore, Williams & Wilkins, 1985, pp. 426–435.
10. Marshall E: Looking backward. *AJOT* 39:297–300, 1985.
11. Bettencourt C, Carlstrom P, Brown SH, Lindau K, Long CM: Using work simulation to treat adults with back injuries. *AJOT* 40:12–18, 1986.
12. Gliner JA: Purposeful activity in motor learning theory: an event approach to motor skill acquisition. *AJOT* 39:28–34, 1985.
13. Ayres A: *Sensory Integration and the Child*. Los Angeles, Western Psychological Services, 1979, pp. 135–156.
14. Broderick T, Glazer B: Leisure participation and the retirement process. *AJOT* 37:15–22, 1983.
15. Arnetz BB: Gerontic occupation therapy—psychological and social predictors of participation and therapeutic benefits. *AJOT* 39:460–465, 1985.
16. Seplowitz C: Technology and occupational therapy in the rehabilitation of the bedridden quadriplegic. *AJOT* 38:743–747, 1984.
17. Kielhofner G: A heritage of activity: development of theory. *AJOT* 36:723–730, 1982.

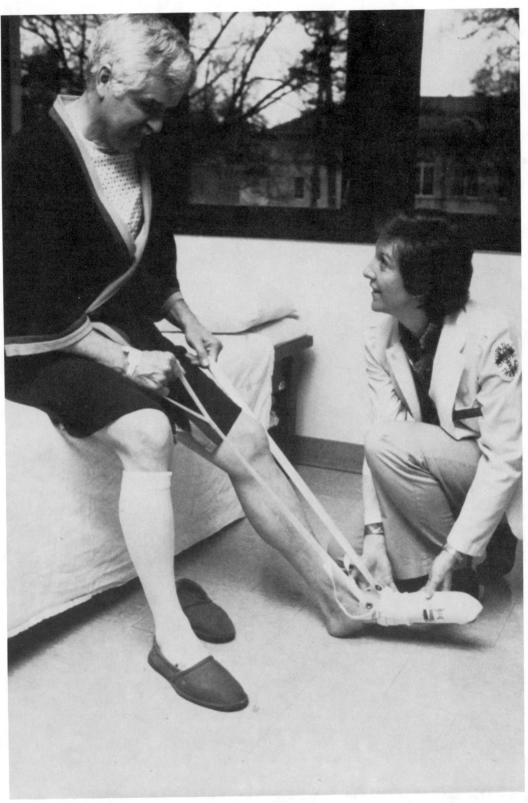

THREE

Historical Development of the Field

Although occupational therapy is a relatively new field, beliefs concerning the curative value of occupation are found in the records of many civilizations. Dr. Sidney Licht, in his *Occupational Therapy Source Book* quotes from the writings of Asclepiades, the early Greek physician, who advocated the use of music, exercise, and occupation for the treatment of mental illness (1). There are references in Egyptian records from 200 BC describing large temples dedicated to Saturn to which people afflicted with melancholia were brought in search of a cure. Groves and gardens were cultivated in which they could exercise, and boating excursions on the Nile and other pleasurable activities were arranged to distract individuals from their troubles and offer them alternative occupations (2).

It is generally agreed that the progressive ideas of Dr. Philippe Pinel, who was medical director of the Bicêtre hospital in Paris in the late eighteenth century, provided inspiration for the use of organized programs of activity and occupation in institutions for the mentally ill in Europe and in America. Pinel could not accept the neglect and cruelty commonly found in asylums for the insane at that time and shocked many of his contemporaries by releasing 50 "maniacs" from their chains at his institution in 1792. He experimented by replacing physical restraint with the use of physical exercise and manual occupations with these inmates, and in 1801 he described his results in a book. Pinel recommended the use of such activities in all mental hospitals "as a means of securing good morale and discipline" (1). Johann Reil in Germany agreed and added his own verification of the effectiveness of such methods in a paper published in 1803 (1). Other enlightened thinkers in Europe had begun to make similar efforts.

In England, Samuel Tuke, an English Quaker, established an asylum for the insane at York and began to implement a new philosophical approach to the problems of mental illness. Tuke described his approach as "moral treatment," and reasoned that natural methods should be used to remedy diseases of the mind. At the York Retreat inmates were encouraged to participate in the ordinary activities of daily life. Such activities as gardening, sewing, knitting, and helping with the work of the institutional farm were actively encouraged. Tuke believed that occupation for the mentally disturbed helped the individual achieve better self-control and provided habit training, which had a normalizing effect. No physical restraint or coercion was used, although quiet seclusion of manic patients was sometimes employed. Special events and entertainments were organized for the patients, at which normal behavior was expected. Patients, staff, and visitors mingled at teas, church services, and outings. Every kind of "rational and innocent employment" was encouraged, and visitors were much impressed to see the effectiveness of this program in action. Tuke's work was much admired by several American visitors who came to observe the new methods.

Thomas Scattergood, a Quaker minister, became convinced of the value of Tuke's approach after a visit to the York Retreat, and on his return to Philadelphia in 1800 he actively worked to establish a similar institution there. Thomas Eddy, another Quaker, pressed for the introduction of moral treatment methods in the Lunatic Asylum of New York Hospital in 1815. The first American physician to endorse and supervise a program of planned occupation for mental patients was probably Dr. Rufus Wymann, who in 1818 opened the McLean Asylum near Boston. Wymann wrote:

The treatment of insanity chiefly depends upon the connection between the mind and the body. If there be inflammation of the brain or its membranes, it is to be treated as an inflammation of those parts. But in mental disorders without symptoms of organic disease, a judicious moral management is more successful. It should afford aggreeable occupation ... engaging the mind and exercising the body [1].

During the second quarter of the nineteenth century there was growing acceptance of the use of occupation as a treatment method for the mentally ill in Europe, but there was much less interest in the United States. Some American physicians claimed that American citizens equated "occupation" with paid employment and that American patients would refuse to participate in "work therapy" programs unless they were paid. Whether this was the real reason or not, American physicians did not press for large-scale occupation programs in their mental hospitals. One notable exception was the Asylum at Utica, New York, at which full-time instructors were hired to teach the patients academic subjects and to organize a wide variety of recreational and work activities for them. A hospital newspaper was published, and "occupation therapy" flourished under the direction of Dr. Aramiah Brigham.

Another early supporter of occupation therapy was Dr. Thomas Kirkbride, superintendent of the Pennsylvania Hospital for the Insane during the 1840s. Kirkbride had visited asylums in England and the United States to acquaint himself with the methods currently in use and became a strong advocate of "activity treatment." He introduced a planned program of patient occupations at the Pennsylvania institution between 1840 and 1842 and wrote: "The value of employment in the treatment of insanity is now so universally conceded that no arguments are required in its favor. Its value cannot be reckoned in dollars and cents. The object is to restore mental health and tranquilize the restlessness and mitigate the sorrows of disease" [1]. Kirkbride later helped to form an association of asylum medical superintendents that eventually became the American Psychiatric Association. For the rest of his life, Kirkbride actively supported the concepts of patient occupation in the treatment of mental disease.

The final quarter of the nineteenth century was not an auspicious period for occupational therapy. Successive waves of immigrants from Europe had swelled the population in mental hospitals with people who spoke little or no English and whose values and customs were strange and different from those of the native-born population. As hospitals were larger and more crowded, programs of therapeutic occupation grew less practical to organize and run. Widespread prejudice against the newly arrived immigrants provided additional rationalizations for neglect of such persons who became mentally disturbed. A more important factor that influenced change in the treatment of mental illness, however, was that medical concepts about the causes of mental illness were changing. Medicine had embraced the scientific method employed by the physical sciences and had applied it to the study of disease. This method tended to reduce everything to its lowest common denominator for purposes of study. Thus the brain was viewed in terms of cellular structure and pathology. Physical pathology of the brain was believed to be the basis for mental illness, and since there was no known cure or remedy for brain pathology, the mentally ill were considered hopelessly incurable and any form of treatment to be useless. A period of pessimism and neglect set in, and mental institutions reverted to their former status of custodial facilities. The activity programs so enthusiastically begun were largely abandoned during this era (3).

Early in the twentieth century, however, reformers began to agitate for improvements in conditions in mental hospitals and for active treatment of mental disorders. Dorothea Dix and Clifford Beers publicized the poor conditions that prevailed in many asylums and documented the mistreatment of patients confined to them. Public sentiment for improvements was aroused and some instititions began to make changes.

OCCUPATIONAL THERAPY PIONEERS

In 1906 a progressive physician, Dr. Herbert Hall, was awarded a grant by Harvard University to study "the treatment of neurasthenia through progressive and graded manual occupation" (1). Hall patterned his experimental program after one he had observed in Switzerland and set up a workshop for industrial therapeutics. Craftsmen were hired to work side by side with neurotic patients to improve their adjustment and ability to function in daily life. After four years of operation, Hall reported that the manual and intellectual work his patients had participated in had indeed had a normalizing effect on their behavior (1).

At about the same time, Susan Tracy, a nurse who taught nursing students at the Adams Nervine Hospital in Boston, began teaching a course in "invalid occupations" to her students. Tracy is often considered the first "occupational therapist," since she had observed as a nurse the positive effects that occupation could have on bedridden hospitalized patients. She emphasized to her students that the goal of patient occupation was to improve the patient's condition, not to produce beautiful handiwork. In 1910 her lectures were published in book form and were available to hospital nurses as a guide to patient activities (1).

In the spring of 1911 a course in occupation treatment was offered for nurses at the Massachusetts General Hospital. At about the same time, Dr. William Rush Dunton, Jr., was teaching a course in patient occupation for nurses at the Sheppard and Enoch Pratt Hospital in Towson, Maryland. Dunton's lectures were also published in book form and included guidelines on how occupational therapy should be prescribed and utilized.

Dr. Adolph Meyer, a Professor of Psychiatry at Johns Hopkins University in Baltimore, was another early promoter of the use of occupation for the mentally ill. Meyer viewed mental illness as a manifestation of problems in living and believed that "systematic engagement of interest and concern about the use of time and work was an obligation and a necessity" in the treatment of mental disorders (4). He pointed out that human beings operate on the basis of rhythmic cycles of work, play, rest, and sleep. For the individual to function well, Meyer suggested that a balance was required between these different activity states. He proposed organizing patients' activities in a balanced daily schedule of work, play, and rest. Meyer stressed that opportunities must be created for mentally ill persons to engage in learning activities, manual occupations, and creative pastimes to regain their ability to function as integrated individuals in their environment (4).

Another person much interested in the therapeutic uses of occupation was George Barton. Barton was an architect who developed tuberculosis and underwent several hospitalizations for this disease. He later had gangrenous foot amputated and developed a left hemiplegia. During his long convalescence, he discovered the value of activity in helping him to overcome his feelings of depression and taught himself to garden and do structural work within his physical limitations. He became a keen advocate of "occupation therapy." In 1914 Barton organized Consolation House, a school and workshop for convalescents in Clifton Springs, New York. Its program emphasized adjustment to disability and the use of occupations to train the disabled for a productive life. To develop his program, Barton initiated a correspondence with other people who were also using occupation as a form of treatment. He contacted Dunton and Tracy, whose work we have already described. Another contact was with Eleanor Clarke Slagle. Slagle had completed one of the

early courses in curative occupations at the Chicago School of Civics and Philanthropy. She then worked in the field of psychiatry and in 1913 became Director of Occupational Therapy in the Henry Phipps Psychiatric Clinic in Baltimore under the supervision of Meyer. Later she served as director of the Chicago school (now called the Henry Favill School of Occupations) until it closed in 1921. Barton also corresponded with Susan Johnson, an arts and crafts teacher who was one of the early educators and practitioners of occupational therapy. Thomas Kidner was another person whom Barton got in touch with to discuss occupation therapy. Kidner was an English architect who had organized a system of vocational rehabilitation for the disabled veterans of Canada during World War I and later served as a consultant to the United States government when the United States wished to establish reconstructive services for their own veterans of the war.

In 1917 Barton invited these six persons to meet with him in Clifton Springs to discuss forming an organization to promote and publicize this new field of occupation therapy. Slagle, Johnson, Kidner, Dunton, Barton, and his secretary, Isabel Newton, met and agreed to develop such an organization. The fledgling group was called the National Society for the Promotion of Occupational Therapy, and Barton agreed to serve as its first president. In 1921 the group changed its name to the American Occupational Therapy Association and continues to function under that title today (1,5).

During the early periods of development of occupational therapy, this new form of treatment was called by many different names. *Activity therapy, moral treatment, the work cure,* and *ergotherapy* were all terms used to identify the new approach. Dunton is credited with originating the term *occupation therapy,* which was later modified by Barton to *occupational therapy*. This became the generally accepted term, although there have been periodic movements to change the name of the field to something more readily recognizable.

IMPACT OF WORLD WAR I

World War I provided a major impetus to the development of the young field. As the United States mobilized for war, the military organized field hospitals near the battle lines for the treatment of casualties. Dr. Frankwood Williams was an army psychiatrist who was responsible for organizing base hospital 117. He was familiar with the use of occupation with mentally disturbed patients and asked his superiors for occupational workers to accompany his hospital unit to France. His pleas fell on deaf ears, since his request was interpreted as a request for workers for vocational training and this was believed inappropriate. Williams was undeterred, however, and convinced a small group of women who had some training in crafts to join the hospital unit under the unglamorous job title of "scrubwomen." The women were classified as civilian aides, with no military rank or uniform and very minimal pay. Their training consisted of three lectures in neuropsychiatry. These intrepid women sailed on a troopship for France, bringing their own tools and such minimal supplies as they could collect on short notice to outfit their workshops. Upon landing in Le Havre, they traveled by train to the location of base hospital 117. They were assigned to a drafty, unused barracks in which the hospital barber, the carpenter, and a gardner were already installed. The women rolled up their sleeves and went to work, cleaning up the area as well as they could and wangling usable items of furniture from sympathetic officers. Make-

shift workbenches were constructed from old hospital beds, and large tin cans from the kitchen were transformed into charcoal furnaces for heating of soldering irons. The kitchen dump proved to be a treasure trove of discarded tin cans that, when cleaned, became the raw material for many craft projects. Soon the workshop was a reality, and soldiers flocked to it, out of curiosity at first and then out of interest in the craft work that was available. Metal work, woodworking, weaving, block printing, wood carving, and toy making were among the crafts used. Later the Red Cross assisted by supplying the needed raw materials and a more suitable building to house the workshops.

Visiting medical officers, who were impressed with the effects of constructive activities on the neuropsychiatric patients who participated, began to make urgent requests of Washington for similar workers for their own field hospitals. By 1918 there were 116 reconstruction aides, as they were now called, and they had become a recognized category of hospital worker. After the armistice, these workers returned home to find that their wartime work had been much publicized in the civilian press. To their surprise, they found themselves in demand by civilian hospitals. Cordelia Meyers, who led the initial group of reconstruction aides to France, later established a therapeutic workshop in the Panama Canal Zone at the request of Williams and trained workers to staff it (6).

Canada was the first country to organize occupational therapy in its military hospitals. Two early graduates of the Chicago school were among those who served in Canadian military hospitals. When the United States entered the war, it sought the assistance of Thomas Kidner, who had helped to organize the Canadian reconstruction program for its wounded veterans. Several emergency training programs were hastily established during the war years to train reconstruction aides for army hospitals (6).

1920–1940

In 1922 the American Occupational Therapy Association voted to hold annual meetings in conjunction with the American Hospital Association and to publish an official journal. The new journal was titled *Archives of Occupational Therapy* and was published from 1922 to 1924. In 1925 its name was changed to *Occupational Therapy and Rehabilitation*, a title felt to be more in keeping with the broad scope of the field. The journal had by now become one of the membership benefits of the organization. Eleanor Clarke Slagle accepted the position of Executive Secretary of the Association in 1923 and provided strong leadership to the growing organization. Slagle was instrumental in starting a national registry of qualified occupational therapists, thus assuring employers of a reliable listing of trained workers who held a professional standing comparable to that of registered nurses.

In an editorial that appeared in a 1922 issue of the *Archives of Occupational Therapy*, Thomas Kidner (then president of the Association) noted that 67 hospitals had sent exhibits of occupational therapy work to the 1921 meeting of the organization. Over half of these were tuberculosis hospitals, followed by a number of hospitals for nervous and mental cases. Orthopedic and general hospitals were less well represented, and Kidner urged that therapists make more effort to promote occupational therapy in these types of institutions. He advised occupational therapists to follow the lead of political reformers whose motto was "Organize, Agitate, Educate" in order to further the goals of the new profession (7). Members of the association must have done so, for during the 1920s and 1930s occupational

therapy gradually expanded from its initial focus on mental and nervous diseases to orthopedic and general hospitals and even to private practice.

The period from 1910 to 1929 was one of significant medical advance. The war, a serious polio epidemic in 1916, and increasing numbers of industrial and automobile accidents resulted in larger numbers of chronically disabled people who required long-term care and rehabilitation. Conditions in hospitals were improving, making them safer places for patients to recover. Freud's psychoanalytic theory was revolutionizing many physicians' ideas about the roots of mental disturbances and was providing new tools for treatment. Behaviorist theory was developing and offered an alternative explanation and treatment approach for aberrant behavior. The concept of occupational therapy as a way of reactivating the minds and motivation of the mentally ill and of restoring function to the physically disabled was gaining momentum. The literature of this period reflects much concern over craft modalities to be used for specific types of disabilities and a strong work orientation. The goal of occupational therapy was seen as a return to productive employment, and the craft activities employed were viewed as tools to help the patient advance step by step toward that goal.

The 1920s and 1930s saw a steady growth of educational programs preparing registered occupational therapists. It was also a time in which some of the enduring traditions of the field were established. Because many of its early practitioners were nurses, teachers, and social workers, occupational therapy developed as a female profession. Nurturing attitudes, then felt to be largely a female characteristic, were believed to be the essential in working with the sick and the mentally ill. Early training programs in the field were open only to women, and this set a pattern that was modified very slowly. In the 1920s and 1930s more women began to enter the work force, and occupational therapy, along with teaching and nursing, was considered a respectable field for a woman to enter. This tradition of female dominance has engendered much concern and discussion in recent years; salary levels in this field and opportunities for independent decision making are viewed by many occupational therapists as lagging far behind other fields that are less female oriented.

Another tradition established during this period was that of close association and identification with organized medicine. Much of the early progress in the field was due to dedicated physicians who recognized the limitations of currently used medications and technology to improve the condition of patients with long-term disease or disability. The support they provided for occupational therapy as a new approach to improving mental and physical abilities was crucial in gaining acceptance by the conservative medical establishment of the time. When the American Occupational Therapy Association joined forces with the American Medical Association in 1935 to accredit educational programs for the registered occupational therapist, close links were forged that firmly connected occupational therapy with organized medicine. This alliance has been questioned seriously in recent years, and the debate continues as occupational therapy moves through the 1980s.

By 1930, occupational therapy was becoming known as a field. It had established a viable professional organization and was increasingly recognized as a contributor to medical care of the sick and injured. Because of its ties with medicine, occupational therapy was beginning to accept the need for a more scientific approach to the problems presented by the mentally ill and the physically handicapped. Increasingly, occupational

therapy practice focused on the subcomponents of functional performance—muscular function, neurophysiology, biomechanical principles, and specific abnormal behaviors—rather than the holistic view of the individual that had been prevalent in the earliest years of the field.

The professional progress of occupational therapy in the 1930s was severely limited by the great economic depression that affected the United States from 1929 to 1941. Health care in general suffered massive setbacks during this period, and occupational therapy was directly affected along with the other health care fields. Spending on medical care dropped 33% from 1929 to 1933, even though physicians and hospitals lowered their fees. Many hospitals refused to accept patients unless payment of the bill was guaranteed. The American Medical Association acted to protect the financial interests of its members by reducing the number of medical schools, limiting admissions, and tightening up licensure provisions. It was a period of no growth for medical education or medical services. Many hospital occupational therapy clinics were forced to close during this period, and those that survived were forced to new heights of creativity in the use of scrap materials and donations.

Rerek (8), in her review of the effect of this period on the development of occupational therapy, lists three major influences. First, future leaders of the field, who were growing up during this period, were strongly influenced toward caution and conservatism because of their experiences with economic instability. Second, the federal government entered the health care arena during this period, and its influence on funding mechanisms and regulation of health care took root and became a major factor in the delivery of health services. Third, the public developed a pervasive attitude of suspicion and skepticism toward elected officials and the federal government; this suspicion would last for decades. No longer would the population give its leaders the unquestioned support and trust that pre-depression leaders had enjoyed.

WORLD WAR II AND THE REHABILITATION MOVEMENT

The United States was rescued from the economic depression by new government policies and by the outbreak of a second world war. Again the military sought occupational therapists to organize and run rehabilitation programs for wounded and disabled veterans. Emergency training courses were again developed to meet the urgent need for occupational therapists. As ever larger numbers of veterans with severe physical disabilities and mental impairments were returned home, it was increasingly apparent that services to meet their needs were totally inadequate. Although many new medical techniques were being developed to save the lives of wartime casualties, few facilities were available for the rehabilitation and long-term care of wounded veterans. Families had become more mobile during the war years, and housing was in short supply. Most families were unable to provide the kind of care needed by disabled veterans. Educational institutions were not prepared to deal with the needs of war veterans for job training and reintegration into civilian life. The medical establishment was more concerned with the treatment of acute illness and injury and was unconvinced of its role in long-term care. Families and veterans groups pressed hard for services, and their needs could no longer be denied. Government support was made available for the construction and operation of rehabilitation facilities, staff training, and research. Organized medicine rather reluctantly accepted rehabilitation as a legitimate medical responsibility but never awarded

it the kind of prestige that some of the other medical specialties enjoyed (9).

The era from 1942 to 1960 is often referred to as the period of the rehabilitation movement. During this time the needs of the handicapped population were increasingly recognized and new facilities and methods for improving functional abilities were developed. Occupational therapy took its place as a rehabilitation field and therapists became involved in such areas as prosthetic training, the development of orthotic devices, training of patients in activities of daily living, use of progressive resistive exercise to increase muscle strength, evaluating patients' vocational aptitudes and abilities, and the use of neuromuscular facilitation and inhibition. The use of antibiotics increased the survival rate of patients with serious illnesses and resulted in greater numbers of handicapped adults. In psychiatric settings, therapists were involved with the therapeutic use of self, dealing with patients' unconscious needs, analysis of patients' artwork in psychodynamic terms, and group techniques to improve self-awareness and interpersonal communication. Occupational therapists continued to practice primarily on a technical level. There was little attempt during this period to relate treatment approaches to a theoretical framework or to seek the underlying principles of treatment. Therapists tended to work with specific diagnostic categories and were becoming more specialized. Educational programs preparing the registered occupational therapist were including more medical content in their curricula and programs were becoming more comprehensive. During the 1950s another occupational therapy staff member emerged: the certified occupational therapist assistant (COTA). The COTAs were employed to supplement and expand occupational therapy services and provide additional personnel for existing programs. By 1960 a number of schools had been established to prepare COTAs, and their contributions to the practice of occupational therapy were increasingly recognized (10).

1960–1980

The 1960s ushered in a turbulent period in the United States. Politically and socially it was a time of great change. The country's intervention in Viet Nam and other unstable governments gave rise to widespread political unrest and the polarization of attitudes concerning the country's role in international politics. Economic inflation made for a growing gap between the "haves" and the "have-nots" of society. Traditional values and institutions were being challenged. The traditional family was weakening, and many experimented with alternative family arrangements and life-styles. Early retirement was encouraged, and the elderly were becoming a larger proportion of the population. Technology was forcing many workers from their jobs, and ideas about what competencies were necessary to exist in society were rapidly changing. Enrollments in colleges and technical schools boomed, as students tried to prepare for the changing job market. The incidence of drug and alcohol abuse, crime, and suicide rose sharply. On the positive side, progressive civil rights legislation was enacted and enforced, the problems of poverty were discussed and solutions proposed, and there was greater recognition of personal responsibility in matters of health and disease prevention. People were paying more attention to diet, exercise, methods of reducing stress, and constructive use of leisure time. There was a new search for spiritual values among the younger generation, and religious groups attracted many new members.

The technological advances seen in society as a whole were reflected in health care and in occupational therapy practice.

Medicine was becoming highly specialized, since new information was proliferating so rapidly that no one could hope to remain current with broad areas of medical practice. The same trend was seen in occupational therapy, with some therapists now identifying themselves as "hand therapists" or "specialists in sensory integration, spinal cord injury, or burns." The kinds of medical conditions that occupational therapists were treating had changed since the 1940s and 1950s. Devastating epidemic diseases, such as poliomyelitis, were now things of the past thanks to the development of effective vaccines. Tuberculosis was no longer common, as preventive measures and effective drug treatment controlled its incidence. On the other hand, stress-related diseases and dysfunctions were on the increase. Drug and alcohol abuse had become a national problem, as had the incidence of some forms of cancer. The growing population of elderly persons brought about a recognition that new services were needed to maintain their health and provide for a reasonable quality of life. Because of improvements in prenatal care and delivery, more handicapped children were surviving with more severe handicapping conditions.

The medical community was seeing the need to educate the public about disease and injury prevention and was advocating the use of methods and technology to safeguard the public's health. Occupational therapy also was reviewing its role in health care and was becoming more involved in education, prevention, screening programs, and health maintenance. Therapists were seeking new ways of delivering their services to meet these needs and were entering new markets, such as public school programs for handicapped children, community mental health centers, agencies promoting independent living for the elderly and the handicapped, hospital outreach programs, and private practice.

Traditional medical institutions were undergoing major changes as they moved into the 1970s and 1980s. Many mental hospitals and residential institutions for the mentally retarded were closed across the country as the concepts of deinstitutionalization gained acceptance. It was believed that patients in such institutions could live more normal and more productive lives in community settings than in large state and private residential institutions where they had traditionally received care. There was growing concern over protection of civil rights for such individuals and a belief that the civil rights of many may have been violated by long-term confinement to an institution. As a result, large numbers of mental patients and mentally retarded persons were discharged or transferred from institutional to community facilities. Unfortunately the development of adequate community programs lagged far behind the need for such facilities, and many chronically mentally ill and retarded persons were reduced to life on the streets or in slum housing with no adequate resources to maintain health and prevent serious deterioration. Steps were taken to correct the situation, but its effects remain to haunt us today.

Along with the closing of custodial institutions, health care in general was moving from a hospital base to a community base. By the 1980s, hospital costs were so high that hospitalization was feasible only for the most severe illnesses and injuries. Routine medical care continued to be delivered by private physicians but also by new forms of medical practice, such as community health centers and outpatient surgical facilities. Occupational therapy was again part of this trend, with increasing numbers of therapists and therapy assistants employed in public and private schools, outreach programs, community service agencies, and private or group practices.

In the late 1970s and early 1980s, many occupational therapists were voicing concern over their traditional role as an associate or an assistant to the physican. There was a growing opinion that the medical model no longer served occupational therapy well. Many therapists now believed that they had a role to play in the prevention of disability and the maintenance of health as well as fulfilling their traditional role in treating existing limitations of function. Occupational therapists were beginning to see themselves as fitting better into an educational or a social model of practice, rather than a model that emphasized pathology and illness (11,12).

Graduate programs had begun in occupational therapy education in the 1960s, but the 1970s and 1980s saw a steady growth in the number of graduate programs available. With knowledge expanding at an ever increasing rate, advanced education was becoming more and more necessary for the occupational therapy practitioner. The need for research in occupational therapy had long been recognized, but in the 1970s it became a major issue for the field. There was an urgent need to test basic occupational therapy concepts, to explore the value of assessment and treatment techniques, and to determine whether occupational therapy was cost-effective. A sound theoretical base was believed to be needed to explain why occupational therapy worked and to provide unifying concepts for occupational therapy practice. During this period the *American Journal of Occupational Therapy* changed its focus from that of occupational therapy practice to research. It was now publishing more scientific investigations into aspects of occupational therapy; several other new journals were also contributing to the research literature of the field.

The 1970s and 1980s saw greater involvement of occupational therapists and their professional organization in legislative activities. It was recognized that the field and its clients must be represented when health care legislation was being proposed, and lobbying activities and testimony to various legislative bodies became an important priority for the profession during this era. Many states enacted licensure laws for occupational therapists and therapy assistants during the 1970s. By 1986 a total of 34 states, the district of Columbia, and Puerto Rico had occupational therapy licensure laws and two additional states had "trademark" laws. This trend continues and has been encouraged by the national organization. State licensure has enabled legal recognition of occupational therapy services in those states and provides legal recourse when abuses occur by unqualified practitioners.

BEYOND 1980

In the mid-1980s the health care system in the United States is undergoing a great deal of change in an attempt to contain health care costs while still maintaining quality services. Whether this effort will be successful remains to be seen. Would the founders of occupational therapy recognize the field today? One wonders what they would make of biofeedback training, computer programs for cognitive retraining, or use of electronic equipment for the severely handicapped. In a 1977 paper reviewing the evolution of occupational therapy, Kielhofner and Burke (13) pointed out that early occupational therapy was based on a humanistic philosophy that reflected beliefs about the nature of man in the eighteenth and nineteenth centuries. Moral treatment, and subsequently occupational therapy, arose out of a holistic view of individuals in the context of their environment. Later a competing scientific school of thought gained dominance in medicine and in occupational therapy. This viewpoint focused on pathology and the study of function and

dysfunction at the cellular level. This became the medical model that continues to dominate organized medicine today. Kielhofner and Burke suggested that by accepting the medical model, occupational therapy became fragmented and less cohesive. Therapists under this model tended to focus on muscles, psychic mechanisms, or sensorimotor interactions rather than taking a broad view of the individual. In doing so, these authors claimed, occupational therapy became scientifically respectable but lost its original broad concepts of occupation and its contributions to health and well-being. These authors and others have proposed an occupational behavior frame of reference for the field that would recapture some of the founders' original concepts of occupation and its contributions to health. They suggest retaining the technology that has been developed within the medical model, but reorganizing occupational knowledge under its original philosophy of occupation.

George Barton, Dr. William Rush Dunton, Eleanor Clark Slagle, and the other pioneers of the field might marvel at some of the techniques used today in occupational therapy and at the broad scope of practice, but they would also recognize that humanistic values continue to guide the practice of occupational therapy. The field has come a long way from its early beginnings and from the concepts so well stated by its pioneers. Its future depends to a great extent on the decisions that the profession and its organization make in the 1980s.

DISCUSSION QUESTIONS

1. Do you think that occupational therapy's close relationship with organized medicine helped or hindered the development of the profession?

2. Is occupational therapy still a female-oriented field? Justify your answer.

3. How did political and social conditions influence the nature of occupational therapy practice during its developmental periods?

4. How did the client population of occupational therapists change in the different eras of its development?

5. Did the movement to deinstitutionalize mentally retarded and mentally ill persons result in improved care for these groups? Justify your answer.

6. Are the humanistic values of occupational therapy compatible with the modern view of health care as a business or industry? Why or why not?

REFERENCES

1. Licht S: *Occupational Therapy Source Book.* Baltimore, Williams & Wilkins, 1948, pp. 1–17, 41–56.
2. Slagle EC, Robeson HA: *Syllabus for Training of Nurses in Occupational Therapy,* ed. 2. Utica, New York State Department of Mental Hygiene, 1941, pp. 3–75.
3. Bockoven JS: The Legacy of moral treatment. *AJOT* XXV:223–225, 1971.
4. Meyer A: Philosophy of occupational therapy. *Arch Occup Ther* I:1–10, 1922.
5. Licht S: The founding and founders of the American Occupational Therapy Association. *AJOT* XXI:269–277, 1967.
6. Meyers C: Pioneer occupational therapists in world war I. *AJOT* II: 208–215, 1948.
7. Kidner TB: Editorial. *Arch Occup Ther* I:499–501, 1922.
8. Woodside H: The development of occupational therapy, 1910–1929. *AJOT* XXV:226–230, 1971.
9. Rerek M: The depression years—1929–1941. *AJOT* XXV:231–233, 1971.
10. Mcsey A: Involvement in the rehabilitation movement—1942–1960. *AJOT* XXV:234–236, 1971.
11. Diasio K: The modern era—1960–1970. *AJOT* XXV:237–243, 1971.
12. Reilly M: The modernization of occupational therapy. *AJOT* XXV:243–246, 1971.
13. Kielhofner G, Burke J: Occupational therapy after 60 years: an account of changing identity and knowledge. *AJOT* 31:675–690, 1977.

SUGGESTED READINGS

Bing R: Occupational therapy revisted: a paraphrastic journey. *AJOT* 35:499–518, 1981.
Brainerd W: O. T. and me: early days at the sanitarium, Clifton Springs, NY. *AJOT* XXI: 278–279, 1967.
Cromwell F: Eleanor Clarke Slagle, the leader, the woman. *AJOT* 31:645–648, 1977.
Johnson J: Nationally speaking: humanitarianism and accountability: a challenge for occupational therapy on its 60th anniversary. *AJOT* 31:631–637, 1977.

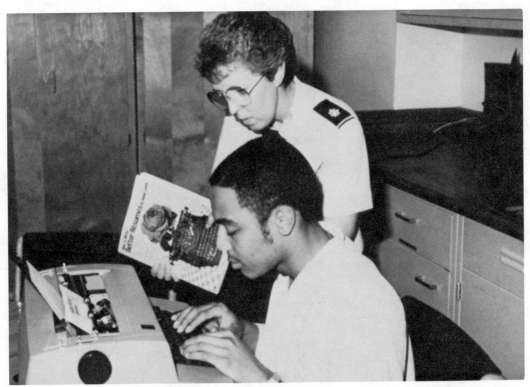

Courtesy AOTA

FOUR

Education and Certification Patterns

Three different levels of personnel are involved in the delivery of occupational therapy services. The registered occupational therapist (OTR) is a graduate of a baccalaureate, certificate, a master's degree program. This education prepares the individual to plan and direct occupational therapy services and to supervise the work of employees with less training. The certified occupational therapy assistant (COTA) is a graduate of a certificate or associate degree program of technical education. The COTA performs many of the daily treatment activities in occupational therapy programs and may direct programs aimed at helping clients achieve independent living skills. The occupational therapy aide usually has no formal education in the field but receives on-the-job training that equips him or her to assist with routine procedures in occupational therapy programs. These three types of personnel work cooperatively to help clients achieve their treatment objective. In addition, an occupational therapy department may include volunteer workers who provide important supplementary services to the program. In this chapter the type of educational preparation required

of the OTR and the COTA is discussed and the certification process is described.

The OTR is probably the best known, having been on the scene the longest time. As early as 1906 Susan Tracy, a nurse, was teaching a short course to nursing students on invalid occupations that emphasized the value of activity for bedridden patients. Later, Julia Lathrop, Dr. William R. Dunton, Eleanor Clarke Slagle, and others conducted training programs to prepare personnel to work in "occupation therapy." By 1918 there were four schools offering an education in occupational therapy in Milwaukee, Philadelphia, Boston, and St. Louis. By 1949 all occupational therapy education programs were required to be located in colleges or universities and to be authorized degree programs. In 1932 the American Occupational Therapy Association (AOTA) began its registry of qualified occupational therapists who had completed the required program of study and were prepared to practice in the field. In 1935 the AOTA together with the American Medical Association, began to accredit educational programs in order to maintain minimum educational standards and assure some uniformity of educational preparation. Educational programs for the OTR have continued to develop; in 1986 there were 61 such programs, with more being actively encouraged (1).

EDUCATION OF THE REGISTERED OCCUPATIONAL THERAPIST

To be admitted to an educational program preparing OTRs, a prospective student must meet the admission requirements of the college or university to which he or she is applying. A high school diploma is required, and there may be specific requirements for high school preparation in mathematics, English, science, and social studies. A high school background in speech and English composition is helpful, since communication skills are highly valued in occupational therapy. Also desirable is a foundation in the biological and behavioral sciences so that the student may build on these areas in college course work. A background in liberal studies is beneficial, as these subjects will contribute to the student's overall preparation for working in a helping relationship to others.

A listing of all educational programs for OTR and COTA education in the United States in 1986 may be found in the Appendix on pages 239–243. Students are advised to contact the program of their choice for specific information about entrance requirements, the educational program offered, and the time and financial resources needed to complete the program.

Once accepted by a college or university, the student will embark on preprofessional course work. A common pattern in many baccalaureate degree programs is two years of preprofessional education, two years of professional education, and six to nine months of supervised fieldwork. Some colleges offer certificate or master's degree level education for entry into occupational therapy. Such programs are designed for persons who hold a baccalaureate degree in another field and are usually more intensive than the standard baccalaureate program. They may also require that certain courses be completed before entry into the professional program, so students should be careful to inquire about prerequisites for admission. Although all accredited programs meet AOTA's minimum standards, they may differ in their emphasis and in their course sequencing patterns. One accredited program may stress biomedical studies, while another may emphasize the human development process or human learning theories. These differences are to be expected, since AOTA's educational standards are intentionally broad to allow for individual differences between colleges. Students are advised to inquire about the program's philosophy and emphasis when they seek information about educational programs so that they are fully informed about the nature of the education they will receive.

The most recent revisions to AOTA's *Educational Essentials for Accredited Educational Programs for the Occupational Therapist* were completed in 1983 and adopted by AOTA and the American Medical Association, who jointly accredit these programs. According to this document, the goal of entry level education for the OTR is to prepare practitioners who are able to do the following:

1. Provide occupational therapy services to prevent deficits, maintain or improve function in daily living skills and their underlying components (sensorimotor, cognitive, psychosocial).

2. Manage occupational therapy service.

3. Incorporate values and attitudes congruent with the profession's standards and ethics (2).

The document also points out that entry-level professional education lays a foundation for other roles of the experienced therapist, such as those of consultant, educator, researcher, and health planner.

The *Educational Essentials for the Registered Occupational Therapist* require that the educational program include content in the following areas:

1. Liberal arts, sciences, and humanities
2. Biological, behavioral, and health sciences
3. Occupational therapy theory and practice
4. Research concepts and applications
5. Values and attitudes congruent with the profession
6. Supervised fieldwork
   Level I: related to didactic learning
   Level II: a minimum of six months of supervised practice

Educational programs arrange these content areas in different ways; however, it is fairly common to find the liberal arts, sciences, and humanities included in the preprofessional part of the curriculum. This content may include courses in English composition, literature, psychology, sociology, biology, speech, anatomy, physiology, kinesiology, and philosophy. The preprofessional program may also include a number of electives so that students may pursue other studies of personal interest to them. Near the end of the preprofessional program, the student may apply for admission to the professional part of the educational program. Admission requirements and methods differ considerably from one program to another; the student should seek information about the admission process directly from the program of his or her choice.

Once admitted to the professional program the student studies subjects directly related to occupational therapy theory and practice. Aspects of human performance are studied in detail, looking at both the normal and abnormal aspects of function. Human occupation throughout the life cycle is analyzed, and the student learns activity processes that can be used to maintain existing functions or to improve deficiences in function. Students are exposed to concepts of health and disease, health maintenance, and prevention of disability. A variety of physical and psychosocial disorders that may interfere with normal occupational performance are studied, and students learn intervention or management techniques for use with these disorders. Learning experiences are not limited to the classroom. Level I fieldwork provides observational and practice experiences in clinical settings, introducing students to the application of occupational therapy concepts and procedures. Such fieldwork is usually supervised by the course instructor or by experienced occupational therapists employed in clinical settings. Level I fieldwork is a vital part of the curriculum and gives the student a better idea of how occupational therapy is used in client care. Students gradually learn how to carry out assessment and treatment procedures with clients and become more comfortable in the therapeutic relationship.

Professional education in occupational therapy is not intended to prepare specialists. Rather it is aimed at giving the student general knowledge and skills that are the basis of all occupational therapy practice. Because of this general focus, both physical and psychosocial disorders are studied, as well as developmental disabilities and limitations related to the aging process. It is only after students have mastered the general concepts and shown the ability to apply them clinically that they may wish to limit their practice to one disability or age group. Specialization usually occurs after some years of clinical practice and requires advanced study of the specialty area through continuing education, advanced clinical experience, or graduate education.

The professional curriculum also includes content on the management of occupational therapy services, research concepts and applications, and values and attitudes related to work in a helping profession. The student who has completed all or a significant portion of the professional coursework then enters the level II fieldwork phase of education. Level II fieldwork is student participation (usually on a full-time basis) in a clinical program or programs that offer supervised experience in occupational therapy practice. The AOTA's *Educational Essentials for the Registered Occupational Therapist* require a minimum of six months of level II fieldwork, but many educational programs exceed this minimum. During this phase of education the student gains further experience in the use of occupational therapy assessment and treatment methods, working with a wide variety of physical and psychosocial disorders and with a broad age range of clients. The student's work is closely supervised by an experienced therapist who is available to consult with the student, answer questions, and assist when needed. The fieldwork student is gradually assigned more responsibility for the care of clients and is expected to complete all of the documentation related to client care that the clinical setting requires. By the end of the fieldwork period, the student is expected to be functioning at the level of an entry-level occupational therapist and should be able to assume full clinical responsibilities. The supervising therapist carefully assesses the fieldwork student's clinical abilities and prepares a detailed report that is discussed with the student. This report is returned to the educational program that prepared

the student and is scored on a pass-fail basis. Students who pass their level II fieldwork successfully are then declared eligible by their educational program to take the national OTR certification examination. Students who fail level II fieldwork may reschedule additional fieldwork (within the regulations of their specific educational program) until they are declared eligible to write the certification examination. (The examination is discussed later when we look at the certification process.)

EDUCATION OF THE CERTIFIED OCCUPATIONAL THERAPY ASSISTANT

The history of COTAs is more recent than that of OTRs. Occupational therapy service programs grew and expanded, until in the 1950s there were simply not enough occupational therapists to meet the needs of the public. In attempting to deal with this situation, some states and private institutions began to train workers to assist in occupational therapy clinical programs. The first training programs were short courses that provided some limited background in occupational therapy concepts and specific training in the use of therapeutic activities. The AOTA recognized the need for another type of worker in the field—technical staff members who could assist the OTR and provide expanded client services. In 1959 AOTA amended its bylaws to permit the credentialing of COTAs and began to approve training programs designed to prepare such workers. Many of the educational programs for COTAs were located in community colleges or technical schools. At first programs tended to be 9- to 12-month certificate courses, but the need was soon recognized for more in-depth education to meet the needs and maintain the professional quality of services. Most COTA educational programs are now two-year associate degree programs. In 1986 there were 58 such programs in the United States, with more continuing to develop.

Just as with educational programs for the OTR, the AOTA developed *Educational Essentials* (standards) for COTA educational programs. These standards closely paralleled those for OTR education, but with some differences that reflected the differences in function of the two types of workers. One major differences was in the depth and complexity of the curriculum. Technical programs generally placed less emphasis on knowledge of occupational therapy theory and did not provide in-depth study of the biomedical and behavioral sciences. They tended to emphasize instead the "doing" aspects of the field—occupational therapy methods and procedures used in daily practice.

According to AOTA's 1983 *Educational Essentials for Accredited Programs for Occupational Therapy Assistants*, technical education in the field was intended to prepare workers who could do the following:

Collaborate in providing occupational therapy services with appropriate supervision to prevent deficits and to maintain or improve function in daily living skills and underlying components

Participate in managing occupational therapy services

Direct activity programs

Incorporate values and attitudes congruent with the profession's standards and ethics (3).

In the 1983 revision, content requirements for COTA educational programs included the following:

1. General education
2. Biological, behavioral, and health sciences

3. Occupational therapy concepts and skills
4. Values, attitudes, and behaviors congruent with the profession
5. Fieldwork education
   Level I: related to didactic course work
   Level II: a minimum of two months of supervised practice

Just as with educational programs for the OTR, technical education programs tend to vary in their approach and emphasis, although all are expected to meet AOTA's minimum educational standards. Thus some programs stress preparation for employment in long-term care facilities, while others focus to a greater extent on home health care or employment in community agencies. The philosophy and emphasis of a program should be investigated by prospective students, since it pervades the educational program and influences the type of education provided.

In a two-year associate degree program, the first year is often spent in general studies that prepare the student for the study of occupational therapy concepts and methods in the second year. Observation and practice experiences in clinical settings (level I fieldwork) are required in COTA education just as at the OTR level, and these experiences are tied in with classroom learning. Two months of level II fieldwork is required; however, many schools exceed this minimum. Level II fieldwork is usually done on a full-time basis and provides the student with direct clinical experience under the close supervision of an experienced OTR or COTA. This practice experience enables the student to apply the knowledge learned in the classroom to actual cases and is an important part of the curriculum. Just as with the OTR student, the COTA fieldwork student is observed and a written performance assessment is completed by the supervisor. This report is sent back to the student's school and is scored pass or fail. Students who pass the level II fieldwork and who have completed all other educational requirements are declared eligible to take the national certification examination for occupational therapy assistants.

THE CERTIFICATION PROCESS

Certification is an official recognition by an authorized body that individuals have completed the necessary academic and examination requirements to qualify for practice in a given field. In occupational therapy, certification is provided by a certification board, which operates independently from the AOTA and which administers a national qualifying examination. Membership in the organization is separate from certification, and one may be certified as an OTR or COTA without becoming a member of the organization.

The certification board controls the certifying examinations and is responsible for their content. Monitoring and scoring of the examinations are the responsibility of a private testing agency, and examinations are scheduled twice a year for OTR and COTA candidates. No two examinations are exactly alike. Each year new questions are added and out-of-date or nondiscriminating questions are withdrawn so that the examination reflects the current thinking and practice of the field.

When OTR and COTA candidates have been declared eligible by their educational programs to take the appropriate examination, the testing agency sends candidates information on the location of testing centers and application forms for the examinations. A testing fee is charged to students who apply, and general information on examination content is given. Both examinations are intended to objectively measure the knowledge and skills required by beginning OTRs and COTAs

in clinical practice and are based on role delineation studies of OTR and COTA roles and functions. A multiple-choice format is used for both examinations. After the examinations have been scored by the testing agency, candidates are notified of whether they passed or failed, along with their total score and subscores on specific parts of the examination. Candidates who fail the examination may retake it. Candidates who pass the examination are then certified as qualified to practice and are added to the list of certified OTRs and COTAs. The individual is then entitled to use the initials OTR or COTA after his or her name and may represent himself or herself as a qualified practitioner. Graduates of foreign educational programs in occupational therapy that are approved by the World Federation of Occupational Therapists may apply to take the national occupational therapy certification examination if they wish to qualify for practice within the United States (4).

STATE LICENSURE

A growing number of states require state licensure for OTRs and COTAs. Licensure is a process by which an agency of the state government grants permission to persons who meet established qualifications to engage in a given occupation or to use a particular title. Licensure is intended to protect the public from unqualified practitioners who may cause harm through improper or inappropriate services. Licensure attempts to guarantee a minimum educational standard for practitioners and to provide a minimum quality of services. In 1986, 36 states as well as Puerto Rico and the District of Columbia licensed or otherwise regulated occupational therapy practice (5).

The majority of states with licensure acts require that practitioners be graduates of an accredited or approved educational program in occupational therapy, show evidence of successful completion or fieldwork requirements, and pass a qualifying examination in the field. Candidates who seek employment in states demanding licensure may request that the testing agency forward their examination results to the appropriate state licensing board for review. Applicants may also be asked to complete an application form and pay a state licensing fee. Currently all states with occupational therapy licensure laws accept the results of the national certification examinations, so there is no need to pass a separate qualifying examination when moving from one state to another.

WHICH EDUCATIONAL PROGRAM IS RIGHT FOR ME?

Students are often uncertain which level of occupational therapy practice may suit them best. Both OTRs and COTAs perform valued services to clients. The OTR educational programs require more time to complete and are usually more costly, since they are located in colleges and universities. The COTA programs are shorter, introduce the principles of the field, and graduate workers who are immediately employable in direct service programs. Students who choose the COTA route may later continue their educational level at the OTR level. This laddering process is encouraged, and more COTAs are entering OTR programs each year.

For several years AOTA sponsored a career mobility project, whereby COTAs could undertake an intensive program of individual study and supervised fieldwork to become eligible to take the OTR certification examination. A number of persons earned their OTR certification through this process, but it was recognized that this was a very difficult way to qualify. Relatively few who undertook it completed the process. The program was abandoned in favor of encouraging COTAs to qualify for the next practice level through completion of an OTR educational program. College programs were simultaneously urged to eliminate barriers to COTA graduates who wished to enter an OTR educational program. Most colleges have made genuine efforts to achieve this and try to make the transition from COTA graduate to OTR student as smooth as possible. Although many COTAs are very happy with their work and are satisfied to remain at the COTA level, others wish to continue their professional education and should be given every opportunity to do so. Students are advised to discuss their career goals with faculty members of both educational levels if they are in doubt about which program to enter. Visiting occupational therapy clinical programs and observing the roles of the OTR and COTA can also be helpful in deciding which level of practice will be the most satisfying.

HIGHER EDUCATION IN OCCUPATIONAL THERAPY

There are two other educational levels in ocupational therapy that should briefly be mentioned. Graduate education is becoming ever more important in the field, and most occupational therapy personnel agree that there are some types of jobs where specialized knowledge and skills are needed. Many areas of practice are becoming highly technical, and practitioners find that they need more knowledge in these areas than their entry-level education has given them. To meet such needs, occupational therapists may seek continuing education on an informal basis or may enter a master's or doctoral degree program.

In 1986, 20 colleges and universities in the United States offered postprofessional master's degree programs in occupational therapy [1]. These programs are open to persons with a baccalaureate degree or equivalent in the field and offer advanced study of specific aspects of occupational therapy. Two universities offered doctoral programs in occupational therapy in 1986; many others offered doctoral programs in related fields (1). There has been a great deal of concern in recent years over the lack of occupational therapists who hold doctoral degrees. Such people are needed urgently to teach at the college level and to conduct research and generate and test theory in the field. These functions require knowledge gained at the doctoral level, and the AOTA is encouraging more students to enter doctoral programs. When embarking on an education in occupational therapy, it is well to think ahead. Not all occupational therapists remain clinicians. Many become teachers, administrators, researchers, writers or editors, health planners, or consultants. It is important that beginning students consider all of these roles when planning their professional education. Shortages exist in occupational therapy at all levels, but the need for people with advanced knowledge and skills is particularly urgent.

Students are sometimes surprised to learn that graduation from an OTR or COTA program is not the end of their professional education. The truth is that at this point the real education is just beginning. In any profession that is growing and changing, it is vital that practitioners keep up with new developments and new knowledge in the field. This can be achieved in many ways: through professional reading, through participation in professional meetings and conferences, through discussion and communication with colleagues, through attendance at continuing education programs and workshops. However one chooses to do it, all colleagues in a professional field must accept the responsibility to keep their skills sharpened and their knowledge up-to-date

so that they can provide optimal services to their clients. This means a lifelong commitment to professional education. There is always more to be learned; this process of continued learning makes for a competent professional who is able to make significant contributions to health care and to the advancement of the profession.

DISCUSSION QUESTIONS

1. If you are enrolled in an OTR curriculum, is there a COTA curriculum in your area? Obtain a copy of each curriculum and discuss the similarities and differences between the two. If you are a COTA student, compare your curriculum with that of an OTR program.

2. Are there some personal characteristics that might be desirable in one who wishes to pursue a career in occupational therapy? Discuss some of the personal traits that might be desirable in an OTR and a COTA.

3. Discuss the areas of advanced study that interest you. What are some areas of academic study that would be related or complementary to occupational therapy?

REFERENCES

1. Research Information and Evaluation Division. American Occupational Therapy Association: *1986 Education Data Survey, Final Report*, 1986.
2. American Occupational Therapy Association: Essentials and guidelines of an accredited educational program for the occupational therapist. *AJOT* 37:817–823, 1983.
3. American Occupational Therapy Association: Essentials of an accredited educational program for the occupational therapy assistant. *AJOT* 37:824–830, 1983.
4. American Occupational Therapy Association: *Reference Manual: Certification Examination for OTR and COTA*. 1985.
5. State regulation of occupational therapy personnel update 1986 *Occup Ther News* 40(6): 5, 1986.

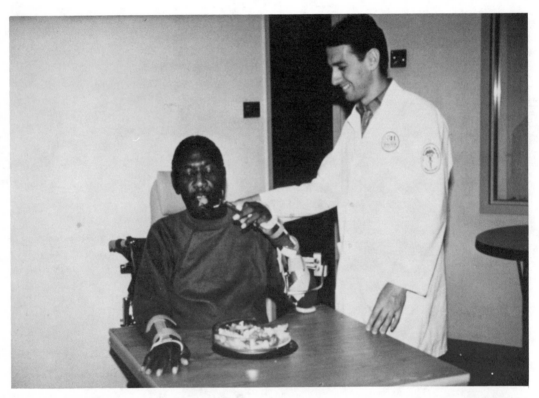

Courtesy AOTA

FIVE

Clinical Roles and Functions of the OTR and COTA

In chapter 4 the similarities and differences in the education of registered occupational therapists and certified occupational therapy assistants were discussed. In this chapter we examine how these two levels of personnel function in the work setting. When training programs for COTAs were first developed in the 1950s, the curriculum was designed to prepare people for work in psychiatric hospitals, since these hospitals had the greatest shortage in personnel at the time. Later nursing homes were also found to be in need of personnel to direct activity programs for their residents. Another curriculum was developed to meet this need, and COTAs were trained in one of these two programs. By 1965, AOTA's Delegate Assembly had voted to combine the two educational programs into a single curriculum, which combined study of psychiatry and general practice. The first group of graduates from the combined curriculum worked in general hospitals and provided diversional activities, ordered equipment and supplies, and made adapted equipment designed by the OTR (1). From this time on, COTAs were given general preparation for occupational therapy practice.

By the early 1970s, a number of OTRs were expressing concern over the roles and functions of COTAs. Some OTRs felt that COTAs were assuming roles that properly belonged to the OTR and were performing functions for which they were not adequately trained. Many more COTAs were practicing without direct OTR supervision than had been anticipated when the assistant level was established. Some highly competent COTAs were indeed performing at levels equal to that of some OTRs, and administrators who were facing increasing operational costs were likely to hire the least costly person to fill positions. In 1973 the AOTA identified six levels of occupational therapy positions: aide; entry-level COTA; exerienced COTA; entry-level OTR; experienced OTR; and specialized practitioner, administrator, researcher, or instructor. In 1976 data were collected for a role delineation study of COTAs and OTRs. This study, which attempted to clarify the functions of the two groups, was published in 1981. It provided some guidelines for how the two levels of personnel could be utilized in delivery of occupational therapy services but was criticized for its methods and its small sample size. An additional weakness of the study was that it focused only on entry-level workers (workers in their first year of clinical practice). Critics pointed out that experienced COTAs and OTRs could legitimately assume higher levels of responsibility and that this was not addressed by the 1981 document (2). In 1985 this problem was corrected by the publication of another occupational therapy personnel classification that described the roles of both entry-level and experienced personnel. This document provides much of the information contained in this chapter (3). The 1985 personnel classification looked at entry, intermediate, and advanced levels of function for both the OTR and the COTA. It also included the roles of occupational therapy supervisors and department managers or directors. Because of these additional levels of function, it more clearly showed the differences between levels of experience and job functions. The functions for three levels of COTA jobs and five levels of OTR jobs are summarized next.

COTA ROLES AND FUNCTIONS

According to the 1985 document (3), the primary function of the entry level COTA is "to *implement* occupational therapy services for patients and clients under the supervision of an occupational therapist (OTR)." *Entry level* is defined as less than one year of practice experience as a COTA. The entry-level COTA is expected to have competency skills in the delivery of occupational therapy treatment, and the document describes a number of critical performance areas for the entry-level COTA (see Table 5.1). Close supervision is required for the entry-level COTA in clinical performance, and general supervision by an OTR or an experienced COTA is recommended for administrative functions.

An intermediate-level COTA has one or more years of clinical practice as a COTA. This more experienced worker is expected to possess all of the entry-level competencies as well as the ability to implement programs to improve independent living skills and the ability to use a variety of treatment activities. The intermediate-level COTA may also be developing advanced skills in areas of special interest. This staff member is expected to perform all of the entry-level COTA functions and additional functions that are consistent with the additional experience and training. General supervision by an experienced OTR or an advanced level COTA for administrative functions.

The advanced-level COTA has three or more years of experience in a specialized area of practice. At this level, COTAs function in staff positions but demonstrate a higher level of performance than that of intermediate-level COTAs. Assigned job responsibilities vary from one facility to another, but these highly skilled staff members have advanced competencies in their specialty area and are capable of sharing their knowledge through education, publication, or participation in clinical studies. The advanced-level COTA is a skilled practitioner who requires only general supervision in clinical service and in administrative functions. The advanced-level COTA may function more independently in some types of clinical practice, but when the client's condition is unstable, supervision by an OTR is recommended (3, 4).

Frequently COTAs are employed by nursing homes, group homes, and residential settings as directors of resident activities. In this type of position the COTA is able to function fairly independently in

Table 5.1[a]
COTA

	Entry	Intermediate	Advanced
Experience	Less than 1 year of practice experience as COTA	One or more years of practice as a COTA	More than 3 years experience
Competencies	Competencies in delivery of OT services under the direction of an OTR	Entry-level competencies plus skill in implementing a variety of independent living skills and treatment activities	Demonstrates advanced clinical, educational, or administrative skills; shares knowledge through education, publication, or clinical studies
Examples of performance areas	Transmits requests for service to OTR; contributes to client assessment; assists OTR in planning and implementing treatment; reports client observations to OTR; maintains necessary documentation as directed by supervising OTR	Entry-level competencies plus greater independence in performing selected assessments, reports observations to OTR and other team members; assists in the documentation of treatment protocols, department records and procedures; provides inservice and community education; supervises entry-level COTAs, OT aides, volunteers, and COTA students	Performs assigned tasks at a higher level than an intermediate COTA and demonstrates greater knowledge of areas of practice; may contribute to a variety of department functions
Supervisory support	Close supervision of clinical performance and general supervision of management functions by experienced OTR or COTA	General clinical supervision from intermediate or advanced-level OTR and general management supervision by experienced OTR or advanced-level COTA	General clinical supervision from intermediate or advanced-level OTR; general management supervision by an experienced OTR

[a]Adapted from Schell BA: Guide to occupational therapy personnel. *AJOT* 39:803–810, 1985.

providing an ongoing program of meaningful activities to promote the overall health and well-being of residents. As an activity director the COTA is directly responsible to the administrator of the facility and administers as well as implements the activity program. Keeping records of programming and resident participation are part of the COTA's role in this setting, as are ordering supplies and equipment, supervising volunteers, aides, and students, and managing the program budget. Activity programs of this kind are not considered occupational therapy, because they meet general rather than specific needs. If a COTA activity director finds a resident with specific functional problems who could benefit from occupational therapy intervention, an OTR should be consulted to evaluate the resident and develop a treatment plan.

ROLES AND FUNCTIONS OF THE OTR

The entry-level OTR has less than one year's practice experience as an OTR. According to the 1985 personnel classification (3), the primary function of this worker is "to provide occupational therapy services to patients/clients, including assessment, treatment planning and implementation, related documentation, and communication." Competencies as a general practitioner of occupational therapy are required. The personnel classification lists a number of critical performance areas for the entry-level OTR. This staff member is viewed as having greater responsibility for assessment and documentation of client problems than the entry-level COTA (see Table 5.2). There are also greater responsibilities for administrative functions, and the entry-level OTR may be given some supervisory duties. Close supervision of the entry-level OTR's clinical performance and direct supervision of administrative functions should be given by an intermediate or advanced-level OTR.

An intermediate-level OTR has had one or more years of practice experience as an OTR. This staff member must demonstrate all of the established entry-level OTR skills and should be able to use a variety of treatment approaches independently. This practitioner may be developing advanced skills in one or more areas of occupational therapy and may be assigned higher level departmental functions. General supervision by an experienced OTR is recommended for clinical performance, and administrative supervision by an OTR with administrative experience is suggested.

The advanced-level OTR holds a graduate degree in occupational therapy or a related area and/or certification by an organization or group that offers continuing education, examination, or advanced practice requirements in a specialty area of practice. These practitioners must have three or more years of practice experience in a specialty area of occupational therapy practice. Their skills should reflect a broad range of experience and a greater depth of knowledge than the two previous OTR levels. At the advanced level, OTRs should show ability to integrate clinical theory and practice at a high level, resulting in evaluation and treatment services that are innovative, complex, and efficient. Advanced practitioners are expected to share their knowledge through staff and

student education, publications, clinical studies, or research. The duties are likely to be diverse, and advanced practitioners should serve as a resource to their occupational therapy colleagues and to members of related professions in their areas of expertise. No supervision is required for these staff members when they are working in their specialty area of practice and only occasional supervision when working in nonspecialty areas. General supervision for administrative functions is recommended.

Two additional positions that require specialized skills were described for the OTR in the 1985 personnel classification: occupational therapy supervisor and department manager/director. The primary duties of a supervisor are to "supervise OTRs, COTAs, students, volunteers, and aides." Supervisors may also provide direct client service, but this may be omitted if they are responsible for supervising a large group of people. Coordination of occupational therapy fieldwork may be another role for the OTR supervisor. Additional education related to supervision is recommended for this job classification, and at least three years of clinical experience is considered necessary before assuming a supervisory role. This position requires an understanding of personnel and department policies, demonstrated leadership skills, good communication skills, and the ability to organize time, material, and personnel effectively. An occupational therapy supervisor should possess intermediate or advanced clinical skills. General supervision in clinical and administrative functions is recommended.

The final OTR position described in the 1985 document is that of occupational therapy department manager or director. This function includes "planning, organizing, directing, controlling, and coordinating all aspects of the department or service." Continuing education relevant to

Table 5.2.[a]
OTR

	Entry	Intermediate	Advanced	Supervisor	Manager/Director
Experience Competency	Less than 1 yr experience Competencies as general OT practitioner	More than 1 yr experience Demonstrated independence in use of varied treatment approaches	More than 3 yr Broad range of experience and depth of knowledge; innovative, complex and efficient clinical practice; shares knowledge with others	More than 3 yr Thorough understanding of department policies and procedures; leadership potential; intermediate or advanced clinical skills	More than 3 yr Thorough knowledge of OT and management principles and practices; understands department's objectives and functions and can communicate them to others
Examples of performance areas	Receives referrals for service; performs screening and assessments, plans and implements treatment procedures; documents services; complies with agency standards; supervises COTAs, aides, volunteers, and students.	All entry-level tasks, plus greater involvement in the development and provision of record-keeping systems, continuing education; review of service program; of documentation of treatment protocols and procedures	Integrates clinical theory and practice at an advanced level; participates in providing student and staff education; publication, clinical research	Participates in staff selection, evaluates job performance, coordinates education and work schedule; implements departmental policies; assists with documentation of department goals and objectives; assists department manager	Hires and evaluates staff; develops and implements department policies and procedures; participates in organizational planning; represents department to other units of organization, ensures compliance with government and professional standards
Supervisory support	Close supervision of clinical performance; general administrative supervision by experienced OTR	General supervision of clinical performance; and general administrative supervision by experienced OTR	General clinical supervision as required; general administrative supervision by experienced OTR	General supervision of clinical performance by department manager and also of administrative responsibilities	General supervision by administrative personnel of the organization

[a]Adapted from Schell BA: Guide to occuaptional therapy personnel. AJOT 39:803–810, 1985.

management and administration is a prerequisite for this position, and some practitioners may hold graduate degrees in administration and management. The amount of experience required to assume such responsibilities will vary with the size and scope of the department, but three years of clinical experience is suggested as a minimum requirement, with at least one of those years being spent in a supervisory role. Individuals who assume management positions must have "a thorough knowledge of occupational therapy and of management principles and practices; demonstrate understanding of department objectives and functions; and conceptualize, interpret, and integrate occupational therapy services into the relevant organizational context." The occupational therapy department manager works under the general supervision of the administrative personnel of the organization.

Tables 5.1 and 5.2 identify some of the key differences between the different levels of occupational therapy personnel. Generally the COTA is viewed as an implementer of occupational therapy services—the frontline worker who carries out vital client interventions. The COTA is viewed as having less responsibility for specialized assessment of client deficits, treatment planning, and independent delivery of services. Supervision is required for all three levels of COTA personnel, although the advanced-level COTA may need only minimal supervision. This document suggests that the OTR is expected to carry greater responsibility for assessment, treatment planning, supervision of treatment services, documentation, and administrative functions. At higher levels, responsibilities steadily increase, with additional education being needed to help the practitioner master more complex clinical and administrative skills. An entry-level OTR, however, might rely heavily on the experience and skills of an intermediate- or advanced-level COTA and might consult with that individual on many clinical and administrative matters.

In both OTR and COTA positions there is a need to develop a high degree of skill in one's daily job functions. This process of professional growth and development strengthens the clinical program and provides personal satisfaction to practitioners as their competence increases. Both OTRs and COTAs have relevant skills to contribute to the total occupational therapy program and should strive to work in a complementary fashion for the maximum benefit of the clients they serve.

CURRENT AND FUTURE TRENDS

Elnora Gilfoyle, president of the American Occupational Therapy Association in 1986, commented on the changing roles and functions of OTRs and COTAs when writing about the future of occupational therapy (6). Gilfoyle noted that health care and occupational therapy are changing in response to social changes that have taken place within the last several decades. Some of these changes have influenced the roles and functions of occupational therapy personnel. She believes that occupational therapists will assume independent health care roles in the future and will provide their services through consultation, monitoring, and supervision. They are also likely to be more active in research, theory development, education, and administration. Gilfoyle also believes that COTAs will provide much of the direct patient care and become more involved in independent practices. Gilfoyle notes that occupational therapy expanded its services significantly in public and private schools as a result of legislation that defined occupational therapy as an education-related service. In education-related practices there will be an increase in the need for consultation and supervisory skills, ability to participate in research, and ability to manage resources effectively. The COTAs are likely to become the major deliverers of service in schools, with the indirect service functions being carried out by OTRs.

Practitioners who continue to function in medically related settings will need to learn to deliver services outside the domain of the hospital and demonstrate the cost-effectiveness of occupational therapy. In these settings, OTRs are likely to become more involved in research and management of cost-effective services, while COTAs will expand their direct service role to agencies outside the traditional medical institution.

Gilfoyle warns that as OTRs assume greater responsibility for consultation and supervision, research involvement, and management roles, graduate education is likely to become necessary. In a similar way, COTAs will need more education to adequately assume expanded clinical roles. Gilfoyle predicts that a minimum of four years of higher education (including a liberal arts component) will be necessary for the expanded COTA roles.

Part II of this text presents case examples that show how job responsibilities are divided between the OTR and COTA in some clinical settings. When teamwork between OTR and COTA is working well, exemplary occupational therapy services can be provided.

DISCUSSION QUESTIONS

1. Contact several OTRs and COTAs in your area and find out about their roles and responsibilities. What similarities or differences did you find between the two groups? Does the setting make a difference in the job responsibilities or the amount of supervision needed?

2. What promotional opportunities are there for OTRs and COTAs in your area?

3. Are there civil service classifications in your state for OTRs and COTAs who are state employed? If so, how are these positions described?

4. Read some job descriptions of OTR/COTA positions in your area. What roles and functions are described, and what level of experience is required for the positions?

5. Many students enter occupational therapy because of its direct service opportunities. For the experienced practitioner, however, there are likely to be supervisory or administrative responsibilities as well. How do you feel about assuming these roles later in your career?

REFERENCES

1. Hirama H: A chronological review. In Ryan S. *The Certified Occupational Therapy Assistant: Roles and Responsibilities.* Thorofare, NJ, Slack, 1986, pp. 23–24.
2. Shapiro D, Brown D: The delineation of the role of entry-level occupational therapy personnel. *AJOT* 35:306–311, 1986.
3. Schell BA: Guide to occupational therapy personnel. *AJOT* 39:803–810, 1985. (Approved by the Representative Assembly, April, 1985).
4. Ryan S: Therapeutic intervention: an overview. In Ryan S *The Certified Occupational Therapy Assistant: Roles and Responsibilities.* Thorofare, NJ, Slack, 1986, pp 149–152.
5. Ryan S: The role of the COTA as an activities director. In Ryan S (ed): *The Certified Occupational Therapy Assistant: Roles and Responsibilities.* Thorofare, NJ, Slack, 1986, pp 295–304.
6. Gilfoyle E: The future of occupational therapy: an environment of opportunity. In Ryan S (ed): *The Certified Occupational Therapy Assistant: Roles and Responsibilities.* Thorofare, NJ, Slack, 1986, pp. 399–406.

The Practice Arena of Occupational Therapy

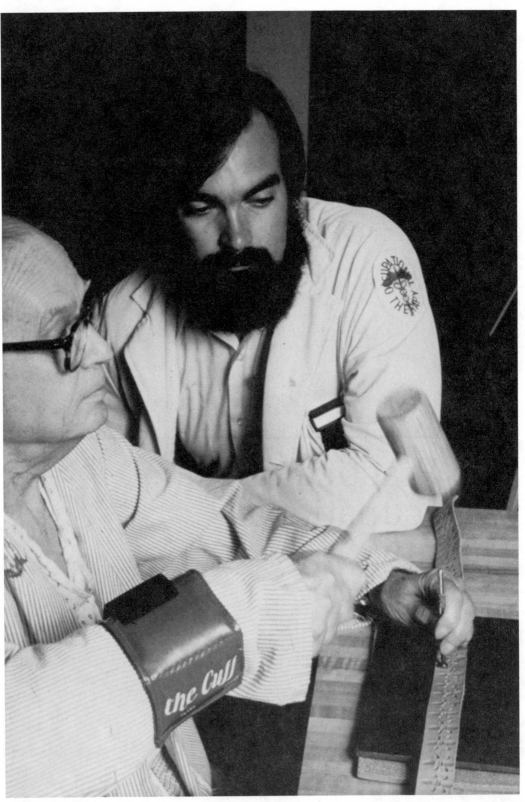

SIX

Health Care Funding and Services in the United States

Health care is the nation's third largest industry, with a labor force of over six million people and expenditures of over $247 billion per year. It accounts for 9.4% of the gross national product. Americans have come to expect exemplary medical care and rely on health care services to be there when they need them, both for routine care and for catastrophic illnesses or injuries. Americans average four physician visits per year, and 14% of the population is hospitalized annually.

Hospitals are the largest part of the health care network of services. They employ 75% of the health care work force. The 7100 hospitals in the United States account for about 40% of all health care expenditures. Over 70% of those employed in the health care industry are women. Another large component of the health care industry is composed of nursing homes and long-term care facilities. Over one million aged, disabled, and chronically ill persons are cared for in nursing homes (1). In addition to these institutions, there is a vast array of health services and products available to the American public. One might expect that health care would be a highly organized and integrated system of services, but in the United States that is far from true. There is no single, unified American health care system. Think of a large shopping mall with an enormous variety of restaurants, department stores, specialty shops, and offices. One can compare health care in America to this shopping mall model. It includes a bewildering variety of institutions, clinics, laboratories, government agencies, business organizations, and independent practitioners. In the United States, health care has developed along the lines of private business, with fee-for-service being the traditional pattern of payment. To understand the status of health care in this country, it is necessary to review how health care services developed and how they reached their present form.

PREINDUSTRIAL PHASE

In discussing the evolution of health care in America, Ehrenreich (2) describes two phases of development: the preindustrial phase that went up to the 1930s and the industrial period from the 1930s to the present. This is a useful distinction, since health care services in the nineteenth and early twentieth century resembled a cottage industry and functioned quite differently from those of today. In the early years of the nation, health care was largely the responsibility of each individual or family. Doctors were rare, so people had to care for most illnesses or injuries on their own. Books on home medical care provided some guidance, and in many communities persons with a special talent for healing developed reputations as lay practitioners. The few physicians who were available had a minimal education. Their real training occurred primarily during an apprenticeship to an experienced doctor. What medical services there were rested in the hands of these independent practitioners, and the few hospitals that existed were custodial institutions (hospices) for the destitute or the mentally ill.

In 1910 the Flexner report brought to light the poor quality of many medical schools that were then in operation. The report helped to establish higher educational standards for medical education, and many substandard medical schools were forced to close as a result of this tightening of educational requirements. Those that survived were substantially modernized and improved.

By 1910, hospitals had begun to play a more important role in health care. In Europe, hospitals had evolved from charity institutions to public facilities staffed by physicians who were employed by the hospital. In the United States, however, a mixed economy of hospitals developed. Some hospitals were public, tax-supported institutions; others were nonprofit institutions run by religious or charitable organizations (voluntary hospitals); still others were private, for-profit institutions (proprietary hospitals). Hospitals were financed through patient fees; they charged the individual on a fee-for-service basis. With

the development of nursing as a trained profession, the division of labor in health care began. By the end of the nineteenth century, hospitals had developed into a sizable industry that was organized along business lines. As standards of cleanliness and personal care improved, hospitals overcame their previous reputation as "pest houses" and became an important adjunct to medical care. Gradually hospitals began to limit their care to the acute phases of illness rather than to its full course. Other institutions began to develop to serve the needs of patients who required long-term nursing care. These included nursing and convalescent homes as well as sanitariums for the treatment of specific diseases such as tuberculosis.

As hospital budgets increased, new patterns of financing hospital care were inevitable. The number of charity cases treated declined as hospitals became more business oriented. Although state and local governments operated their own hospitals and accepted patients who were unable to pay for their care, these institutions were unable to keep up with the health care needs of the poor, the chronically ill and disabled, and the unemployed. Gradually a two-tiered system of health care evolved: a highly developed private sector for those who could afford to pay for care and an underdeveloped public sector that provided care for the poor and those with chronic medical problems. Public institutions were filled with patients who had tuberculosis, alcoholism, mental disorders, diseases of social disorganization (3). Public health in America was relegated to a secondary status and lagged far behind private medicine in prestige and financial resources. The underfinanced public health establishment was never able to assume a leadership or coordinating role in health care.

In the early years of the twentieth century, hospitals functioned fairly independently with local trustees, physicians, and administrators deciding on the policies and procedures for their particular institution. There was little attempt to integrate services in hospital care, ambulatory care, or public health. Group practice (the organization of a group of physicians into a clinic), which could offer a broader array of medical services than the individual practitioner, began to develop in the 1880s. The Mayo Clinic in Rochester, Minnesota, was the prototype for this type of practice. Typically, doctors financed such clinics and became their owners while other doctors became their employees. Thus a new type of profit-making organization entered American medical practice. Group practices gradually spread throughout the country, although many physicians continued to practice independently. By the 1920s, other health-related industries were developing, such as the pharmaceutical industry and hospital equipment industries.

As the demand for medical services grew, doctors were forced to delegate some of their responsibilities as health care providers. They did this in three ways: 1) by using young doctors in training to help provide hospital care; 2) by encouraging responsible professionalism in a number of related health care fields; and 3) by employing women in auxilliary health care service roles. Professionalism was encouraged to free the physician from the need to directly supervise every aspect of care. Doctors, however, maintained their position of authority over other health care workers and never relinquished their role as direct intermediary between the patient and the health care system. The subordinate health care professions eventually became rigidly stratified, with a large gap between their status and that of the physician.

Throughout the preindustrial period of development, physicians had been able to maintain control of the health care market and services. Even in the nineteenth century, however, a small number of Americans had begun to carry some insurance against sickness through an employer, a fraternal order, a trade union, or a commercial insurance company. The need for health insurance centered around four basics types of costs:

1. Individual loss of income
2. Individual medical costs
3. Indirect costs of illness to society
4. Social costs of medical care

By the end of World War I, all of the European countries had developed some form of coverage of health care costs for their citizens. Most of these plans were part of a general program of social insurance against the risks that interrupted the income of workers: industrial accidents, sickness and disability, old age, and unemployment. Such plans were worker oriented and were intended to stabilize incomes and offer some degree of protection against catastrophic events. In the United States, however, government was highly decentralized and there was much less government involvement in programs of social welfare. There was no national sponsor for the types of programs developed in the European countries and no structure on which to build such programs.

From the beginning of the twentieth century, various types of national health insurance plans had been proposed, but each time they were defeated. Labor organizations did not favor the concept. Employers saw compulsory health insurance as contrary to their interests. The private insurance industry, which was beginning to do a flourishing business in private sickness insurance, was strongly opposed to a national health insurance plan. The most vehement opposition came from the physicians themselves and their national organization, the American Medical Association (AMA). Doctors feared that they would lose their autonomy under such a system, and they also believed that national health insurance would place limits on their income.

By the 1920s and 1930s a concern was developing over the cost of medical care. As the middle class began to feel the effect of higher costs for health care services, they began turning in larger numbers to private insurers who offered at least partial coverage of costs. With the impact of the Great Depression of the late 1920s, then was renewed interest in a program of national health insurance. Unemployment insurance, however, was considered to be an even higher priority and took precedence. Old age benefits were also a major concern, and in 1935 Congress passed the Social Security Act, which provided a minimum income for retired persons and some additional welfare health care costs, although that had not originally been part of the package.

EARLY INDUSTRIAL PHASE: 1930–1950

The severe economic depression resulted in a sharp drop in spending for medical care. Doctors and hospitals, whose income had fallen abruptly, no longer felt that they could provide free services to the poor and began to ask state and local welfare departments to pay for the cost of health services for this population. Welfare departments began to do so on a temporary basis, and this set the precedent for government financing of health care for low-income groups. In the mid-1930s the AMA softened its opposition to private health insurance, as more and more people began to take advantage of such plans. Physicians were now seeing that private insurance coverage could increase rather than decrease their incomes and need not substantially interfere with the doctor-patient relationship. In 1946 the AMA created the Associated Medical Care Plans, the precursor of Blue Shield, and entered

into their own version of private health insurance (4). Another type of insurance plan, Blue Cross, was developed by the hospital industry.

After World War II, Truman included a program of national health insurance in his election platform, but the AMA and other health care interests opposed the plan and it was abandoned, except for some funding to expand hospitals and allow new hospital construction. The strong fear of "socialized medicine" prevented compulsory health insurance from developing, and the groups that had formed an alliance to support it eventually drifted apart. By 1952 over half of all Americans had purchased some health insurance. Labor unions had now entered the arena and had successfully bargained for health care benefits for their members (5). The extent of coverage was highly variable, however, and the persons most likely to be insured through employer plans were workers living in urban industrial areas. The unemployed, those living in rural areas, the elderly, and the chronically ill—those who needed it most—remained uninsured.

Private health insurance plans offered three different types of benefits.

1. Indemnity benefits (in which the insurer reimbursed the consumer for partial costs of medical care)
2. Service benefits (in which the insurer paid the physician or hospital for services rendered, often in full)
3. Direct services (in which the insurer directly provided health care services to the consumer in return for prepayment)

Each type of insurance plan contained some mechanism for cost control and limitation of services.

In the 1930s and 1940s, indemnity and service-benefit plans predominated. Slowly, however, a few direct service plans began to appear. These early health cooperatives enrolled members for a set monthly or annual fee and provided a full range of health services. They built their own clinics and hospitals and employed their own staff to provide ambulatory care. Popularly known as Health Maintenance Organizations (HMOs), they emphasized prevention and health maintenance in addition to offering sickness care. Their coverage was usually more comprehensive than indemnity or service-benefit plans; however, start-up costs were high and, since no government aid was available to them in the 1950s, they were largely local ventures. They attracted widespread interest, however, since they seemed to be effective in controlling health care costs by stressing prevention, providing maximum ambulatory care services, using physician extenders, and minimizing hospitalization (3,6).

INCREASING INDUSTRIALIZATION: 1950–1970

With the increased use of health insurance, the industrial phase of health care delivery had begun. By the early 1950s, commercial insurance plans were gaining ground over the service-benefit plans of Blue Cross and Blue Shield. As commercial health insurance expanded, the nature of the health care industry changed. Individual policies were still being sold, but the bulk of health insurance was now being marketed for groups as employee health benefit plans became one of the standard fringe benefits of employment. Starr, in his book *The Social Transformation of American Medicine* (3), sums it up by saying:

America had taken a different road to health insurance than the one taken by European societies, and it arrived at a different destination. The original European model began with the industrial working class and emphasized income maintenance. From that base, it expanded in both its coverage of the population and the range of benefits. . . . But in America, there was no institutional structure for health insurance when the middle class encountered problems in paying for hospital costs during the 1920's and when the hospitals encountered problems in meeting their expenses during the depression. . . . . America developed an insurance system . . . to improve access of middle-class patients to hospitals; an insurance system developed under the control of the hospitals and doctors that sought to buttress the existing forms of organization.

The evolution of health insurance was a direct outcome of the private enterprise system that had developed in America.

In the years that followed World War II, an immense medical research establishment developed in the United States. From the early part of the twentieth century, the chief sources of mortality had been shifting from infectious to chronic disease. Research into the causes of cancer, heart disease, and other life-threatening diseases had become a high priority. The public was also concerned about some of the behavioral problems that were being seen with greater frequency: alcoholism, drug use, and delinquency. The federal government generously supported medical research in many areas, and private foundations supplemented this effort by providing private funding for health research and projects. Hospitals had benefited from increased governmental support as well. The Hill-Burton Act of 1946 had provided construction funds for community hospitals in underserved areas, and many small hospitals were able to expand under this program. Medicine was becoming highly specialized and more and more young doctors were choosing to enter lucrative specialty practices rather than general practice. The higher levels of education required for specialization helped to raise health care costs even further.

By the early 1960s it was recognized that large segments of the population did not have access to adequate medical care. Congress had provided funding to educate greater numbers of health care workers and had encouraged the development of community-based mental health services and ambulatory care clinics; despite this, health care resources were unevenly distributed and not readily available to the underprivileged. The antipoverty and civil rights programs, begun during the Kennedy administration and continued by President Johnson, helped to focus awareness on the health needs of the poor, the elderly, and minority groups. By 1965 there was adequate Congressional support for passage of the Medicare and Medicaid programs. Medicare provided both compulsory hospital insurance (part A) for persons over the age of 65 under the umbrella of the Social Security Act and a government-subsidized voluntary insurance program to cover physician's bills (part B). Medicaid provided for federal grants to the states for programs of medical assistance for the poor. States were given considerable discretion in how Medicaid funds would be applied, and eligibility requirements varied widely. The objective of both programs was to enable the poor and the elderly to "buy into" the private health care system. Despite these measures, the gap between health care services available to the middle-class and low-income groups actually widened. By the 1970s a large group of people still lacked financial protection for periods of illness or disability. Part-time workers, the recently unemployed, and the working poor who earned too little to afford private insurance but too much to qualify for public assistance were still left out of the picture.

COST-CONTAINMENT MEASURES: 1970–1985

The 1970s brought a wave of disillusionment with the health care system in general and with physicians in particular. Health care costs had soared out of control, and the government was forced to intervene in a direct way. In 1970 a federal program was authorized that provided funding to establish health maintenance organizations (HMOs). State governments began to enact tougher laws regulating the health care industry and requiring state approval (certificates of need) for the construction of new hospitals and nursing homes. In 1973 a federal law was passed requiring businesses with more than 25 employees to offer at least one qualified HMO as an option in employee health insurance coverage. In 1974 a new health planning law established 200 Health Systems Agencies (HSAs), which were given responsibility for drawing up three-year plans, reviewing proposed new health projects, and recommending action to the states and the federal government on certificates of need and the use of federal funds. Health care planning was now seen as an urgent need and as the responsibility of the public sector. A proposal for national health insurance came very close to being introduced by the Nixon administration, but, as in the past, other needs took priority and it did not reach Congress.

By 1979 there were 217 HMOs operating throughout the country, and they were providing health care at significantly lower costs than traditional medical practices. With the election of Ronald Reagan to the presidency, a wave of political conservatism swept the country, which affected health care as well as other segments of the economy. The Reagan administration believed that America's health care problems could best be resolved by reducing government involvement to a minimum and relying instead on competition and the incentives of the marketplace to contain health care costs and restructure services. Consumers, doctors, hospitals, and even the insurance companies were reluctant to lose the benefits of federally funded programs and the public programs of medical assistance and voiced their opposition strongly. The Reagan administration was forced to modify its position and left the Medicare and Medicaid programs in place; however, substantial cuts in funding were made in public health services and medical assistance for the poor. There was also much less inclination for the government to continue its efforts to regulate the health care industry.

RISE OF HEALTH CARE CONGLOMERATES

During the 1980s a new type of health care organization appeared. This was the large health-care corporation that bought up hospitals and other health service organizations and proceeded to operate them along corporate lines. These large corporate enterprises in health care have become common and are extremely attractive to private investors. Relman (7) writes that we are seeing the rise of a "medical-industrial complex" in the United States, with the large health care conglomerates becoming a central element in the delivery of health services. About half of the proprietary hospitals in the United States are now owned by large corporations that specialize in hospital ownership and management. Proprietary nursing homes are an even bigger business, with many owned by small investors or physicians. About a third of the diagnostic laboratories are now owned by profit-making companies. The Naisbitt Group, which published projections of future trends, refers to this development as "the privatization of health care" and says "the era of corporate medicine is here. Large hospital corporations enjoy $16 billion annual revenues and the numbers keep growing" (8). The Naisbitt Group predicts that the health care industry will be deregulated not through formalized government control but through cost controls imposed by third-party payers—the federal and state governments through Medicaid and Medicare and the commercial insurers.

Other health services are also being taken over by business interests. Home care services, formerly provided by public health programs or community agencies, are growing rapidly and include such services as nursing care, homemaking assistance, physical and occupational therapy, respiratory therapy, and pacemaker monitoring. Other health-related services such as mobile computerized tomography (CT) scanning, cardiopulmonary testing, industrial health screening, rehabilitation counseling, dental care, weight-control clinics, alcohol- and drug-abuse programs, and fitness centers are being aggressively marketed by private entrepreneurs. Two areas of special interest are hospital emergency room services and long-term hemodialysis programs for patients with end-stage renal disease. Large corporations have taken over these services in some areas and provide them to hospitals on a contract basis.

The move toward corporate control and management of health services may have both positive and negative effects. On the one hand, it may result in slowing down health care cost increases through strong central management of the corporate structures and increase the efficiency of health care delivery. On the other hand, health care may not respond to the classic laws of supply and demand, since the consumer of health care is often not really free or knowledgeable enough to shop around for the best bargain in health care services.

Also, private enterprises exist to sell their services. The more they sell, the more profit they make. This sales emphasis has the potential for consumer exploitation in health services and will require some type of regulation. Relman (7) also points out that since profit is the bottom line for corporate health care giants, they are unlikely to want to provide services for the poor or for low-income groups. They may also be reluctant to involve themselves in the costly process of educating physicians and other health professionals. (Teaching hospitals are in a double bind, since they are expected to compete with other hospitals while carrying out their teaching mission.) It is too soon to say what impact corporate health organizations will have on health services in the United States, but it is worthy of close monitoring and study in the next decade.

MULTIPLE HEALTH CARE SYSTEMS

American health care evolved in a free-enterprise system as a network of private business enterprises. Government has played a role when necessary to guarantee health services for the underprivileged in society, to promote research, and to regulate the health care industry. According to Torrens (9), there are at least four health care systems operating in the United States today. First, there is the system of health care used by middle and upper income groups (frequently referred to as the American health care system). Each individual or family puts together a set of services to meet their needs and pays for them out of their own resources or through private insurance. This service system revolves around the physician, who coordinates services to some degree and calls on specialized services as needed. Local community hospitals are used most frequently

by this group of consumers. Their only contact with a public institution may be when long-term care is needed for mental disturbances. The individual services used have little formal connection with one another, and the only thread of continuity in care is provided by the physician or by the consumer.

A second system of health care is used by the poor, the inner-city dwellers, and minority groups. Again there is no formal system but rather a loose network of services that the individual or family uses to meet immediate needs. These groups tend to have no continuity of care through a single provider. Some routine prevention services such as immunizations are available through local health departments, and the hospital emergency room is often used as a source of treatment for acute illness or injury. City or county hospitals are most frequently used when hospitalization is required, and outpatient clinics of public hospitals may provide some ambulatory care. To some extent these patients are now beginning to enter private hospitals and nursing homes because of reimbursement through Medicare and Medicaid funds. Health care is generally unplanned and unmonitored for these groups.

A third system of health care is that provided by the military services. Extensive health care services are available to all active military personnel and their families. This is a highly organized system and is available everywhere military personnel are found. This system emphasizes total care, with a particular emphasis on preventing illness and injury.

A fourth health care system is that of the Veterans Administration, which was designed to provide medical care for retired, disabled veterans. It is a hospital-based system, with 171 hospitals located within the continental United States, and now provides some outpatient care as well. Torrens notes that the two civilian systems are informal and somewhat haphazard in their organization. There are many health situations that may fall between the cracks, and entry into each system requires a certain amount of know-how. These multiple systems of health care make for areas of overlap and areas of scarcity of services. No one authority plays a coordinating role.

Mechanic (10) agrees that physicians in the United States have concentrated on developing private, entrepreneurial medicine rather than on building a rational system of health care. Because demands for care have always exceeded the resources available, various forms of rationing have existed. The most basic form is fee-for-service medicine. Care has only been available to those who could purchase it, and this was in effect a method of rationing resources. A second method is by implicit rationing. In countries that have a government-sponsored health insurance system, health care is rationed through centralized budgeting for health expenditures or by limiting the resources available to insured consumers. Today most societies are moving toward the explicit rationing of health care, in which limits are set on total expenditures for health services but rational decisions are made as to which services will be supported. Mechanic contends that under the latter system the physician's role shifts from that of expert to that of bureaucrat. "The locus of control for medical decision-making is a key variable in examining the implications of medical care for social life more generally.... In a bureaucratic structure, physicians are rewarded more for being good managers and researchers ... than for providing interested and humane care." According to Mechanic the bureaucratization of medicine is inevitable, and he warns that the humane aspects of health care may be neglected in the effort to make the technology of health care work.

HEALTH CARE TRENDS IN THE UNITED STATES

What are some of the problems that American health care faces in the 1980s? A number of realities must be confronted, including a surplus of physicians, hospital beds, and centers for tertiary care. Ginzberg (11) has noted that planning is a major need, but there is almost a complete lack of mechanisms within the United States for planning and operating health care resources on a regional basis. He predicts that there will be continuing pressure for more money and more resources by health care facilities and speculates that there will continue to be a wide gap between expenditures for health and actual accomplishments. Baum (12) predicts that too many professionals will be competing for limited health care dollars. She notes that there will be more people with chronic conditions and an increasing population of elderly people who will need services. Even today some types of health professionals are in short supply, particularly in the rehabilitation fields. This shortage will continue in the foreseeable future. Baum also points out that technology is now capable of sophisticated life-support systems and predicts that there will be more ethical and legal questions over the prolongation of life for seriously ill individuals.

What trends can we expect in the health care services in the next decade? A number of writers have made some predictions, and they fall into several major areas.

1. *The shift from inpatient to outpatient care.* As hospital costs have continued to rise, there has been rapid development of outpatient services. The Naisbitt Group refers to these programs as the McDonald's of health care. Such services as outpatient surgical centers,

walk-in clinics that provide urgent care, shopping mall clinics, women's health centers, and expanded physician office services provide "fast-food" types of health care. The main attraction of such programs is that minor ailments and emergencies can be treated quickly and at a price considerably lower than their hospital counterparts. Continuity of care may be sacrificed, however.

2. *Shorter hospital stays.* For those conditions requiring hospitalization, shorter stays are the rule. Under a new formula of diagnostic-related groups (DRGs), hospitals are paid a fixed rate for Medicare patients. The rate depends on the patient's diagnosis, age, and condition. If the hospital treats patients for more than the standard Medicare rate, it must absorb the loss in revenue. If it treats them for less, it can keep any savings accrued. Medicare has established 471 different diagnostic categories of disease and surgical procedures and now pays for all Medicare hospital charges on this basis. Although it has resulted in considerable savings in cost for the government, doctors criticize the system for discharging patients "quicker and sicker." As a result, patients often need a period of convalescence in a nursing home or home health services after hospital discharge. If this prospective payment system is found to be effective as a cost-saving measure, a similar system may be adopted by private insurance companies as well.

3. *New cost-saving concepts.* Employers who provide health care coverage for their workers are beginning to look for new ways of saving money on health care. In 1983 one large company experimented with a plan that gave every employee a fixed amount to spend as he or she wished for health care costs. Employees could keep the money they didn't spend. As a result, hospital stays became shorter and medical claims declined by more than 6% (13).

4. *Increased competition among hospitals.* To keep their beds filled, hospitals are being forced to compete with one another for patients. Some hospitals have offered all-expense "package deals" for some types of surgery or discount rates to members of related health care plans. Others have opened units where a family member can provide direct care at a lower cost to the patient. In an effort to keep solvent, some hospitals are diversifying into new areas and are becoming the supermarkets of the health care industry. There are hospital-related HMOs, and some hospitals provide laboratory services to other agencies. Sports medicine clinics, rehabilitation services, home care, hospice programs, and dialysis centers are among the services offered. Some hospitals have become involved in consumer health education. In addition, some of the more expensive hospital services (emergency rooms, pathology, radiology, and psychiatric services) have been contracted out to corporate providers. To maintain flexibility some hospitals are now designating a certain number of beds as "swing beds," which can be used as skilled nursing care beds if the need arises.

5. *New ways of packaging and paying for health care.* It is likely that the traditional physician in an independent private practice will become extinct. Group medical practice is becoming the norm. The HMOs are well accepted and are being joined by a new type of organization, the preferred provider organization (PPO), which is a relatively new idea that is spreading rapidly. The PPOs provide a channel by which health care providers can bid for the right to serve the health care needs of a particular group or organization. The PPOs and

HMOs have become so successful that they may well become the standard way in which most people receive their health care.

6. *Multihospital systems and health care corporations.* More hospitals will become part of a multihospital system. Many local health facilities may be unable to survive in the highly competitive health care market of the 1980s. They will either be forced to close or will be acquired by one of the large hospital corporations. There will be a corresponding loss of autonomy by physicians and by local communities; however, cost-control benefits may be achieved through tighter management practices. Fiscal controls are expected to become even tighter in the years ahead.

7. *New health care partnerships and alliances.* The Naisbitt Group predicts that there will eventually be a climate of cooperation between the doctors who operate the freestanding outpatient services and the hospitals. Hospitals may grow to depend on these clinics for referrals for care of serious illnesses or injuries. Competition may be replaced by cooperation between these two segments of the health care industry, if enough growth occurs that there is room (and profit) for both.

8. *New voluntarism in health care.* As awareness grows of the many people who fall through the cracks of the health care system, new voluntary programs of care may develop. Some health care professionals and medical societies are organizing free health care services to meet the needs of the poor and the underemployed. The Naisbitt Group predicts that, to some degree, voluntarism will replace inadequate private and public health care, filling in the gaps where services are missing or not easily accessible (8,12–14).

In reviewing where American's health care has been and speculating on where it might be going, Starr (3) says that the large health-care corporation will dominate in the 1980s. He predicts that public planning will be replaced by corporate planning and that the rate of return on investments will be the chief determinant in organizing new or expanded services. Starr foresees greater disunity, inequality, and conflict throughout the health care system in the immediate future. The Naisbitt Group is less pessimistic. They suggest that while the new competitiveness may be uncomfortable it is not detrimental to health care services. They foresee that the primary challenge in the future will be to provide quality health care while also addressing the needs of low-income groups.

Only time will tell how the changes now taking place in health care will affect both consumers and providers of care. One thing is certain, however. Health care will continue to be big business in the 1980s and 1990s. The health care industry will continue to develop and will adapt complex new technologies to its purposes. It will be part of our responsibility as service providers to make sure that the *care* elements in health care are not lost in the effort to streamline services and make them cost-effective.

DISCUSSION QUESTIONS

1. Is health care a right or a privilege? Do you believe that every person has an inherent right to health services?

2. What is the middle- and upper-income health care system like in your area?

3. Is the health care service system different for low-income groups? How?

4. What health services exist in your area to serve the needs of the poor, the unemployed, and the elderly?

5. Is health care an industry in the sense of the automobile industry or the aerospace industry? If so, can it be managed according to the same business principles?

6. Should health care policies and decisions be made by the federal government to ensure the public good, or should they be left to private provider organizations?

7. What type of health insurance do you and your family have? Do you know what it covers? Are there any services that are specifically excluded?

8. Does your state have a health plan that lists the state's priorities for allocation of funds to health services? If so, what are the top priorities?

9. Can we as a nation afford the high-tech, high-cost private health industry that has developed?

10. How can consumers influence public policies on health care?

REFERENCES

1. Shortell SM: The organization of health care. In *The Nation's Health*, ed 2. San Francisco, Boyd & Fraser, 1984, pp. 219–222.

2. Ehrenreich B: The health care industry: a theory of industrial medicine. In *The Nation's Health* ed 2. San Francisco, Boyd & Fraser, 1984, pp. 187–195.

3. Starr P: *The Social Transformation of American Medicine.* New York, Basic Books, 1982, pp. 30–198, 235–449.

4. Numbers RL: The third party: health insurance in America. In *The Nation's Health*, ed 2. San Francisco, Boyd & Fraser, 1984, pp. 196–204.

5. Munts R: *Bargaining for Health: Labor Unions, Health Insurance, & Medical Care.* Madison, University of Wisconsin Press, 1967, pp. 81–100.

6. Luft HS: Definition and scope of the HMO concept. In *The Nation's Health*, ed 2. San Francisco, Boyd & Fraser, 1984, pp. 243–250.

7. Relman AS: The new medical-industrial complex. In *The Nation's Health*, ed 2. San Francisco, Boyd & Fraser, 1984, pp. 233–242.

8. Naisbitt Group: *Health: a look to the future. Occupational Therapy Newspaper* 38(10): 1, 15–16, 1984.

9. Torrens PR: Overview of the health services in the United States. In *The Nation's Health*, ed 2. San Francisco, Boyd & Fraser, 1984, pp. 223–232.

10. Mechanic D: The growth of medical technology and bureaucracy: implications for medical care. In *The Nation's Health*, ed 2. San Francisco, Boyd & Fraser, 1984, pp. 205–215.

11. Ginzberg E: Health reform: the outlook for the 1980s. In *The Nation's Health*, ed 2. San Francisco, Boyd & Fraser, 1984, pp. 361–372.

12. Baum C: The evolution of the U.S. health care system. In *The Occupational Therapy Manager.* Rockville, MD, American Occupational Therapy Association, 1985, pp. 3–25.

13. Robinson D: We can stay healthy for less. *Parade Magazine.* Dec. 15, 1985, pp. 4–5.

14. Greifinger RB, Sidel VW: American medicine: charity begins at home. In *The Nation's Health*, ed 2. San Francisco, Boyd & Fraser, 1984, pp. 176–186.

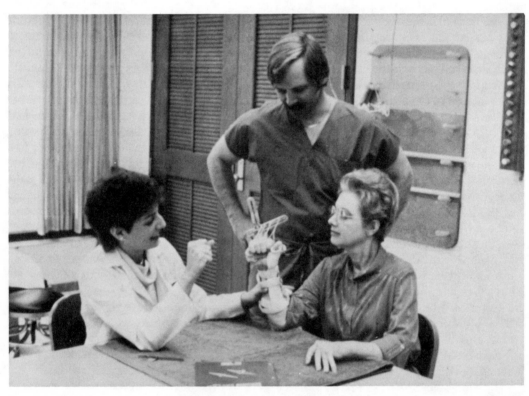

Courtesy AOTA

SEVEN

Working Together: The Health Care Team

MARTHA K. STAVROS, MSW, ACSW
DARALEEN SITKA, OTR

Today interdisciplinary health care teams are made up of many professionals who are experts in the management of one aspect of patient care. These professionals collaborate closely to provide a comprehensive level of care that was not possible when treatment was managed solely by a physician and a nurse.

Health care is shifting away from the narrow medical model that viewed the patient much like a machine with a faulty part that responded to the physician-technician's manipulation. A greater awareness of the *whole human*, who is not only a physical being but a social, psychological, cultural, and spiritual one has increased the number of specialists who are trained to work together to respond to the variety of needs of clients on their path to wellness. Ideally these professionals work in health care teams that offer the benefits of specialization and a unified comprehensive care program that has continuity from onset of illness to reintegration into the family and community (1).

Occupational therapists are integral members of these teams in hospitals, psychiatric settings, schools, home health agencies, industry, and residential facilities. As such they are challenged to learn effective consultation, supervision, leadership, and communication skills (2), as well as the unique knowledge of the occupation therapy discipline.

This chapter describes some of the teams that might be assembled to meet the needs of clients in various settings, discusses the mechanics of team function, and suggests skills that promote successful team participation. A case study is presented that demonstrates a successful multidisciplinary approach to a head-injured patient who was able to return to a meaningful life in a manner that no single discipline or a few disciplines collectively could have achieved.

TEAM MEMBERS

The membership of a health care team is determined by the setting, requirements of the patient, and family. In a hospital the occupational therapist is routinely joined by the following and an effective health care team is formed:

Physicians: In the hospital, physicians usually lead the health care team. An attending physician is ultimately responsible for medical outcome; physician residents, under the direction of the attending physician, provide much of the day-to-day care.

Nurse: Many interdisciplinary teams now use a nursing system, in which one nurse accepts primary responsibility for the development of a treatment plan that carries out team decisions and reinforces therapies on the patient unit.

Physical Therapists: These professionals work closely with occupational therapists but focus primarily on gross motor functions such as strength, range of motion, ambulation, transfers, balance skills, and mobility.

Speech and language pathologists: These team members outline the nature of communication problems and work to improve auditory-reading comprehension, verbal expression, writing skills, nonverbal communication skills, memory, and cognition (3).

Social workers: The patient and family are assessed by the social workers and treated for their emotional reaction to disability. Social workers facilitate family function and investigate concrete issues related to health care, such as finances and resource needs. The social worker is also concerned with mobilizing the human as well as durable resources needed to develop carryover in the discharge plan.

Psychologists: These team members work with social workers to enable families and patients to adjust to disability. Psychologists administer and interpret appropriate psychometric tests when indicated and treat psychological issues that impact on service delivery.

Specialized vocational counselors: Vocational counselors interface with health care teams, the community, and government funding sources to assist clients to return to work.

Also present on many inhospital health care teams are dietitians, who monitor nutritional needs, and biomedical engineers, who assist with the assessment and acquisition of equipment, especially when it is highly specialized. Respiratory therapists assess respiratory needs and prescribe respiratory support mechanisms. Pastoral care personnel offer spiritual support and counseling.

In school health care teams, the occupational therapist will normally interface with classroom teachers and special educators, who need to carry over treatment recommendations from clinic to classroom experience. School social workers and school psychologists interface with team, family, and community mental health resources. School administrators and principals are also regular members of the team, as are student counselors (4).

Many other professionals expand or change the makeup of the health care team, depending on the setting and team goals: the psychiatrist in a psychiatric setting; lawyers, judges, and police, when legal matters are involved; funding personnel such as insurance representatives, social security and department of social services personnel, visiting nurses, community mental health workers, and private industry staff, when community reentry or work-hardening programs are underway; residential placement staff and personal care attendants (who are trained with the clients).

Today's successful health care teams are models of interdisciplinary rather than multidisciplinary practice. *Multidisciplinary* is a term that refers to the efforts of many different disciplines operating independently of a team with orientations specific to each profession. *Interdisciplinary activity*, on the other hand, is aimed at achieving a common goal. Health care professionals on interdisciplinary teams must know the group goal as well as the goal of each of the other disciplines on the team. "This requires a high level of group interaction and knowledge of how to transfer integrated group activities into action that is greater than the sum of many parts" (5). The occupational therapist, like the other professionals involved, uses the team as a source of information and support for therapy (4).

TEAM MEETINGS

Performance of health care teams depends greatly on communication among team members. A significant amount of time is spent in structured meetings at which participants contribute their individual discipline's finding and note the assessments of other team members in order to increase their understanding of the treatment of the patient/family. Each setting in which the occupational therapist practices may call interdisciplinary meetings something different, but the smooth development and operation of a comprehensive treatment plan requires a structure that includes at least three components: 1) a collaborative assessment (initial staffing); 2) a follow-up evaluation of the treatment plan (rounds); and 3) the involvement of patient and family (family meetings).

Initial staffing brings together each member of the basic health care team as early as possible after the patient, student, or client has been identified for service. It generally assumes each professional involved has made an initial individual assessment and is prepared to contribute to joint problem identification, data collection, problem evaluation, goal setting, outcome prediction, and determination of activities to achieve this outcome (3). Each setting outlines the exact parameters of individual team member's participation in assessment and development of a treatment plan, but ordinarily the team will expect the occupational therapist to have information regarding the following:

Performance of daily living activities
Possible equipment needs
Preliminary cognitive/perceptual evaluation
Information on accessibility of home, school, work setting
Vocational information
Preliminary suggestions concerning use of resources, such as onsite work evaluators and personal care attendants
Some estimation of time required for intervention

Rounds, or some other type of follow-up evaluation of the health care team's treatment plan, is the tool that best shows the dynamic characteristics of team practice. Having established initial goals and a treatment plan, team members reconvene regularly to evaluate these and adjust them according to new information. Because each member shares in the responsibility and accountability for outcome, the meetings involve collaborating, communicating, and consolidating knowledge that changes the treatment plan as appropriate (1). The occupational therapist, like all other team members, must be prepared to cite specific examples of change and recommend continuation or alteration of goals or the treatment initially established.

Some health care teams expand the concept of rounds to include on-site clinic or classroom visits. In such cases the team members go to the treatment area to watch therapy procedures in order to better understand the treatment recommendations. In the occupational therapy clinic, the therapist uses such occasions to increase team members' awareness of actual client performance. In the clinic of another discipline, occupational therapists increase their understanding of that professional's goals and interventions in order to modify or improve their own goals and interventions.

Family meetings are common to almost all health care team efforts, since the family's involvement is generally indispensable to the carryover and maintenance of achievements made by the intervention of the team with the client. The value of team-family meetings depends largely on the clarity of reporting done by each therapist and the projection of a unified set of goals and expectations by the team. The team that is well practiced at active listening attends closely to the questions and suggestions of family members to enhance the treatment plan or to improve communication regarding its goals. Very often the therapeutic area that is the responsibility of the occupational therapist is of great practical value to the patient and family. The following are typical questions: "Will my son need someone with him all the time?" "Can my wife maintain her job?" "Will my mother be able to manage personal care?" The occupational therapist provides the information in the presence of the other discipline specialists, who support or modify it with their own reports. For example, an occupational therapist, physical therapist, and physician might report good functional skills, while the neuropsychologist reports cognitive deficits that increase care needs beyond what a family may have expected.

Family involvement is so critical to most treatment plans that family and patient can be considered members of the health care team. The family and patients'

understanding of professional jargon and the quality of their emotional involvement in the issues being discussed is, however, different. Family-team meetings should be stripped of medical terminology and conducted with a simplicity and clarity that does not reduce the quality of information shared with other team members. Anxiety in family members who are in the presence of many professionals reporting huge quantities of information may interfere with comprehension. Every effort must be made to reduce the formality of the occasion and ensure the participants that the team values their involvement. Because the client is very often present, the occupational therapist can build on his or her rapport with that individual to increase the comfort level of the family. This can be done most effectively by referring questions regarding certain interventions to the client and requesting the client's acknowledgement or opinion.

Team meetings are based on client needs as well as the mandates of individual settings. In a school situation the occupational therapist will participate in team meetings that fulfill the state laws requiring the assignment of special education labels and resources. Legal procedures may involve preliminary meetings with attorneys to prepare for court hearings. Community services ideally require interdisciplinary meetings with referring health care teams to develop carryover plans consistent with treatment already performed inside hospitals or institutions.

In each setting the team meetings bring together professionals with individual expertise to apply to a common goal or purpose. Although there is an organized division of labor, each person must accept the responsibility for making and implementing decisions in his or her own area of expertise. The team sessions support each person's formal and informal involvement for an integrated delivery of service (1).

SKILLS NEEDED FOR GOOD TEAMWORK

The old adage, "a chain is as strong as its weakest link," fits the challenge of interdisciplinary health care team practice very well. Not only must the occupational therapist and each other member of a successful team bring a high level of personal competence to the group, but he or she must develop communication skills that facilitate group process. Furthermore, as a team member, the individual therapist is challenged to develop special characteristics that support the group's ability to set team goals and develop team programs that are superior to individual interventions.

Because the complexity of modern health care has given rise to a vast network of professions, each of which specializes in a segment of the person's total care needs, the totality of the health delivery system depends on the quality of each professional's individual contribution to the whole. Because no one discipline can master all parts of the care plan, each professional is expected to have particular expertise in his or her own area. This is not only true because the client needs each unique intervention but because all members of a health care team tailor their involvement according to information they have gathered from the work of every other member. Thus the whole depends largely on the parts. The quality of each person's contribution greatly affects the quality of the total service delivery.

The complexity of the health care system establishes the need for excellence among the members of the team who serve the client in hospitals, schools, and community services. That same complexity mandates a commitment on the part of each professional to continue to learn and grow after formal education requirements have been met. Not only must occupational therapists develop their skills in occupational therapy by means of continuing education programs, in-service education, and regular reading of professional journals and literature, but they must pursue and improve their skills in team participation as well. Duconis and Golin (6) suggest that this is done in three ways: 1) preprofessional training done in school before certification, involving curriculum-integrated courses of specific training in team skills; 2) continuing education programs after college, such as workshops, seminars, and formal postgraduate courses offered to individuals or groups; and 3) team development with the help of hired consultants trained to facilitate team practice.

The team skills that need to be added to the occupational therapy expertise are many, but the most essential is communication. If an interdisciplinary team is going to do good work, the members must develop their ability to speak, listen, write, and read effectively. In order to express occupational therapy issues and learn about the evaluation of client needs by other disciplines, the therapist's communication must be as clear as possible.

The spoken word in formal and informal settings is the heart of the team process. Because most teams function with limited time, the expression of findings, recommendations, and questions needs to be brief, precise, and objective. The responsibility to listen to what is shared is equally important. Because not all members will be effective speakers, the good listener is active, asking questions that clarify information or requesting repetition or examples to ensure that the facts are understood. There is an important distinction between passive and active listening. Passive listening is the noninvolved relaxed listening one might use at a concert or in a light social exchange. Active listening, which is required on a health care team, involves an active effort to not only hear what is being said but to analyze it in relation to other information one has on a case. This other information could be the occupational therapist's own assessment or a treatment goal previously established by the team.

Not only must team members speak and listen well, they must also read and write accurately. No matter what the setting, the occupational therapist, like every other staff member, will be required to document assessments, interventions, and recommendations in some written form. Documentation responsibility has always been a serious charge for the professional, but it is especially so today when the written word has powerful legal significance. Beyond that, however, the information charted by members of a health care team provides ongoing guidelines for other team members who are providing complementing interventions or piggybacking their own plans for the client with that described by another therapist. The written documentation must be up-to-date, precise, and brief. Lengthy or unnecessarily anecdotal charting is often distracting and overlooked because of the time it takes to read it.

The responsibility to read the documentation of other team members parallels the responsibility to actively listen. Because interdisciplinary practice is an integration of multiple efforts, the charge to know what each team member is doing is very serious. Because there is a professional as well as a legal mandate on each team member to write down assessments and care plans, there is an equally serious responsibility for other team members to read what is written.

Given and Simmons (7) cite eight other personal and team characteristics that support effective health care team function:

1. Open-mindedness, or the willingness to accept differences and the perspective of others.
2. Independence, because the ability to function independently is required to achieve team goals.
3. Negotiation skills, because team members need to assert their perspective but remain willing to achieve a consensus by practicing give and take.
4. The willingness to accept new values, attitudes, and perceptions as appropriate.
5. Tolerance of constant review and the challenges of other team members.
6. The ability to risk.
7. Personal identity and integrity.
8. The ability to accept and assume a team's philosophy of care after it has been established by consensus.

Given and Simmons also suggest that good team players can tolerate frustration, because team process is often arduous and always more time-consuming than individual effort. The professional on a team not only has to be flexible so as to adjust to new situations but must also operate from a basic personal security that allows open-mindedness without experiencing a sense of threat (7).

Team function depends on each member's ability to state his or her opinions positively to assert recommendations with assurance. Furthermore, each member needs to participate in the group process that is identified in each setting to resolve inevitable conflict and then proceed with a spirit of cooperation and flexibility to carry out the plan that is the result of consensus.

According to Etzioni(2) and Thompson(4), the movement away from multidisciplinary to interdisciplinary practice for health care teams has allowed a departure from traditional hierarchal patterns that is stimulating new insights, perspectives, and innovative therapy. Nevertheless the change requires not only the development of a new set of skills for the participants but new and important group skills as well.

The team members must know each other's roles in order to avoid making unreasonable demands. They need to recognize that at times there will be a blurring of traditional roles and therefore a need to accept shared responsibility. The development of expertise in one area does not rule out an opinion or skill in another. In good team process, the occupational therapist may be the most appropriate person to assist with some psychosocial intervention that might ordinarily be seen as the social worker's task. The social worker may be able to help a client with adjustment while he or she participates in activities of daily living (ADLs) that are usually the province of the occupational therapist. Such sharing requires a high level of trust among team members, not only to allow participation in one another's area of expertise but to accept the appropriate guidance of the more expert member when doing so. Teams, therefore, have to accept shifting leadership. There has to be a spirit of cooperation instead of competition, and resolution of issues should follow consensus, not coercion or compromise (3).

Health care team practice is still more of an ideal than a reality in many places where occupational therapists practice. Nevertheless, paralleling the growing recognition that occupational therapy, like many other areas of professional expertise has mastered an important segment of the whole health care system, there is a movement toward group intervention. Duconis and Golin (6) polled 175 professional schools in the late 1970s. Of the 124 schools that responded, only 34% offered specific course work in team process. However, 90% responded that they recognized the growing need and most said that the concepts of team practice were an integrated part of the existing curriculum.

CASE STUDY WITH TEAM INTERVENTION

The following case study dramatically exemplifies the team approach to health care. This team was formed in a specialized rehabilitation unit of a large teaching hospital, but it grew and changed as it moved with the patient into the community and toward the resumption of the patient's normal life. The success achieved here resulted from the careful inclusion of appropriate professionals (as well as laymen), many interdisciplinary meetings of various kinds, a high level of professional and personal skills, and good team dynamics. It is described from the perspective of the occupational therapist, but the therapist acted here as an integral member of a well-functioning team. Therefore, the therapist's intervention not only influenced the work of fellow team members but it was greatly influenced by the team as well. (Medical terms used in this case study are defined in the glossary at the end of the text.)

CASE HISTORY: INTRACEREBRAL CONTUSION

Vreni, a 57-year-old female, sustained an intracerebral contusion as a result of 5-foot fall from a ladder in her home. The patient had no loss of consciousness at the scene, but within 4–6 hours her mental status deteriorated and she was taken to the emergency room, where a craniotomy was performed to remove a subdural hematoma. Once the patient's physical status stabilized, she was transferred to the rehabilitation unit, where an extensive and coordinated treatment program was developed by the interdisciplinary team. Once a referral for occupational therapy services was written by the physician, the occupational therapist's responsibilities included establishing patient contact, performing a chart review, and obtaining preliminary information from other team members (nurses, physical therapists, speech pathologists) regarding the patient's status. Vreni had many deficit areas as a result of the accident. There was focal as well as diffuse damage to the brain. Deficits included visual field cuts, a right homonymous hemianopsia, visual perceptual disorders, language problems, memory deficits, decreased upper extremity coordination, and impaired balance and equilibrium responses. Active range of motion and strength were within normal limits throughout.

During the initial evaluation phase, the registered occupational therapist (OTR) obtained baseline information concerning the patient's physical functioning, sensorimotor integrity, and performance during activities of daily living via direct observation, review of cardex information, and discussion with the nursing staff. Initially the patient was observed in her room performing her morning self-care tasks. She was evaluated for performance, and recommendations for cuing strategies and an overall approach for self-care were made to the nursing staff and to the certified occupational therapy assistant (COTA). The nursing staff was then able to follow through with a consistent and effective program to facilitate appropriate patient response during self-care activities when the COTA was not able to work with the patient. In the clinic, further assessment by the OTR was made of the patient's performance components, e.g., neuromuscular integrity, sensory awareness and integration, and cognitive skills.

Using the preliminary information obtained through the evaluation phase, an occupational therapy treatment plan was devised by the OTR and carried out by the COTA. The preliminary information and treatment program was reported by the OTR to the team members during the initial staffing. Each team member provided valuable information at this staffing that helped to refine the existing

occupational therapy treatment plan. For example, because of the patient's severe language deficits, the speech pathologist recommended strategies for the occupational therapist to utilize for communication with the patient during therapy sessions. The psychologist performed psychometric testing that enabled him to obtain valuable information regarding the patient's cognitive status. Through psychological testing and a review of the patient's psychological history, he was able to recommend to the team and occupational therapist, consistent and effective treatment for the patient. The social worker's ability to analyze the family system and report on the family's dynamics was especially helpful, as this family system was very complicated and revealed long-standing hostility between the patient and her siblings. Because of the severity of this patient's head injury, many approaches and interventions were suggested and utilized by each team member to help remediate the patient's problem areas.

As the occupational therapy program progressed, weekly notes were written and placed in the patient's medical record for other team members to review. This phase of the occupational therapy treatment program focused on extensive remediation techniques to improve the patient's performance of daily living tasks. It was vital for the COTA to clearly document what patient performance she had observed during the weekly treatment sessions because, prior to placing the note on the medical record, the supervising OTR had to review the documentation with the COTA and made modifications as needed to improve clarity. In addition to weekly notes, weekly chart rounds were attended by all team members assigned to the case to discuss patient progress and to promote consistency of treatment techniques among team members.

Family meetings were held regularly with the medical team and the patient and her family. To facilitate communication (the family was from Europe and spoke Swiss-German), a translator joined the team. These meetings were conducted regularly to keep all concerned parties informed of Vreni's progress during rehabilitation.

During the rehabilitation phase, it was important for the occupational therapist to consider the discharge situation. Vreni was adamant about returning to her own home. Therefore the team focused on preparing her for that discharge plan. It was the responsibility of the OTR to evaluate the deficit areas and make recommendations to the team. As a result of the inital evaluation and continuous reassessment, the occupational therapist believed that many core problem areas needed intervention before discharge could be recommended. The patient's severe visual field cuts and visual perceptual deficits needed to be treated in the occupational therapy clinic environment prior to allowing the patient to be discharged home. A determination regarding the extent of physical assistance and the amount and type of cuing strategies the patient required needed to be made by the occupational therapist so that family members and support staff would know how to manage the patient. The family needed to know and understand that at that time the patient could not manage her household independently. She could not prepare simple meals because of her visual field cuts, perceptual problems, and memory deficits. She could not manage her financial affairs independently, and she demonstrated poor judgment during stressful situations. The family needed to know that the patient would require assistance from others if she returned to her home and previous life-style. The occupational therapist needed to inform the family and other team members of the cuing strategies that worked and the ones that did not. One method of informing the family and other team members was through a demonstration of Vreni's performance during a kitchen activity. The family and team members observed that Vreni did not have the cognitive abilities or the visual perceptual skills to locate items in the kitchen to prepare a meal for herself. This method of vertification (observation) for the family and staff was useful for everyone to understand the depth of problem areas Vreni faced. Vreni's family resided in Europe and planned to return home; they clearly understood that a support system from friends and neighbors would be necessary before Vreni could be discharged.

The occupational therapists' final evaluations indicated continued visual perceptual deficits, visual field cuts, cognitive problems, and poor balance responses. The OTR and COTA pointed out problems to the team and family members that resulted in her inability to function independently at home. Vreni continuously bumped into walls and furniture in her environment, because her visual field cuts and perceptual deficits prevented her from seeing accurately. She also had not successfully mastered visual compensatory strategies. Because of the visual and cognitive problems, the team recommended a temporary legal guardian and a 24-hour personal care attendant (PCA). Both the OTR and COTA informed the physician and social worker of the deficit areas so that legal procedures could be initiated. The court's decision to appoint a conservator for legal and financial matters was based on the statements made by the physician and social worker, who received information regarding the patient's functional status from the occupational therapist and other team members.

Another role the occupational therapist played in discharge planning was in the evaluation of the home environment. Two home visits were conducted by the OTR to assess the safety of the patient's home and her functional capacities within her home. The patient was better able to maneuver in her own environment than in the occupational therapy clinic. Despite this, her deficit areas continued to impede independent performance of tasks. For example, she was now able to locate items in her kitchen to prepare a simple meal, but she had difficulty using appliances correctly and safely. She frequently forgot to turn the stove burners and oven off after use. The OTR consulted rehabilitation engineering regarding an electronic, emergency backup system to ensure safe oven and stove use. Several other modifications to the home were recommended by the occupational therapist and rehabilitation engineering installed these devices.

The patient's personal care attendants (PCAs) also joined the team. They were assigned to assist the patient in her everyday routine of self-care and home management tasks and to accompany her on community outings. These attendants were secured after collaboration with a local community agency, the Center for Independent Living. Applicants for the PCA position were interviewed by the family. An attorney and the court-appointed conservator arranged for payment of the PCAs. Once the PCAs were selected, they were formally instructed by the OTR and COTA regarding the patient's ability to perform daily activities within her home. The OTR and the COTA collaborated on the information they presented to the PCAs to ensure complete understanding. The occupational therapist was instrumental in providing individualized training to assist the attendants in learning effective behavioral management techniques and cuing strategies to ensure optimal patient performance during functional tasks. Initially, 24-hour PCA supervision was recommended. However, the team monitored these hours and ultimately reduced PCA participation as the patient's functional status permitted.

Because the patient was an active member of her community, it was important for the team to encourage continuation of these activities. However, the deficit areas that the occupational therapist identified at discharge (visual perceptual deficits, severe visual field cuts) prevented her from actively pursuing these activities in the community, because the physician prohibited her from driving. The social worker, with assistance

from the occupational therapist, immediately developed a plan for concerned friends and neighbors to provide a system of transportation so that the patient could participate in her community activities. Both the social worker and occupational therapist provided information to friends, neighbors, and support staff on effective techniques and methods to use (and what not to use) to promote optimal patient performance during transportation. For example, the occupational therapist recommended that the patient initiate and make the arrangements (i.e., locating phone number, making the call) if she wanted to participate in any community activity.

The patient was discharged from the hospital but was seen by the occupational therapist on an outpatient basis for continued work toward goals that were developed during her hospitalization. The occupational therapist's focus was on improvement of balance and equilibrium responses, improvement of daily living skills, and remediation of visual perceptual deficits. Individual consultations and team staffings with the interdisciplinary members (the physician, neuropsychologist, social worker, and speech pathologist) continued on a regular basis. Occasionally the conservator and the PCA would attend these staffings during the patients' outpatient treatment. From these staffings the PCA was instructed by the occupational therapist on any changes in the patient's therapy program and was provided the opportunity for further education on how to manage the patient during certain situations.

The patient was seen by the occupational therapist on an outpatient basis for nine months. At the end of that time, it was determined by the team that the patient had reached a recovery plateau. She continued to have visual field cuts and a right homonymous hemianopsia; however, the visual perceptual impairments, cognitive deficits, and the balance responses had improved to a functional level. The patient resumed her community involvement, participating in various civic and cultural events and taking an active role in her physical conditioning by joining a local health club. The PCA time was reduced from 24-hour supervision to 6 hours of care a day. Each reduction of PCA time was a result of the team's reevaluation of patient status. For example, the neuropsychologist reevaluated and determined an improvement in cognitive status, and the social worker was able to report a functional support system from the patient's neighborhood friends that effectively replaced the PCA. The patient did not recover her ability to drive. However, with minimal supervision she was able to plan and prepare her daily meals, go shopping for personal items, utilize the telephone on a daily basis, and manage simple money transactions (e.g., using a checkbook, paying for items).

With the assistance of the occupational therapy staff and other team members, the patient became an independent and autonomous individual within her community, despite the traumatic head injury she experienced the preceding year.

DISCUSSION QUESTIONS

1. What are the advantages of an interdisciplinary team as opposed to a multidisciplinary team?

2. Because communication is significant to the success of interdisciplinary practice, suggest ways in which communication can be facilitated in various settings in which occupational therapists work.

3. How could the interpersonal skills required for interdisciplinary team practice be developed?

4. How might Vreni's case have been handled differently had she been treated in

a multidisciplinary setting rather than by an interdisciplinary health care team?

REFERENCES

1. Melvin JL: Interdisciplinary and multidisciplinary activities and the A.C.R.M. *Arch Phys Med* 8:379–380, 1980.
2. Etzioni A: *A Comparative Analysis of Complex Organizations.* New York, Free Press, 1961, pp. 1–22.
3. *Roles: Policies and Procedures Manual.* Ann Arbor, University of Michigan Hospitals, 1985, pp. 1–15.
4. Thompson JO: *Organization in Action.* New York, McGraw-Hill, 1967, pp. 51–65, 132–143.
5. Hopkins, H, Smith HD (eds): *Willard and Spackman's Occupational Therapy.* Philadelphia, JB Lippincott, 1983, pp. 380, 686–688.
6. Duconis A, Golin A: *Educating for Team Work: The Interdisciplinary Health Care Team.* Germantown, MD, Aspen Systems, 1979, pp. 153–166.
7. Given B, Simmons S: Interdisciplinary health care team: fact or fiction? *Nurse Forum* 2:165–184, 1977.

SUGGESTED READINGS

Bailey DB Jr: A triaxial model of the interdisciplinary team and group process. *Exceptional Children* 51:17–25, 1984.
Bailey D, et al.: Measuring individual participation on the inter-disciplinary team. *Am J Ment Defic.* 88:247–254, 1983.
Bailey DB, et al: Participation of professionals, paraprofessionals, and direct care staff members in the interdisciplinary team meeting. *Am J Ment Defic* 89:437–440, 1985.
Bryand J: The health team. In *Health and the Developing World.* Ithaca, NY, Cornell University Press, 1969, pp. 139–199.
Duncombe LW, et al.: Group work in occupational therapy; a survey of practice. *AJOT* 39:163–170, 1985.
Feiger SM, Schmitt MH: Collegiality in interdisciplinary health teams: its measurement and its effect. *Soc Sci Med* 13A:217–229, 1979.
Johnston A, Cummings V, Pooler L: Teammates are equal partners. *Canadian Nurse* 64:36–41, 1968.
Wagner RJ: Rehabilitation team practice. *Rehabil Couns Bull* 20:206–217, 1977.

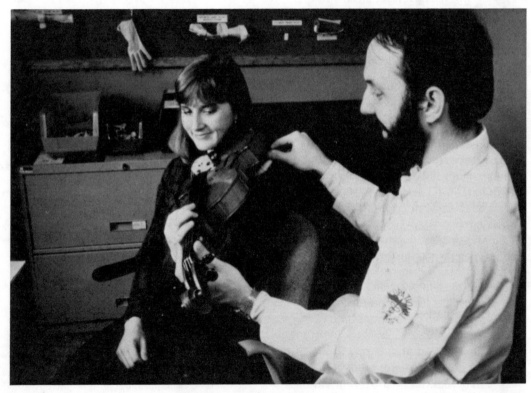

EIGHT

Concepts of Occupational Therapy Practice

Occupational therapists and therapy assistants work with a diverse population and practice in a variety of settings. This chapter introduces some of the specialized areas of occupational therapy practice. Some typical settings in which occupational therapists practice and trends in occupational therapy service delivery today are discussed.

In the early years of occupational therapy, practice tended to fall into only two specializations. Practice might be focused on mental disturbances and be located in an institution for the mentally ill, or it might be focused on physical illnesses and disabilities and be located in a general hospital. In developing countries, this broadly based type of practice is still typical, and therapists must be prepared to work with a variety of diseases or disabilities. In the United States, however, and in other countries with highly developed medical resources, occupational therapists have begun to limit their practices to specific types of disabilities or to specific age groups. This is partly an attempt to cope with an ever increasing knowledge explosion in science and med-

icine. It is also an effort on the part of occupational therapists to offer their clients the benefits of advanced study and training in complex procedures and theoretical aspects of practice. Today the American Occupational Therapy Association (AOTA) recognizes seven specializations within the field: physical disabilities, mental health, developmental disabilities, sensory integration, gerontology, work programs, and administration and management. Other specialties will no doubt develop. To facilitate communication between members who practice in a given specialty area. AOTA has created special interest sections in these seven areas. Members of these groups meet at state and national conferences, sponsor continuing education in their area of interest, promote research, publish materials related to their interest area, and serve as an information resource on practice within the area of specialization.

The OTR and COTA have the choice of remaining general practitioners or of specializing in a more limited area of practice. Specialization is usually achieved through graduate education, work experience in the specialty area, or continuing education. The AOTA has considered establishing a system for specialty certification that would require that a practitioner meet certain criteria to achieve the status of specialist. In 1986 this program was only in the planning stages, however, and is not likely to be implemented for a number of years.

In subsequent chapters, some of the specialty areas of occupational therapy practice are examined. Case examples are

included to illustrate each practice area and to provide a feel for the work of OTRs and COTAs in clinical settings and for the therapy process.

The employment sites where occupational therapists and therapy assistants work are as varied as the client populations. In 1985 an AOTA commission published a report on occupational therapy manpower and found that the practice of occupational therapy had undergone great change in the past 15 years. The AOTA

Table 8.1.
Primary Employment Sites of OTRs and COTAs, 1973–1986[a]

	OTRs				COTAs			
	1973	1977	1982	1986[b]	1973	1977	1982	1986[b]
College, 2 yr	1.4	1.2	0.8	0.6	0.8	0.9	0.6	0.9
College/university, 4 yr	5.6	4.9	4.1	3.4	0.7	0.6	0.9	0.1
Community mental health center	4.2	4.3	2.4	1.7	.0	3.5	3.1	4.3
Correctional institution	0.2	0.2	0.1	0.1	0.3	0.3	0.1	0.2
Day care center program	1.4	1.1	1.0	1.0	1.2	2.4	2.0	4.4
Halfway house								
HMO (including PPO/IPA)	0.3	0.2	0.2	0.3	0.7	0.3	0.3	0.1
Home health agency	0.9	2.2	3.8	4.5	0.2	0.4	0.8	0.9
Hospice			0.0	0.1			0.0	0.0
General hospital—rehabilitation				4.5				5.3
General hospital—all other	20.5	19.8	25.3	22.5	15.1	12.7	17.8	14.1
Pediatric hospital	2.9	2.0	1.6	1.8	1.5	1.2	0.8	0.4
Psychiatric hospital	13.8	11.2	7.4	6.6	22.6	14.3	9.7	8.6
Outpatient clinic (free-standing)			2.5	2.4			1.7	0.6
Physician's office				1.0				0.2
Private industry			0.7	0.7			1.0	0.7
Private practice	1.3	2.1	3.5	6.0	0.3	0.4	1.2	1.3
Public health agency	1.6	1.5	0.8	0.6	0.5	0.5	0.3	0.4
Rehabilitation hospital/center	13.4	10.9	8.9	11.6	9.5	11.0	8.4	9.1
Research facility	0.3	0.3	0.4	0.2	0.2	0.3	0.1	0.0
Residential care facility, including group home, independent living center		4.4	4.2	3.5		8.5	7.6	7.0
Retirement or senior center				0.3				1.0
School system (includes private school)	11.0	14.0	18.3	16.3	3.6	6.2	11.3	13.9
Sheltered workshop	0.7	0.7	0.7	0.3	1.4	0.9	1.9	0.9
Skilled nursing home/intensive care facility	6.2	7.9	6.0	5.5	22.8	26.1	22.5	21.2
Vocational or prevocational program				0.6				1.7
Voluntary agency (e.g., Easter Seal/U.C.P.)		1.7	1.7	1.3		0.4	1.2	0.8
Other	14.2	9.4	5.4	2.6	14.7	9.3	6.7	1.9
Total, %	99.9	100.0	99.8	100.0	100.1	100.1	100.0	100.0
Total employed	8,487	13,619	22,432	28,611	2,010	3,199	5,373	6,500

[a]Data from Ad Hoc Commission on Occupational Therapy Manpower: *Occupational Therapy Manpower: A Plan for Progress.* Rockville, MD, American Occupational Therapy Association, 1985, p. 55.
[b]Unpublished data from American Occupational Therapy Association, 1986 member survey.
Values are percent of total employed OTRs or COTAs.

identified changes in service delivery sites, in the target population that occupational therapy served, and in the skills and knowledge of practitioners. This report noted that the most common work setting for both OTRs and COTAs was still the hospital. Increasing numbers of occupational therapy personnel were being found in school systems, with this becoming the second most common practice site for OTRs and the third for COTAs (1). The changes in employment sites over a period of 13 years are summarized in Table 8.1. Nursing homes (skilled nursing/intermediate care facilities) continued to be a major work site for COTAs.

Practice areas in occupational therapy that are growing and developing include home health care, private practice, and community-based programs. The AOTA data indicate that there has been a 100% growth rate in the number of home health agencies from 1975 to 1984 and that 49.3% of those agencies offered occupational therapy services. Home health care should become a major employment area for occupational therapists in the next decade. Private practice is another growth area. In 1973, only 1.3% of all OTRs were engaged in private practice. By 1986 this proportion had risen to 6%. Community-based programs have also shown steady growth as an employment site for OTRs and COTAs. As hospitals discharge patients earlier, services are increasingly needed to provide continuing therapy and care in the patient's home or in an extended care facility. This transition from institutional care to community-based care has already taken place in the fields of mental health and developmental disabilities. The AOTA predicts continued growth in the number of OTRs and COTAs working with the developmentally disabled and a slow decline in the number of personnel working in mental health (1).

Table 8.2 shows the changing patterns in the age groups that OTRs and COTAs work with. In the 13-year period shown, a decline occurred in the percentages of OTRs and COTAs who work with mixed age groups, probably indicating greater specialization on the part of practitioners. There is an increase in the number of OTRs and COTAs working with clients from 0 to 19 years, reflecting the larger number of practitioners now working in schools. More OTRs are now working with the elderly (another specialization), whereas the number of COTAs working with the elderly has remained fairly stable.

Table 8.3 lists the most common types of health problems that OTRs and COTAs

Table 8.2.

Age Range of Patients Seen Most Frequently by OTRs and COTAs in 1973, 1977, 1982, 1986[a]

	OTRs				COTAs			
	1973	1977	1982	1986[b]	1973	1977	1983	1986[b]
0–19 yr	25.2	28.8	33.0	32.3	9.6	12.4	17.5	21.2
20–64 yrs	21.6	22.7	33.2	30.5	15.9	18.4	33.1	32.1
65 + yr	9.3	11.7	13.3	14.9	25.3	28.0	27.0	22.2
Mixed ages	43.9	36.7	20.5	22.3	49.1	41.1	22.5	24.4
Total, %	100.0	99.9	100.0	100.0	99.9	99.9	100.1	99.9

[a]Data from Ad Hoc Commission on Occupational Therapy Manpower: *Occupational Therapy Manpower: A Plan for Progress.* Rockville, MD, American Occupational Therapy Association, 1985, p. 56.
[b]Unpublished data from American Occupational Therapy Association, 1986 member survey.
Values are percents.

Table 8.3.
Health Problems of Patients Seen Most Frequently by OTRs and COTAs in 1973, 1977, 1982, and 1986[a]

Health Problem	OTRs				COTAs			
	1973	1977	1982	1986[b]	1973	1977	1982	1986[b]
Adjustment disorders				1.3				0.9
Affective disorders				4.0				2.4
AIDS			0.0					0.0
Alcohol/drug abuse	2.5	2.1	1.4	1.1	5.1	4.5	3.2	2.4
Amputation				0.2				0.3
Anxiety disorders				0.3				1.1
Arteriosclerosis	4.1	2.8	0.7	0.3	13.0	12.2	2.6	0.6
Arthritis/collagen disorder	1.5	2.1	1.5	1.1	3.6	4.1	3.1	1.9
Back injury				1.8				1.3
Behavior disorder	5.4	3.6	2.7		9.0	6.5	4.0	
Burns	0.6	0.7	0.6	0.5	0.3	0.5	0.1	0.1
Cancer (neoplasms)				0.3				0.3
Cerebral palsy	13.2	12.4	12.6	11.7	3.0	5.0	6.6	8.0
Congenital anomalies				0.3				0.3
Cerebrovascular accident (stroke)	25.0	26.7	28.3	28.2	18.8	23.7	27.5	28.2
Developmental delay/learning disabilities				16.5				8.7
Developmental disabilities other than mental retardation	5.8	8.0	12.9		0.9	2.3	4.8	
Diabetes				0.0				0.2
Eating disorders				0.2				0.1
Feeding disorders				0.2				0.2
Fractures				1.2				0.9
Hand injuries	4.4	2.1	4.5	7.2	0.9	0.7	1.7	2.1
Head injuries	0.0	0.5	1.4	3.3	0.0	0.3	0.7	2.6
Hearing disabilities				0.1				0.3
Heart disease	0.7	1.1	1.2	0.7	1.9	1.0	0.9	0.6
Kidney disorders				0.1				0.1
Mental retardation	7.5	10.2	10.1	6.2	9.5	11.6	16.4	14.0
Neuromuscular disorders (MD, MS, etc.)	0.3	0.3	0.7	0.6	0.0	0.1	0.4	0.6
Neurosis	6.2	4.3	2.2		4.6	5.7	2.7	
Organic mental disorders				1.6				5.4
Other mental health disorders				0.6				1.8
Personality disorders				0.8				1.3
Respiratory disease				0.2				0.1
Schizophrenic disorders				6.0				9.8
Spinal cord injury	2.7	2.2	2.0	1.5	1.3	1.8	1.7	1.1
Visual disability				0.3				0.3
Well population				0.3				0.3
Other	5.8	8.5	8.4	0.9	13.3	10.5	13.0	1.0

[a]Data from Ad Hoc Commission on Occupational Therapy Manpower: *Occupational Therapy Manpower: A PLan for Progress*. Rockville, MD, American Occupational Therapy Association, 1985, p. 56.
  Unpublished data from American Therapy Association, 1986 member survey.
  Values are percents. Because of a change in classification in 1986 there are no data available for some health problems in some years.

reported in their practices over the same 13-year period. Trends include an increase in the number of OTRs and COTAs working with the developmentally disabled, a decrease in the number of practitioners working with mental health disorders, and an increase in the number of COTAs working with hemiplegics. The number of OTRs and COTAs working with clients who have arteriosclerosis has declined. The most common diagnostic category that both practitioners reported working with was cerebrovascular accident (stroke).

Geographic distribution of occupational therapists and therapy assistants varies widely within the United States.

Figure 8.1 presents the ratio of OTRs to the population by state according to 1983 data. The north central states appear to a large proportion of OTRs according to this comparison. If the state numbers of OTRs are compared with national figures, it can be seen that there are 15 states (largely located in the South or West) that have less than 0.005% of the national OTR population. The states with the largest OTR proportions were California (13.1%) and New York (8.8%).

The geographic distribution of COTAs shows even greater disparity. Figure 8.2 shows the ratio of COTAs to the population by state using 1983 data. Only four states show a proportion of four or more COTAs per 100,000 population. Twenty-one states have less than 0.005%

of the national COTA population. Nearly 48% of all COTAs live and work in five states: California, Minnesota, New York, Pennsylvania, and Wisconsin. The maldistribution of occupational therapy personnel parallels that in other related fields and presents a serious problem in service delivery.

THE OCCUPATIONAL THERAPY PROCESS

No matter what type of setting the OTR or COTA works in, the process for the delivery of occupational therapy services is very similar. The occupational therapy process is based on a problem-solving approach. When a client enters the

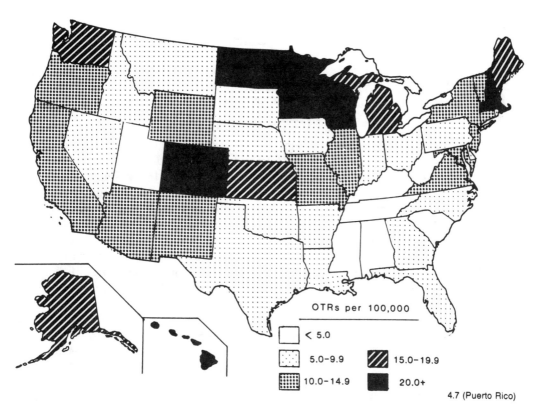

Figure 8.1. Ratio of OTRs to U.S. population, by state, 1983. Overall ratio = 11.7. (From Ad Hoc Commission on Occupational Therapy Manpower: *Occupational Therapy Manpower: A Plan for Progress.* Rockville, MD, American Occupational Therapy Association, 1985, p. 33.)

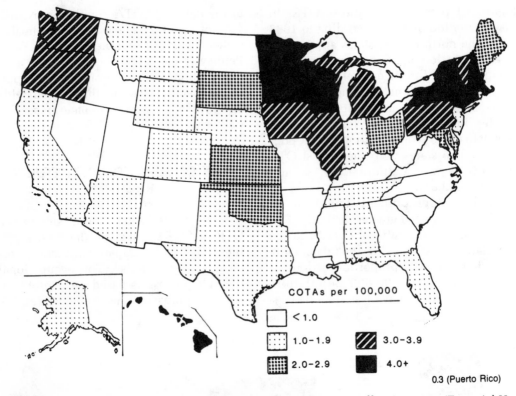

Figure 8.2. Ratio of COTAs to U.S. population, by state, 1983. Overall ratio = 2.8. (From Ad Hoc Commission on Occupational Therapy Manpower: *Occupational Therapy Manpower: A Plan for Progress.* Rockville, MD, American Occupational Therapy Association, 1985, p. 34.

occupational therapy service system, the OTR or COTA sets in motion a series of events intended to determine the nature of the performance problems that the client is experiencing. Once they are identified, the OTR and COTA design a therapeutic program aimed at helping the client regain lost abilities, develop needed skills, retain those abilities he or she has at the desired levels, or prevent further disability. The steps in the process are screening, referral, assessment, program planning, implementation, reassessment, termination, and documentation. The process is diagrammed in Figure 8.3.

SCREENING

A client may enter the occupational therapy service system in a number of ways. Increasingly, occupational therapists are participating in screening programs to identify individuals who may be in need of services. In a school setting, for example, an OTR or COTA might administer screening tests of motor skills and perceptual abilities to determine whether kindergarten children entering the school system have the necessary skills for academic learning. Those found to have deficiencies or developmental delays may be referred for special programs of occupational therapy or other school services. In a hospital setting certain types of diagnoses may be regularly referred to occupational therapy, since patients with these disorders have been found to benefit from the services offered. An OTR might accompany physicians on rounds and suggest that

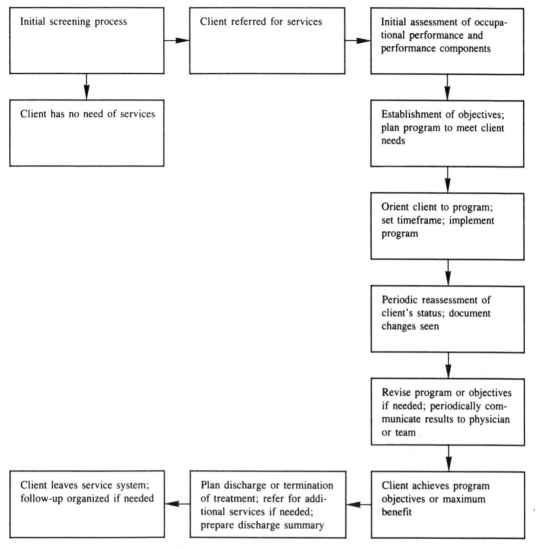

Figure 8.3. The occupational therapy process.

certain patients be referred for help with specific areas of occupational performance. It is part of the OTR and COTA's role to educate those professionals who are part of the health care team so that they recognize patients who are likely to benefit from occupational therapy. Whatever the method, some type of screening takes place that sorts out individuals in need of occupational therapy.

REFERRAL

Those persons who have needs that occupational therapy can help to resolve should be referred, either by their physician or by another professional. Some clients may refer themselves, which is acceptable in many settings. The AOTA has taken the position that a physician's referral is not necessary for all occupational therapy services; however, a facility may require a medical referral if its accreditating agencies, state or federal laws, or third-party reimbursers require it. (Both the Joint Commission on Accreditation of Hospitals and the Commission on Accreditation of Rehabilitation Facilities require a physician's referral for occupational therapy services. Medicare regulations also require a physician's referral as do Medicaid rules in some states.) If there is no physician's referral for service, the therapist assumes full responsibility for determining the appropriate type, nature, and mode of service. The COTAs become involved with clients as authorized by the supervising OTR (2).

ASSESSMENT AND PROGRAM PLANNING

With the referral, the client enters the occupational therapy service system. The first task of the occupational therapist is to gather, analyze, and interpret any available data that can sheld light on the occupational performance problems of the client. The therapist carefully evaluates the overall occupational performance of the client, considering his or her current work, family, and social roles. This area may be delegated to the COTA for evaluation. Data may include material gained from observation, from the client's medical or social history, from reports of prior treatment, and from direct interview of the client. The OTR or COTA may administer specific tests to determine the client's functional abilities and will try to identify areas of strength and areas in need of improvement. The *Uniform Occupational Therapy Checklist* provides a standard format of items to be evaluated (3). A copy of the checklist may be found in the Appendix. Once the data have been collected, the therapist analyzes the available information and begins to formulate priorities for the treatment proc-

ess. If the results of a developmental test of motor abilities show that a child is delayed in acquiring motor skills, the therapist will conclude that motor skill development must be a priority in the treatment program. The therapist plans a program that begins at the child's current functional level and gradually progresses until the child approaches a level of motor development compatible with his or her age or physical status.

An important part of treatment planning is the prioritizing of specific areas as a focus for treatment. Often both long-term and short-term objectives are identified. Long-term objectives describe the desired outcome of treatment and may be quite broad. They depend on the achievement of short-term objectives. The short-term objectives describe the immediate goals— the ministeps that will lead to the desired end result. They are highly specific and are written in measurable terms so that changes can easily be documented. The client may have needs that are outside the scope of occupational therapy, and in this situation it is appropriate for the OTR to refer the client to other professionals for the needed services.

The therapist then begins to plan an organized program of treatment to deal with the identified client needs. A written treatment plan is usually prepared, listing the short-term objectives and the methods to be used to help achieve them. Both the OTR and COTA may contribute ideas to the treatment plan. When the client is an adolescent or an adult, the therapist is likely to involve him or her in the planning process so that personal priorities can be considered. When the client is a child, the family may be consulted. When the client's and family's needs and wishes are taken into account in the planning process, they are much more likely to be active participants in treatment. Motivation and cooperation are usually better when the client and family are fully involved in the program from the beginning and when they know that their personal needs and priorities are respected.

The format of the treatment plan varies from one setting to another, as does the documentation of treatment results. Most treatment plans are brief and succinct, including only critical pieces of information. Some plans must also include a projection of how long the treatment process is expected to take. The initial plan and subsequent documentation of changes seen may be shared with the referring physician or the treatment team. Everyone who works with the patient must understand the total treatment program and coordinate their efforts. Nothing is more disruptive to client care than conflicts among members of the care team.

IMPLEMENTATION

After development of the treatment plan, the OTR and COTA prepare to implement the plan. Decisions are made as to which person will be responsible for the different phases of treatment. A schedule is established for regular client visits, and the actual treatment activities begin. It is important that the person who is to carry out treatment activities preplan each client visit, preparing the necessary materials and setting up any needed equipment so that the client can begin work immediately and no treatment time is wasted. The OTR or COTA may need to orient the client to each stage of the treatment program, teach procedures that are unfamiliar, and closely monitor the client's physical and emotional reactions during treatment sessions. Activities used should be compatible with the amount of time available for the treatment session and with the physical and mental capabilities of the client. Activities may be done individually or within a group environment. Many clients enjoy and benefit from group interaction during ther-

apy sessions, and the pleasant, cheerful ambiance of the occupational therapy clinic can be a powerful motivator to a client who is depressed or discouraged. The OTR and COTA offer emotional support and encouragement to clients throughout the treatment program and try to lead them to higher and higher steps of achievement until treatment objectives are accomplished.

REASSESSMENT

Periodically during the treatment process, the OTR or COTA will reassess the problem areas and compare them with the initial test results and with the stated treatment objectives. If adequate progress is not occurring, the therapist may need to consider changes in the treatment program or adjustments in the objectives. Sometimes the objectives are set too high for the client to achieve in a limited period of time. If the initial objectives are unrealistic, the therapist may modify them to a more reasonable level. In some situations only limited gains may be made. When the client's ability reaches a plateau and no further progress is seen, it may be appropriate to terminate treatment. On other occasions the objective is to maintain existing abilities at their present level, preventing further deterioration of the client's performance skills. This is a valid goal, and in such cases the therapist helps the client to make use of his or her current abilities so that these abilities continue to be functional.

DOCUMENTATION

As treatment continues, the OTR and COTA regularly document changes occurring in the client's abilities or behavior. Formats for reporting progress differ from one facility to another. Usually documentation consists of brief, factual notes on the client's progress, comparing present abilities with the initial status. Documentation of services takes up a great deal of the health professional's time, but accurate written records of the service provided and the client's progress toward objectives are absolutely essential for the service to be reimbursed. In many settings, client records have been computerized; this has greatly facilitated the entry of new data and the retrieval of client information.

TERMINATION OF SERVICE

When treatment objectives have been achieved or when maximum benefit is believed to have occurred, treatment is terminated. At this point, the OTR or COTA prepares a written summary of the occupational therapy treatment process and the results that were achieved. The report may also include recommendations for follow-up services once the client leaves the facility. When the site is a hospital or a skilled nursing facility, the physician or a treatment team may set a date for the client's discharge and make plans for any further services that are needed. Referrals may be made for continued nursing or therapy services to a local community agency. Elderly or handicapped clients may need Meals on Wheels, transportation services, or telephone follow-up A home assessment may be needed to determine whether clients can safely manage living in their own homes. This planning is often critical to the successful independent living of clients after an illness or injury and is an important responsibility of the staff. Because many people today have no family members living nearby to assist them during periods of illness or incapacity, community services are absolutely essential to fill these needs. The OTR and COTA should be familiar with local community resources

so that they can recommend appropriate services for clients when needed.

STANDARDS OF PRACTICE

This, then, is the occupational therapy process. It occurs, with minor variations, in each setting where occupational therapy is available. To encourage quality occupational therapy service, AOTA has developed standards of practice that describe the minimum acceptable standards of service for occupational therapy programs. They may be applied to all types of facilities and all client populations. The standards of practice describe the OTR's responsibility in screening, referral, evaluation, program planning and implementation, discontinuation of service, and maintaining quality care. They also discuss indirect service responsibilities, including supervision of employees, record keeping, maintenance of professional skills, and consultation. Finally, they address the ethnical/legal aspects of occupational therapy service. These standards guide the OTR in the development of an adequate service program and are a resource for employers, reimbursers, and consumers who are concerned with the quality of occupational therapy services. A copy of the standards of practice may be found in the Appendix (4).

LEGAL/ETHICAL CONCERNS

There are many legal and ethical issues that arise in practice that the OTR and COTA must consider and resolve. In some states, occupational therapy licensure laws regulate the qualifications of occupational therapy service providers and the services that they may offer. In states without licensure, there is no formal mechanism for investigating and acting on consumer complaints of inadequate service or service by a unqualified provider. Most state occupational therapy associations have a committee that receives and responds to complaints of unethical conduct, but these groups have no real authority to enforce any penalties or sanctions. The AOTA has established principles of occupational therapy ethics that are intended as guidelines for its members in professional conduct and responsibility (5). A code of ethics defines acceptable relationships between practitioners and their consumers, employers, and the public as a whole. Occupational therapists and therapy assistants strive to conduct their practice under these guidelines. Occupational therapy personnel can be sued for malpractice as other health professionals can, and many carry malpractice insurance to protect them against costly legal actions (6). The AOTA *Principles of Occupational Therapy Ethics* may be found in the Appendix.

REIMBURSEMENT MECHANISMS

Before we begin our in-depth review of occupational therapy practice, we should briefly discuss the reimbursement of occupational therapy services. Services are paid for by a variety of sources: the client's personal funds, commercial health insurers, or state and federal funds. Insurance programs (Medicare, Medicaid, worker's compensation, and private plans) pay service providers after the service has been delivered. Grant programs (the Education for all Handicapped Children Act, Community Mental Health Centers Act, the Older Americans Act, Social Security Title XX) provide ongoing funding for an overall program of which occupational therapy may be a part. There are great differences between these two types of reimbursement systems: insurance programs are highly specific as to what services will be paid for and to what extent; grant programs are more flexible as long as the broad goals of the program are met. All payment systems regulate, to some extent, the way in which services are delivered. Providers must be familiar with the regulations of reimbursement systems that pay for their services so that they know in advance the coverage allowed for the services they provide (7).

The AOTA has developed an occupational therapy product output reporting system to aid practitioners in billing and reporting their services uniformly. This system lists each service provided by occupational therapy and assigns a relative value for each 15-minute interval of service. Costs are calculated based on the service activity, the amount of time spent in the activity, and the therapist-client ratio (8). Occupational therapy services may be billed specifically as occupational therapy or they may be included in a larger service category. A 1982 survey of occupational therapy service programs revealed that 66.9% of the OTRs and 49.6% of the COTAs responding billed their services as occupational therapy; smaller proportions billed their services as physical medicine, rehabilitation, activity therapy, or part of a general service charge. Table 8.4 shows the percentage of reimbursement that came from various funding sources. For both OTRs and COTAs, the largest reimbursement source was state or local programs.

The OTR and COTA need to be knowledgeable about the reimbursement systems in effect at their facility, since they directly participate in the billing process. Grant funds administered by a facility are subject to close scrutiny by federal or state auditors, while insurance reimbursement systems are closely monitored by the insurer. The health care provider needs some knowledge of cost accounting and fiscal management in order for the service department to run smoothly.

Table 8.4.
Percentage of Reimbursement for Services from Various Sources[a]

Sources	OTRs	COTAs
Blue Cross	8.0	7.0
Other private insurance	8.9	8.0
Medicare	20.0	20.8
Medicaid	12.0	15.5
Vocational Rehabilitation Agency (DVR/OVR)	1.5	1.6
Other federal programs	13.0	11.3
State/local programs	27.4,	27.5
Other	9.1	8.4
Total responses, %	99.9	100.1

[a]Dataline: Billing and reimbursement of occupational therapy services. *Occup Ther News* 38(12):6, 1984. Values are percent.

SUMMARY

Occupational therapy practice is in a period of transition as the health care system moves from its traditional fee-for-service reimbursement system to prospective payment. This is discussed in greater detail in chapter 19. According to projections from the AOTA and the United States Bureau of Labor Statistics, the field of occupational therapy will continue to grow and expand in the next several decades. The sites of service delivery may change dramatically, but the need for occupational therapy service continues to be strong and the profession anticipates a period of steady growth and development of occupational therapy clinical programs.

DISCUSSION QUESTIONS

1. What might be some of the advantages or disadvantages of being a general practitioner of occupational therapy rather than a specialist?

2. What are some of the most common work settings for OTRs and COTAs in your area? Are they similar to or different from those shown in national statistics?

3. Why do you suppose that fewer OTRs and COTAs are being employed in mental health programs? Is this trend being seen in your area?

4. The geographic maldistribution of occupational therapy personnel is a serious problem that has slowed the development of services in some areas. What might some of the reasons be for this, and how could it be corrected?

5. The OTR and COTA assess the client's performance skills before treatment is begun and then periodically reassess his or her abilities as treatment proceeds. What is the purpose of this frequent reevaluation of the patient's performance skills?

6. Paperwork is a necessary part of every professional's job. Why is it so important?

7. One of the important ethical issues in health care is protecting the confidentiality of the patient's medical record and respecting the private nature of health information. How can students and staff members help to maintain confidentiality?

8. What are some of the charges billed for occupational therapy services in clinical settings in your area? On what basis are charges calculated?

REFERENCES

1. Ad Hoc Commission on Occupational Therapy Manpower: *Occupational Therapy Manpower: A Plan for Progress*. Rockville, MD, American Occupational Therapy Association, 1985, pp. 32–39, 55–56.
2. I'm glad you asked. *Occup Ther News* 39(5): 4, 1985.
3. Uniform occupational therapy evaluation checklist. *AJOT* 35:817–818, 1981.
4. Shriver D, Foto M: Standards of practice for occupational therapy. *AJOT* 37:802–804, 1983.

5. Principles of occupational therapy ethics. *AJOT* 38:799–802, 1984.
6. Steich T: Malpractice insurance important for occupational therapy personnel. *Occup Ther News* 40(3):7, 1986.
7. Scott SG: Payment for occupational therapy services. In Bair, Gray (eds): *The Occupational Therapy Manager.* Rockville, MD, American Occupational Therapy Association, 1985, pp. 325–340.
8. Task Force, Commission on Practice: *Occupational Therapy Product Output Reporting System and Uniform Terminology for Reporting Occupational Therapy Services.* Rockville, MD, American Occupational Therapy Association, 1980.
9. Dataline: Billing and reimbursement of occupational therapy services. *Occup Ther News* 38(12): 6, 1984.

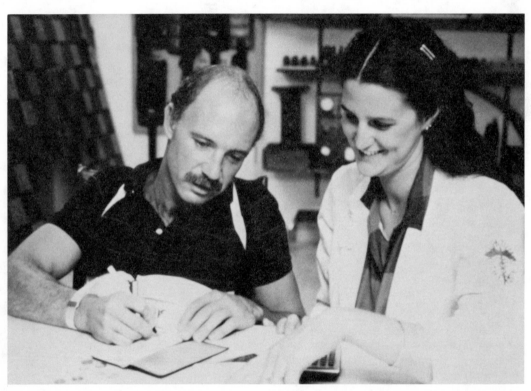

Courtesy AOTA

NINE

Practice in the Acute Care Hospital

Hospitals have always been the largest employer of occupational therapy personnel, and they continue to be. A survey of occupational therapists showed that in 1982, 34.3% of all OTRs and 28.3% of all COTAs were working in hospitals. Not all hospitals offer occupational therapy services, however. According to the American Hospital Association, only 45.4% of all hospitals provided occupational therapy in 1984. Table 9.1 shows the different types of hospitals and the percentage of each offering occupational therapy services (1).

Smaller hospitals were less likely to have an occupational therapy department, with only 25% of the hospitals of 200 beds or less reporting the service. Because these account for over 60% of all hospitals, it is apparent that many hospital patients do not have access to occupational therapy services. That situation may be slowly changing. A 1984 survey indicated that 18% of the hospitals were planning to add or expand occupational therapy departments within the next two years (2). There is a slow decline in the number of acute care hospitals as intense economic competition forces some hospitals to become part of large hospital corporations or go out of business. There is a steady growth in the number of OTR positions in acute care hospitals, but there does not appear to be corresponding growth in COTA positions (2).

The acute care hospital treats patients with immediate medical needs (a serious illness, severe injuries, or a need for a surgical procedure) and provides short-term hospital care. It has always been a challenging place to work. Occupational therapy personnel must be prepared to deal with a variety of diagnostic categories and must be able to quickly plan and implement a treatment program once a patient has been referred for service. The pace tends to be rapid and maximum flexibility is needed, since the caseload changes frequently. Therapists or therapy assistants working in this setting must be particularly good at managing their time, since patient stays are often short. In the acute care hospital, close team relationships help to make treatment of patients much more effective. Often treatment teams are organized to deal with specific diagnostic groups. Table 9.2 shows some of the related services that are typically found in acute care hospitals.

Table 9.1.
Occupational Therapy Services in United States Hospitals in 1984[a]

Hospital Type	Hospitals Offering Services, %
All hospitals	45.4
Federal	56.8
Psychiatric	100.0
General	54.2
Nonfederal	44.7
Psychiatric	84.9
TB and other respiratory diseases	50.0
Long-term general	93.3
Short-term general	40.0
Nongovernment not-for-profit	50.2
Investor-owned (for profit)	27.5
State and local government	23.4

[a]Data from Dataline: Occupational therapy services increase in the nation's hospitals. *Occup Ther News* 40:4, 1986.

Table 9.2.
Services in United States Hospitals in 1984[a]

Service	Hospitals Offering Service, %
Occupational therapy	45.4
Physical therapy	86.8
Respiratory therapy	85.3
Social work	82.7
Speech pathology	44.1
Rehabilitation otupatient services	35.7
Hospice	9.8
Home care	20.6
Organized outpatient department	50.6

[a]Data from Dataline: Occupational therapy services increase in the nation's hospitals. *Occup Ther News* 40:4, 1986.

CHANGES IN ACUTE CARE

As health care delivery changes, the role of the acute care hospital is changing dramatically. In 1983 a prospective payment system was implemented for inpatient care of Medicare recipients. The system was based on the concept of diagnostic-related groups (DRGs). Categories were developed for 471 medical, surgical, psychiatric, and rehabilitation diagnoses. Each DRG was assigned a weighting system that determines the payment that the hospital receives for the care of Medicare patients. Among the factors considered are principal diagnosis, operating room procedures, additional diagnoses and procedures, the age and sex of the patient, and the patient's status at discharge. Under this reimbursement system, the hospital receives a fixed rate of payment for each Medicare patient treated, regardless of the number of services provided or the length of stay. In 1986 psychiatric and rehabilitation units were still excluded from the prospective payment system; however, it is expected that some form of prospective payment will be developed for these units as well (3).

The prospective payment system has caused major changes in health care delivery. Hospital stays are growing shorter, and patients are being discharged not yet able to resume their normal patterns of living. There is an increasing need for extended care facilities, home health services, and outpatient programs that can continue the treatment regimes begun in acute care hospitals. There is a comparable need for hospice programs to provide services and support to the terminally ill. More and more active treatment will be taking place in these alternative care facilities and less in the acute care hospital.

EFFECTS ON OCCUPATIONAL THERAPY

In 1985 the American Occupational Therapy Association (AOTA) conducted a survey to study the impact of the prospective payment system on occupational therapy services. They found that many hospital-based departments were reporting a decrease in the number of inpatient referrals. Referrals for outpatient services, however, were increasing. The survey confirmed that the average length of patient stay was growing shorter, but more discharged patients were being referred to home health agencies or nursing homes for continued care. There seemed to be no loss of occupational therapy positions in acute care hospitals. The diagnostic categories that occupational therapy most frequently worked with were CVA (cerebrovascular accident, stroke)/hemiplegia, hip and knee disorders, arthritis, head injuries, and cardiac disorders. Occupational therapists were beginning to see patients earlier in their hospital stay (often while patients were still in the intensive care unit) and were working with more patients who were medically unstable. Many rehabilitation units had waiting lists, sometimes necessitating an extended wait before a bed became available. Significant growth was occurring in outpatient occupational therapy services. Because of earlier discharge, inpatient occupational therapy was becoming more intense and was compressed into a shorter period of time. Occupational therapists were taking an increased role in the assessment of patients' functional status, both early in the hospitalization and in preparation for discharge (4). More detailed documentation of patient status and progress was being demanded, and computerized record keeping became common in many hospitals. There were increased demands for quality assurance programs in order to be fully accountable to hospital administration and to reimbursers.

RESPONSES TO CHANGES IN ACUTE CARE

Occupational therapy departments in acute care hospitals are responding to these changes in a variety of ways. In some departments, personnel are being reas-signed from inpatient care to the growing outpatient services. Alternative work schedules are being introduced, so that maximum use can be made of facilities, staff, and equipment. Some departments now provide service seven days a week and may be open during the evening as well as the day. Highly specialized personnel may be on call for emergency situations where their expertise is needed. Documentation of services continues to take large amounts of time for all health professionals. Occupational therapy departments are being urged to adopt productivity measures and to practice cost containment in the ordering of supplies and equipment (4).

LONG-TERM EFFECTS

As hospitals engage in intense competition for the health care dollar, some loss of occupational therapy positions may occur. It is likely, however, that such losses will be offset by the development of new positions in alternative care services. Acute care services are not declining. They are only shifting to new locations. Occupational therapy will continue to be a needed service in many of these new programs. In addition, some hospitals are expanding the range of occupational therapy services to meet changing needs. Larger outpatient programs, involvement in home health care, work-hardening programs to prepare the injured worker to resume employment, and health promotion and education are only a few of these expanding service areas.

The acute care hospital is in the vanguard of major changes now occurring in health care. The nature of these changes will challenge the OTRs and COTAs who work in acute care settings for years to come. Creativity and flexibility will be needed to respond to the changing health care economy and the changing patient population. It is expected that occupational therapy personnel will adapt to these changing needs and continue to play an active role in acute care.

What is it like to work in an acute care hospital? Let's look at a typical hospital and follow the case of an occupational therapy client who was seen in an acute care setting.

CASE STUDY:
HEAD INJURY

St. Joseph's Hospital is a community hospital of 517 beds. It was founded by a religious order of hospital sisters in 1890 and is located in a midwestern city of 100,000. There are 2 other hospitals in town and 20 nursing homes. St. Joseph's is a private, not-for-profit hospital that serves as a regional medical center for a multicounty rural area. It offers psychiatric care, rehabilitation services, and short-stay surgery. It reaches out to the community through childbirth preparation classes, home health care services, and educational publications. The hospital is an important community resource and employs 1600 persons.

The occupational therapy department at St. Joseph's consists of 15 OTRs, 2 COTAs, and 2 recreational therapists. Each member of the department is assigned to a team that provides services to an inpatient rehabilitation unit, an inpatient physical disabilities service, an outpatient physical disabilities program, a hand therapy program, a perinatal care unit, an inpatient psychiatric unit, and an outpatient psychiatric day program. The department is administered by a director and an assistant director. A clerk-typist provides clerical support. The department provides services 5½ days a week and works in a close conjunction with nursing, physical therapy, speech therapy, and the department of social services.

In November of 1984, Laurie was admitted to the emergency room of St.

Joseph's. She was an 18-year-old college student who resided in her parents' home. A healthy and active student in high school, she had graduated in the top 15% of her class and had been a member of the women's track team. After graduation she entered a local college as an art major and also took a part-time job at a McDonald's restaurant. On the night of November 5, 1984, Laurie had been out with friends and was returning home in their car when the vehicle was struck head-on by another car. Laurie's two friends were both killed in the accident. Laurie was rushed by ambulance to the emergency room at St. Joseph's where she was found to have sustained a severe closed-head injury and facial trauma. From the emergency room she was transferred to the intensive care unit (ICU), where she spent the next nine days in a comatose state. She developed complications, including respiratory difficulties that required a tracheostomy and placement on a respirator and a cranial blood clot that required opening the skull in the left frontal area for removal of the clot. After nine days in the ICU, she was transferred to the neurology unit and was referred to occupational therapy by her neurosurgeon.

During the first two days on this unit, she was evaluated by an OTR and was found to have the following problems:

1. Abnormal posturing
2. No right-sided movement
3. Flailing movements of the left arm and leg
4. A fixed gaze with left pupil dilation and deviation to the left

Laurie could not move on command and was totally unresponsive to most stimuli. She did withdraw her left hand when a painful stimulus was applied. She had been placed on medications for a urinary tract infection, skin allergy, restlessness, pain relief, and blood pressure regulation.

Laurie was totally dependent in all areas of self-care. Initally all communication was absent; however, after two weeks she was able to respond to yes or no questions with eye blinks. Nutrition was by nasogastric tube, because the swallowing reflex was absent. No movement was observed on her right side. Her left side moved only in purposeless flailing movements. Passive range of motion was normal in both arms; however, there was increased tone (muscle tightness) in the right arm that made moving the arm difficult. Laurie would grimace as if in pain when this was attempted. Within the first week of occupational therapy treatment, Laurie began to focus her eyes momentarily on the therapist and on family members. Eye tracking, however, was absent.

Based on the evaluation results, the OTR established a treatment plan with long-term and short-term goals. The most immediate need was to prevent sensory deprivation and encourage awareness of sensory stimuli. The OTR spoke to the family and the nursing staff about the need to provide frequent sensory stimulation to help rouse Laurie from her coma and to prevent the negative effects of sensory deprivation. Family members and staff were encouraged to talk to her in a normal tone of voice, present her with simple one-step commands, play tapes of family member's voices, and turn on the radio and television periodically. For tactile stimulation, Laurie's skin was rubbed with varied textures, deep touch pressure was applied, and hot and cold temperatures were touched to her skin. For visual stimulation, bright and colorful objects were presented and were moved across her visual field to encourage eye tracking. Pictures of family members and friends were shown to her. To stimulate Laurie's sense of smell, the therapist brought various scents for her to smell. At first, unpleasant odors were used for their arousal effect, but later familiar and favorite scents were used. Taste stimuli were also presented, with various flavors applied to Laurie's tongue with a cotton swab. Sensory stimulation was done frequently but for short periods of time, since care had to be taken not to overload Laurie's nervous system.

Another early goal of therapy was to prevent contractures and deformity, which can result from lying in one position and not using muscles and joints. The OTR provided passive range of motion to the joints of both arms twice a day. She instructed the unit nurses on proper bed positioning for Laurie to minimize muscle tightness and to prevent deformity, and posted positioning diagrams over Laurie's bed so that all staff members could see at a glance how to best position her in bed. During this early phase of treatment, the OTR also constructed a resting pan split for Laurie's right hand so that it would remain in a normal position until some movement returned.

Laurie's family was extremely concerned about her condition and spent a great deal of time at her bedside. They frequently questioned the staff about her condition and what the outcome of her treatment might be. Another goal of the occupational therapy treatment plan was to educate the family about Laurie's condition and provide them with emotional support during this difficult period.

Laurie was seen twice a day by the OTR for 30-minute sessions during the acute phase of her hospitalization. Her status was reassessed daily and goals were upgraded as she began to improve. After two weeks of hospitalization, great improvements were seen in Laurie's general awareness. She could now follow simple commands, move her left arm voluntarily, and track objects with her eyes. Because her medical condition was now considered stable, she was transferred to the rehabilitation unit of the hospital.

The therapeutic programs begun on the neurology unit were continued on the rehabilitation unit. Passive movement of her arms was continued by the OTR, with the physical therapist working to maintain the movement of her legs. Calendars, photographs, and a daily schedule helped Laurie orient herself to time, place, and people. Minimal gains were made during the first two weeks on the rehabilitation unit. The muscle tightness of the right arm actually increased; however, she was beginning to be able to move this arm, although movement was slow and awkward. Laurie now showed some awareness of visual forms and shapes. She was able to place a single form into a formboard. Her attention span was only about 15 seconds, and she was so easily distracted that occupational therapy activities had to be carried out in a less-distracting environment than her hospital room. A splint was made by the OTR to help decrease the tightness of the biceps muscle, and Laurie was encouraged to use her right arm and hand in purposeful activities. During treatment sessions, Laurie was given simple perceptual activities and attempts were made to increase her attention span. During this phase of treatment, Laurie was being seen by occupational therapy, physical therapy, and speech therapy twice a day for 45-minute sessions with each discipline.

Within the next month, Laurie's progress was dramatic. She began talking, eating, and was able to breathe without the tracheostomy. At this point, she began to assist with self-care activities. A COTA was assigned to work with her for 45 minutes daily for self-care training. Initially Laurie and the COTA worked on grooming tasks, such as brushing teeth and washing Laurie's face. Then a bed bath and dressing were added to Laurie's daily program, and later she learned to take a daily shower. The tightness in her right arm had decreased, and she was now able to actively move it through its full range of motion. Its strength and coordination were still deficient. Laurie's attention span and her perceptual abilities showed steady improvement. It was evident, however, that severe cognitive limitations continued to be present. Laurie had great difficulty with problem-solving, judgment, sequencing, following complex directions, and memory. Treatment now focused on active and passive range of motion, gaining improved strength and coordination of her right arm, self-care

training, and perceptual and cognitive retraining.

During this phase of her hospitalization, Laurie was participating in recreational therapy and enjoyed taking part in a swimming program and community outings. She was allowed to go home for a weekend visit, and the visit went well. Laurie admitted, however, that it gave her an increased awareness of the full extent of her injury.

In January, Laurie was discharged from St. Joseph's Hospital after two months of hospitalization. At discharge she was independent in all self-care skills and needed only stand-by assistance for safety in bathing. Both arms had achieved a normal range of motion and normal muscle tone. The strength and coordination of her right arm was still somewhat deficient. Her perceptual abilities were much improved; however, she continued to show moderate to severe cognitive impairment. Postdischarge recommendations included the use of home programs of activity to strengthen deficit areas. Plans were made to have Laurie attend outpatient occupational therapy sessions three times a week for continued treatment. While in the hospital, Laurie had been taught to use a home computer for cognitive retraining. Impressed with the effectiveness of this treatment tool, Laurie's family purchased a home computer to enable her to continue these retraining activities at home. The OTR recommended appropriate software programs for her to use and assigned homework tasks that were checked during her outpatient visits.

Laurie's progress was expected to continue. She had been highly motived throughout her hospital stay and took pride in her growing list of achievements. Outpatient occupational therapy focused on helping Laurie redevelop selected work skills and improve her ability to manage money, keep a checkbook, and improve her cognitive functions. Although she will never be able to draw as well as before the accident and will not return to college because of her cognitive impairment, she will be able to work and enjoy a full range of social and recreational activities.

The team that worked on Laurie's case consisted of physicians (the ICU physician, a neurosurgeon, and a physiatrist), nursing staff, a physical therapist, an occupational therapist, a COTA, a recreational therapist, a speech therapist, and a social worker. The overall treatment program was supervised by the physican responsible for each phase of Laurie's medical treatment. The nursing staff provided ongoing daily care and followed through on a range of motion exercises, positioning suggestions, and the sensory stimulation program as directed by the OTR. A physical therapist provided range of motion exercises for Laurie's legs, muscular stimulation to help her regain movement in her legs, and assisted her to regain her ability to walk and stand. The speech therapist aided Laurie in regaining her ability to speak and communicate. A social worker provided support and counseling to Laurie's distraught family and also assisted them with financial matters related to the hospitalization. Laurie's multiple problems required a strong team approach and a unified treatment plan. Each discipline contributed its special skills to Laurie's recovery process, and the cooperative effort resulted in a good outcome for Laurie.

DISCUSSION QUESTIONS

1. What kind of team skills may have been needed by the team members who worked with Laurie?

2. What kind of knowledge did the OTR and COTA need to have to work effectively to restore some of Laurie's functional abilities?

3. What areas of occupational performance were affected by Laurie's injury?

What performance components were affected?

4. How did the occupational therapy treatment plan change as Laurie's condition improved?

5. How did the OTR and the COTA work together on this case?

6. If St. Joseph's Hospital had not had a rehabilitation unit, where might Laurie have received such services?

7. Is there an acute care hospital in your community? What types of occupational therapy services does it offer?

REFERENCES

1. Dataline: Occupational therapy services increase in the nation's hospitals. *Occup Ther News* 40(4): 6, 1986.
2. Ad Hoc Commission on Occupational Therapy Manpower: *Occupational Therapy Manpower: A Plan for Progress.* Rockville, MD, American Occupational Therapy Association, 1985, pp 35, 37–39.
3. Questions and answers about medicare prospective payment. *Occup Ther News* 38(10):4, 1984.
4. Prospective payment survey shows occupational therapy a healthy profession. *Occup Ther News* 39(10):8, 1985.

Suggested Readings

Cope D, Hall K: Head injury rehabilitation: benefit of early intervention. *Arch Phys Med Rehab* 63:433–437, 1982.

Farber S: *Neurorehabilitation. A Multisensory Approach.* Philadelphia, WB Saunders, 1982.

Gardner H: *The Shattered Mind: The Person After Brain Damage.* New York, Alfred A Knopf, 1975.

Head Injury. Rockville, MD, American Occupational Therapy Association, 1985 revision, pp 1–84.

Jennett B, Teasdale G: *Management of Head Injuries.* Philadelphia, FA Davis, 1981. (Contemp. Neurol. Ser.)

Logue PE: *Understanding and Living with Brain Damage.* Springfield, IL, Charles C Thomas.

Marmo N: A new look a the brain damaged adult. *AJOT* 28:199–206, 1974.

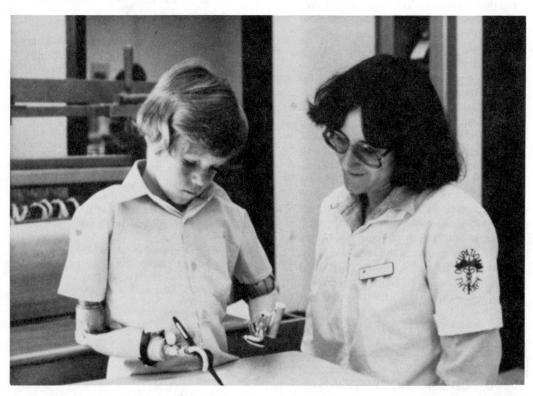

Courtesy AOTA

TEN

Practice with Physical Disabilities

Long-term care and rehabilitation of physical dysfunctions has been a traditional area of occupational therapy practice and represents one of the most common specialty areas within the field. Although practice with physical dysfunctions has undergone many changes in theoretical approach and technique, it continues to be an integral part of the medical management for many diseases and physical disabilities. Table 10.1 shows the major physical dysfunctions treated by occupational therapists and therapy assistants in 1986. (American Occupational Therapy Association, unpublished data).

The types of physical disorders that OTRs and COTAs are working with have not changed substantially in the last 13 years, although there is an increase in the number of COTAs who are working with hemiplegic patients and a decrease in the number of OTRs and COTAs who are working with patients who have arteriosclerosis. The overall number of COTAs working with physical dysfunctions appears to have increased steadily over the last few years. According to AOTA projections, more occupational therapists will be working with cancer patients in the future, as more patients survive the dis-

ease and become candidates for rehabilitation services. The AOTA also predicts an increase in the number of head trauma patients seen by occupational therapy personnel. The incidence of cerebrovascular accident (CVA/hemiplegia) is expected to decline.

One additional trend seen in practitioners who work with physical dysfunctions is that more therapists appear to be specializing. Hand therapy, specialized work in spinal cord injury, and the treatment of burns are all areas demanding advanced knowledge and skills and are attracting greater numbers of therapists.

PRACTICE SITES

Practice locations for the treatment of physical dysfunctions include acute care hospitals, rehabilitation centers, nursing homes and extended care facilities, outpatient services and community-based programs, public and private schools, and private practices. Each contribute a somewhat different type of care for the client with a physical dysfunction. The first place where a patient with a physical disorder is seen by occupational therapy is usually

Table 10.1.
Physical Disorders Seen Most Frequently by OTRs and COTAs in 1986[a]

Health Problem	OTRs	COTAs
AIDS	0.0	0.0
Amputation	0.2	0.3
Arteriosclerosis	0.3	0.6
Arthritis/collagen disorder	1.1	1.9
Back injury	1.8	1.3
Burns	0.5	0.1
Cancer (neoplasms)	0.3	0.3
Cerebral palsy	11.7	8.0
Congenital anomalies	0.3	0.3
CVA/hemiplegia	28.2	28.2
Developmental delay/learning disabilities	16.5	8.7
Diabetes	0.0	0.2
Feeding disorders	0.2	0.2
Fractures	1.2	0.9
Hand injuries	7.2	2.1
Head injuries	3.3	2.6
Hearing disabilities	0.1	0.3
Heart disease	0.7	0.6
Kidney disorders	0.1	0.1
Neuromuscular disorders (MS, MD, etc.)	0.6	0.6
Respiratory disease	0.2	0.1
Spinal cord injury	1.5	1.1
Visual disability	0.3	0.3

[a]Unpublished data from American Occupational Therapy Association, 1986 member survey.
Values are percents.

the acute care hospital. Here the patient's condition is stabilized and immediate medical needs are attended to. If long-term rehabilitation services are needed, the patient may be transferred to the rehabilitation unit of the hospital if such a service is provided. If not, he or she may be transferred to a separate rehabilitation hospital or to a nursing home where long-term residential care and rehabilitative services can be offered. If the client is ambulatory, outpatient service or therapy programs offered by community agencies might be used. For children with physical disabilities, private and public schools provide therapy services as part of the overall educational program. In addition, OTRs and COTAs working in private or group practices may offer therapy on a fee-for-service basis. The occupational therapy services provided will vary with each practice location. Frequently the physically disabled client needs a continuum of rehabilitation services, ranging from acute care of the injury or illness to long-term restorative care and follow-up as his or her condition improves. It is not unusual for a client to be seen by three or four different agencies in the course of treatment, with each providing care at a different stage of recovery.

PSYCHOLOGICAL EFFECTS OF PHYSICAL DYSFUNCTION

A disease or injury that causes severe physical or mental impairment can be devastating to an individual and to the individual's family. When the condition is the result of a sudden occurrence such as an accident, the physical and emotional shock is especially great. Although usually the patient's condition is nonprogressive, the disruption of the individual's life is so extreme that the physical injury can result in serious psychological disturbances as well. Patients may have to face not only changes in their physical abilities but also changes in their family and social relationships, temporary or permanent loss of work roles, and dependence in the most basic areas of self-care. Patients may have been disfigured by the injury or may have lost their ability to communicate with others. All of these losses combine to overwhelm the client who is suddenly disabled (1). Sometimes clients in this situation retire into the "sick role," giving up individual control of their daily life and retreating into invalidism. Clients may withdraw from social interactions and be unable to maintain their former family and social relationships. These psychological reactions are not unusual in people who must face severe physical impairment; the OTR and COTA must be prepared to deal with the patient's psychological reactions just as much as with his or her physical limitations. Verlsuys (2) has noted that normal emotional reactions to severe illness or injury may include depression, mourning, denial, regression, and anxiety. The OTR or COTA working with physically handicapped clients needs to understand these reactions as part of the adjustment process. Sensitivity to the feelings of clients as they move through a long period of adjustment enables the therapist to know when the clients can be safely "pushed" toward further achievement and when their occasional refusal to participate in treatment activities must be accepted.

When the condition is progressive, such as multiple sclerosis or arthritis, clients may experience periods when they feel well and periods of pain and limited function. These clients must be helped to accept the continuing nature of their disability and adjust to the changing status of their health. Often the emotional reactions of clients influence their physical condition. Clients may need to learn to reduce stress and express their frustration and anxiety in nondestructive ways.

ADDITIONAL CONSIDERATIONS

Many injuries or illnesses lead to secondary complications that make the treatment process even more complex. The therapist may have to consider multiple problems when developing a treatment plan. The therapist works with the client to establish priorities and organizes treatment in a logical progression. Some problems may demand immediate attention, while others can legitimately be postponed until a later phase of treatment. By making the client a member of the treatment team, these issues can be discussed and resolved in a way that everyone can accept.

Family involvement is often an important part of the treatment program. To make treatment as relevant as possible to individual client needs, the therapist must be aware of the client's life-style, family relationships, home and work responsibilities, and personal goals. The family can be extremely helpful in sharing information and can also actively participate in treatment activities. The OTR and COTA may teach family members some of the therapy procedures so that they can provide additional practice for the client in treatment activities. Families often need encouragement and emotional support throughout the client's recovery and may wish to remain in contact with the OTR or COTA for a period of time after the therapy program has been completed. The therapeutic relationship between the therapist, the client, and the client's family is critical to success in the treatment process.

The occupational therapy process is the same for treatment of physical disorders as for other types of client problems. In a long-term rehabilitation program, however, therapy may continue for months or even years before adequate functional abilities are restored. Because the delivery of health care services is rapidly changing in the United States, it is likely that more and more rehabilitative care will be provided through nursing homes, outpatient programs, home health care, and community agencies. Good coordination will be needed between agencies involved in rehabilitation services to ensure continuity of care to meet changing client needs.

The OTR and COTA working in physical dysfunction need to have in-depth knowledge of several theoretical approaches that are currently in use to treat physical disabilities. They include the neurodevelopmental approach, the biomechanical approach, orthotics, and the rehabilitative approach (3). Each of these approaches to treatment has its own theoretical framework and body of knowledge. Depending on the nature of the client's disorder, the therapist selects an approach that is relevant to the client's needs. Advanced education in these approaches is necessary to become skilled in their use, and many continuing education programs are available to enable the OTR and COTA to further develop their clinical skills.

THE TREATMENT TEAM

The team approach is often used in rehabilitation settings. The treatment team may be headed by a physiatrist (a physician specializing in physical medicine and rehabilitation) who refers the client for specific therapy services and supervises the medical management of the case. Other members of the team might be rehabilitation nurses, who provide daily nursing care and follow-through on therapy procedures; physical therapists, who work to restore movement and ambulation skills; speech therapists, who deal with speech and language deficiencies; social workers, who provide liaisons with the client's family, the community, and the reimbursement system; psychologists, who may be involved in client counseling; and vocational rehabilitation personnel, who are concerned with the client's eventual employment. Other team members who are called in if needed include the orthotist, who will make customized splints, and the prosthetist, who may evaluate the client's need for an artificial limb and then fabricate or adapt one. Long-term rehabilitation demands a strong team effort, because the problems confronted are often complex and affect so many areas of the client's life. Good communication between team members greatly enhances the effectiveness of the total treatment program, and team members often resemble an institutional "family," all working together for the maximum benefit of the client.

TREATMENT GOALS

Goals in rehabilitation programs may include the restoration or improvement of functional abilities, the maintenance of a client's abilities at an acceptable level, the prevention of further disability, the improvement of the client's ability to function in the home and work environment appropriate environmental adaptations, the adjustment of the client to temporary or permanent limitations, the exploration of the client's vocational or avocational potential, and resumption of a work role. Goals will vary with the nature of the illness or injury, the stage of recovery, and the client's developmental level and personal circumstances. Goals will be changed frequently as the client progresses in the rehabilitation program, and the OTR or COTA will need to reevaluate the client's status often to upgrade treatment goals and activities.

CHALLENGES AND REWARDS FOR OTRs AND COTAs

Work in the practice area of physical dysfunction offers the OTR and COTA challenges and opportunities. Although the physical impairments seen may be severe, occupational therapy can offer clients practical help in dealing with the resulting physical limitations and psychological reactions. In this practice area, progress can be seen and measured objectively and dramatic improvements can occur. Some clients, however, will be unable to recover all of the abilities that were lost and may have to learn to live with a life-long disability. Work in long-term rehabilitation requires patience, sensitivity to client feelings and needs, good interpersonal and communication skills, a strong scientific and medical background in physical dysfunction, and the ability to work closely and cooperatively with other members of the treatment team.

New roles for occupational therapists and therapy assistants are developing in areas such as pain management, cardiac rehabilitation, group approaches to client rehabilitation, the development and dissemination of new rehabilitation technologies, private practice, and public education programs. Practice in physical dysfunction will continue to be a strong specialty area within occupational therapy and will face new challenges as health care delivery continues to change.

CASE STUDY: SPINAL CORD INJURY

Mark is an example of a typical case seen in a long-term rehabilitation program. Mark is a 27-year-old man who was employed as an air traffic controller at the airport of a large midwestern city. He was married but had no children. On July 10, 1984, Mark and his wife were attending a family picnic in a country park beside a large lake. Mark joined other family members who were swimming and dove into the lake from a pier. When he did not come up, family members dove for him and recovered his body in three feet of water. He was quickly brought to shore, where he was found to have no pulse or respiration. While someone called an ambulance, Mark's cousin began cardiopulmonary resuscitation and was able to restore Mark's breathing. Mark was taken to the emergency room of a small rural hospital, where he was found to have a spinal cord injury. He was put into cervical traction and later underwent surgical resection of bone fragments at the level of cervical vertebra 5. Bone grafting was later carried out. Mark remained in this acute care hospital until August 14, when he was transferred to a larger hospital. Here a pulmonary embolism was diagnosed and treated. Mark continued to develop medical complications, including a gastric ulcer, diarrhea, a weight loss of 35 pounds, pressure sores on both heels and his sacrum, and continued pulmonary problems. After these conditions were stabilized, Mark was again transferred. This time he was admitted to Lakeland Rehabilitation Hospital, a 96-bed private rehabilitation facility in his home city. He entered this hospital in January of 1985 for an extensive rehabilitation program. Lakeland Rehabilitation Hospital was the only physical rehabilitation hospital in Mark's state. It provides long-term care and restorative services for a variety of physical disabilities, including spinal cord injuries, strokes, amputations, arthritis, brain injuries, and other neuromuscular disorders. It offers a full range of rehabilitation services and a treatment team is assigned to each patient. The occupational therapy staff consists of 16 OTRs, 3 COTAs, a department chief, and an assistant chief. The physiatrist who was supervising Mark's care referred him to occupational therapy for evaluation and treatment early in his stay. He was seen the same afternoon by the OTR on his treatment team, who explained the goals and methods used by her department and how they would be incorporated into his total treatment program. The OTR completed a preliminary evaluation and found that Mark had the following problems:

1. Paralysis and loss of sensation below the level of cervical vertebrae 5 and 6. Mark had no movement or feeling in his legs or lower trunk.
2. Deficiencies in strength and sensation of the arms at the level of the lesion and lack of functional use of both arms.
3. Poor endurance and upper body balance.
4. Frequent dizziness and faintness due to blood pressure problems.
5. Dependence in all self-care activities: feeding himself, caring for his own hygiene, and dressing. Mark was unable to carry out any home or work tasks.
6. Impairment in bowel and bladder functions.
7. Occasional depression and sense of hopelessness about the future.

A variety of medications were being given to help stabilize Mark's many complications, but with time many of these medications were discontinued. Mark was taught to monitor his own levels of medication so that he could alert the physician to needed changes.

A number of precautions had to be observed in Mark's occupational therapy treatment. When he was admitted to Lakeland Hospital he was wearing a neck brace to protect the bone grafting that had been done. The brace was later removed, but caution was needed to ensure that no damage occurred to Mark's neck that would interfere with the healing of the graft. Because of Mark's pulmonary complications, his respiratory capacity was decreased. He was still prone to respiratory infections and the buildup of secretions, and these had to be guarded against. Mark experienced low blood pressure when sitting and could not be left for long in that position. Because he had no bladder control, any bladder problems that developed could send him into shock. The pressure sores on his heels and sacrum required care, and precautions were necessary to prevent other pressure sores from developing. The occupational therapist recommended that night splints be made for Mark's hands so that they would remain in a curved resting position and would not develop excessive tightness.

Five days after Mark's admission to Lakeland Hospital, the occupational therapist completed a comprehensive assessment of his occupational performance and the performance components that provided the foundation for functional activities. She found that Mark was unable to perform any independent living activities. He could tolerate only 20 minutes of sitting with his hips and trunk at a 90° angle. He could move his arms partially through their range of motion but was unable to hold objects. He could partially extend his wrists but had no adequate grasping action of his hands. He could communicate orally but could not write because of his motor impairment.

At this point in his recovery, the resumption of his home and job respon-sibilities were long-term goals. A great deal of improvement in his physical abilities was needed before these could be realistic objectives. Fortunately, Mark's high level of intelligence, his emotional health, and his positive self-concept gave him many strengths to build on in working toward these end goals.

Assessment of the neuromuscular performance components was conducted jointly by the occupational therapist and the physical therapist. They found that Mark had fair to good strength in the muscles of his arms and shoulder girdle. His wrist extensor muscles were only fair on both sides, although the left was slightly stronger. (Mark was left-handed.) Sensory evaluation revealed that Mark could feel and respond to light touch, deep pressure, sensations of hot and cold and sharp and dull, and he had adequate position sense in his upper chest, upper arms, and forearms. He was unable to identify objects placed in his hands through touch alone (stereognosis), and this, along with his decreased muscle function resulted in limited use of his hands. Mark had only slight tenodesis action (a natural curl of the fingers when the wrist is extended) on which to build active grasp. His endurance was low and pain in his shoulders further limited his movement. Mark's posture was poor because of his weak trunk muscles, his loss of equilibrium reactions, and the inadequacy of his wheelchair back, which was not adjusted for his height of 6 feet 4 inches. Other sensory functions, cognitive abilities, and interpersonal relationships were found to be at normal levels.

The occupational therapist felt that there was an immediate need for some positioning splints to prevent further disability and adapted equipment to promote use of Mark's hands and wrists. Night splints were made for him, and the occupational therapist recommended that a dynamic (movable) wrist-driven flexor hinge splint be made for Mark and fitted to him when he had developed strong enough wrist movements to be able to use it. This splint would help him to achieve a three-point grasp of the fingers and would improve his pinch strength. The OTR also recommended that Mark use a universal cuff into which the handles of utensils and tools could be slipped so that he could begin to work on self-care skills. The immediate goals developed for Mark's occupational therapy treatment plan were for the improvement of performance components that would enable him to move toward independent living. They included strengthening Mark's wrist extensor muscles, increasing his ability to sit in his chair for up to 30 minutes at a time, teaching him substitute patterns of movement for some he had lost, compensating for some of his sensory losses, developing increased independence in self-care tasks, improving his ability to use his hands for functional activities, and helping him adjust to his disability.

Treatment sessions were conducted on a daily basis, with frequent reassessment of abilities. Twice a month the treatment team met to discuss Mark's progress. Mark's team consisted of a physiatrist, who was in charge of the total treatment program, an occupational therapist, a physical therapist, a recreational therapist, a social worker, a nurse, and a psychologist. Mark also attended the team meetings and contributed to the development of new goals for the next two-week period.

After a month of intensive treatment, Mark had achieved the short-term goals and the emphasis of the occupational therapy program had changed to focus on lower extremity dressing, homemaking skills, bathing, and the bowel and bladder program. These areas required a longer training period, but assessment continued to be done twice a month. Mark's general muscle strength and endurance were assessed weekly by the COTA who was in charge of group sessions to increase muscular strength and power.

In carrying out the occupational therapy treatment program, the OTR functioned as primary therapist. She identified the treatment goals, developed the treat-

ment plan, and conducted one-to-one therapy sessions aimed at improving components of Mark's performance skills. Half-hour daily sessions were spent in the development of hygiene, dressing, and self-feeding skills. An additional half-hour daily session was used for range of motion activities (both passive and active), exercise, development of tenodesis action, splint training, development of muscle substitution patterns, and compensatory actions. The COTA worked with Mark in two treatment groups. A strength- and power-building group was used that incorporated progressive resistive exercise to build physical endurance and muscular strength. An adaptive hand skills group was also led by the COTA; this group concentrated on developing the hand skills needed for performance of self-care and work tasks. Each group included five or six patients with spinal cord injuries. The COTA also fabricated adapted equipment for Mark's use, including a hairbrush, shower handle, phone cuff, and knife. A rehabilitation aide who assisted in the occupational therapy department also made pieces of dressing equipment for Mark that did not require special fitting.

Mark's family also became involved in his treatment program. Because the staff encouraged communication, the family felt comfortable asking questions of the team and often came with Mark to his therapy sessions when they were visiting. At first Mark was uncertain of what to expect in the rehabilitation program, but as he became familiar with the philosophy of the staff and the institution he began to take an active part in team decisions about his program. He was able to express his thoughts and feelings well and helped solve some of the difficult problems in his own program. Each discipline involved in Mark's treatment contributed it own expertise to the total program. The occupational therapist focused her efforts on self-care skills, adapted equipment, splinting, and the development of functional hand skills. The physical therapist concentrated on bed and wheelchair mobility. The social worker took most of the responsibility for discharge planning and looked into housing arrangements for Mark. She also kept in contact with the reimbursement agents paying for Mark's care. Mark's physiatrist was concerned with the medical issues in Mark's case and also coordinated the treatment program. The nurse helped develop a bowel and bladder program for Mark and taught Mark how to care for his skin to prevent pressure sores and skin breakdown.

In addition to the individual treatment programs, an education group was conducted for patients with spinal cord injuries by the nursing staff, occupational therapist, and psychologist. Topics such as bowel and bladder care, muscle spasms, sexuality, and assertiveness were discussed and explored. An evening recreational program, jointly coordinated by the occupational therapist, physical therapist, and recreational therapist, offered daily living and recreational activities, such as a homemaking class, wheelchair football, and trips to the shopping mall, laundromat, and miniature golf course.

Mark made steady improvement and his discharge from Lakeland Rehabilitation Hospital was planned for April 1985. A 16-week program of intensive rehabilitation is typical for a person with Mark's injury. A home visit was made by the occupational and physical therapists, along with Mark to see if environmental modifications were necessary. A similar visit that included the vocational counselor was made to Mark's work site. A few minor alterations were recommended, and additional practice was given with the wrist-drive tenodesis splint so that Mark would be able to accomplish his tasks at work.

At the time of discharge, Mark was able to feed himself independently, take care of his own hygiene, put on his own shirt and jacket, and use his splint for typing and writing. He still needed some help with putting on his pants and leg bag (a urinary drainage system), performing some homemaking tasks, and carrying out his bowel program. He was discharged to his parents home, since he was in the process of a divorce. Home health services were initiated to offer him continued therapy in specific problem areas. He returned to Lakeland Hospital one month after discharge for continued help with work skills and some daily living skills. A customized wrist-driven flexor hinge splint had been made for him, and with some practice Mark was able to use this to accomplish fine motor tasks.

Since his discharge, Mark has completed a drivers training program, has passed his drivers test, and has purchased a customized van with a lift and hand controls. He returned to work part-time in his old job as an air traffic controller and worked up to full-time employment. His fellow workers and employer are supportive and have confidence in his ability to perform his work tasks satisfactorily. Mark has received no special favors at work and wants none. On reviewing the course of his rehabilitation program, Mark says "Those first days and weeks weren't easy, but now everything is going OK."

DISCUSSION QUESTIONS

1. What special personal qualities do you think an occupational therapist or therapy assistant would need to work with physically disabled clients?

2. Were Mark's personal relationships affected by his injury?

3. If Mark had been unable to return to his old job, what additional services might have been needed in his rehabilitation program?

4. Discuss the role of the COTA in Mark's rehabilitation. How did the OTR and COTA share responsibilities in Mark's treatment program?

5. How much did Mark's positive attitudes contribute to the success of his rehabilitation program?

6. Discuss the division of responsibility by different members of the treatment team in this case. Were there major areas where services overlapped or duplicated one another?

7. How important was the early treatment of Mark's injury to his eventual recovery?

8. Is there a hospital specializing in rehabilitation of physical dysfunctions in your area? What kinds of disabilities are treated there?

9. Consider the implications that a similar injury would have on your life. What does "coping with a disability" mean to you?

REFERENCES

1. Spencer A: Functional restoration—theory, principles, and techniques. In Hopkins, Smith (eds): *Willard and Spackman's Occupational Therapy*, ed 6. Philadelphia, JB Lippencott, 1983, pp 353–380.

2. Versluys H: Psychological adjustment to physical disability. In Trombly C, Scott A (eds): *Occupational Therapy for Physical Dysfunction*. Baltimore, Williams & Wilkins, 1977, pp 10–27.

3. Trombly C, Scott A: The treatment planning process. In Trombly C, Scott A (eds): *Occupational Therapy for Physical Dysfunction*. Baltimore, Williams & Wilkins, 1977, pp 3–9.

•

SUGGESTED READINGS

Bedbrook G: *The Care and Management of Spinal Cord Injuries*. New York, Springer-Verlag, 1981

Ford J, Duckworth B: *Physical Management for the Quadriplegic Patient*. Philadelphia, FA Davis.

Nixon V: *Spinal Cord Injury: A Guide to Functional Outcomes in Physical Therapy Management*. Rehabilitation Institute of Chicago, 1985.

Special issue on spinal cord injury. *Am J Occup Ther* 39:11, 1985.

Tator C: *Early Management of Acute Spinal Cord Injury*. New York, Raven Press, 1982.

Umphred D: *Neurological Rehabilitation*. St. Louis, CV Mosby, 1985.

Wilson D: *Spinal Cord Injury: A Treatment Guide for Occupational Therapists*. Thorofare, NJ, Slack, 1974.

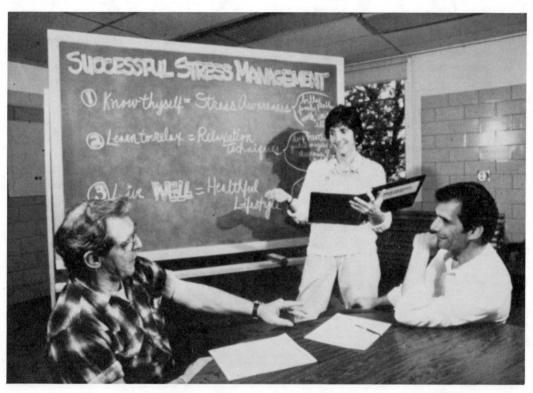

Courtesy AOTA

ELEVEN

Practice with Psychosocial Dysfunctions

Occupational therapy had its origins in the treatment of the mentally ill, and psychiatry and mental health continue to be a major practice area for occupational therapists. Table 11.1 shows the percentages of OTRs and COTAs working with various types of psychosocial disorders in 1986 (unpublished data from American Occupational Therapy Association, 1986 member survey).

The percentage of the occupational therapy work force employed in programs dealing with psychosocial dysfunction has declined gradually over the past 13 years; this decline has been greater for OTRs than for COTAs. The 1985 AOTA Manpower Study points out, however, that the number of personnel working in this practice area has actually increased as the size of the total occupational therapy work force has increased (1). Smaller proportions of OTRs and COTAs appear to be entering practice in this specialty area. There are a number of reasons for this. 1) Occupational therapists have had difficulty identifying their unique contributions to the treatment of psychosocial dysfunction. There has been little consensus among practi-

tioners over the proper role of occupational therapy in mental health settings. 2) There has been a proliferation of other professions working with behavioral disorders. These related professions assumed some of the roles that occupational therapy traditionally fulfilled, and considerable overlap in services resulted. 3) Occupational therapy was somewhat slow to adapt to new modes of service delivery in mental health.

CHANGING PATTERNS OF CARE

With the passage of the Community Mental Health Act in 1963, funding was made available to establish community mental health centers in local "catchment areas." This legislation encouraged treatment programs at the local level rather than in large, impersonal state institutions. Roughly concurrent with this shift in location of services was a corresponding shift in treatment approaches. Long-term therapeutic approaches, such as psychoanalysis, were believed to be too time-consuming and were ineffective for many

Table 11.1.
Mental Health Problems Seen Most
Frequently by OTRs and COTAs in 1986[a]

Health Problem	OTRs	COTAs
Adjustment disorders	1.3	0.9
Affective disorders	4.0	2.4
Alcohol/drug abuse	1.1	2.4
Anxiety disorders	0.3	1.1
Eating disorders	0.2	0.1
Organic mental disorders	1.6	5.4
Other mental health disorders	0.6	5.4
Personality disorders	0.6	5.4
Schizophrenic disorders	6.0	9.8

[a]Unpublished data from American Occupational Therapy Association, 1986 member survey.
Values are percents of total OTR and COTA work force.

clients. Short-term treatment approaches began to evolve that were aimed at helping clients with their everyday problems of living. New approaches were developed to help the chronically mentally ill adjust to community living and provide the necessary day-to-day support. More and more, treatment of acute psychotic episodes and psychological crisis situations took place in small psychiatric units with acute care hospitals.

The introduction of effective drug therapies in the late 1950s caused a revolution in psychiatric care. With the aid of drug treatment, many clients who had previously been out of contact with reality were able to communicate and be in at least partial control of their behavior. The drugs did not cure severe mental illnesses but did reduce symptoms to the point where clients could benefit from other forms of therapy. As knowledge of psychopharmacology increased, an array of drug therapies became available to psychiatrists and drugs became an indispensable part of psychiatric treatment. Occupational therapists were now able to work with clients who had previously been unresponsive, and a new era of psychiatric care began (2).

EFFECTS ON OCCUPATIONAL THERAPY

Slowly a network of services developed to replace institutional care. Occupational therapists found themselves working with (and sometimes competing with) social workers, psychologists, other types of activity therapists (art, music, dance, horticulture, drama, poetry, and therapeutic recreation), and generic mental health workers. These professions shared some commonalities with occupational therapy, and the resulting role confusion was a problem in many mental health settings. In 1975 a Mental Health Task Force was formed by the AOTA to identify issues of concern to occupational therapists working in mental health and to recommend solutions to existing problems. The task force report noted that mental health practice lacked valid and reliable assessment tools, standardized clinical techniques, and a unified theory of practice. Recommendations for change emphasized the need for theory development, research, and refinement of the knowledge base in this area of occupational therapy practice.

Progress has been made in these directions. The theoretical concepts of occupational behavior, as articulated by Kielhofner, Barris, Watts, and others, have provided a model for occupational therapy practice that is compatible with the traditions of the field and that clearly delineates the domain of occupational therapy. This model can readily be applied to mental health practice and complements rather than competes with the services offered by related mental health professionals. Other theoretical approaches have also been proposed, such as the cognitive model offered by Allen (3), but these are more limited in scope and application. It is critical for occupational therapy to carefully define its role in mental health so that its contributions will be respected and seen as substantially different from those of other professions. Without a unique identity, occupational therapy could be submerged in the proliferation of treatment approaches to psychosocial dysfunction.

BODIES OF KNOWLEDGE

In their text, *Psychosocial Occupational Therapy: Practice in a Pluralistic Arena*, Barris, Kielhofner, and Watts (4) offer a review of the bodies of knowledge that have been applied to psychosocial dysfunction. Among them are the psychoanalytic approach, existential-humanistic treatment methods, behavioral approaches, cognitive strategies, reality therapies, communications/interactions theories, social ecological approaches, community mental health concepts, and deviance or labeling theory. The OTR or COTA working with psychosocial dysfunctions needs to have a broad theoretical background in the bodies of knowledge that are applied to psychiatric disorders. Even more important, however, is the knowledge of how to apply concepts of human occupation and purposeful activity to the problems of the mentally ill or disturbed client. Clients with psychological disturbances frequently have difficulty performing their everyday work, leisure, and self-care activities. It is in these areas of occupational performance that the OTR and COTA can make their most meaningful contribution to client treatment. Barris, Kielhofner, and Watts see the role of the OTR or COTA working in psychosocial dysfunction as "an environmental manager, a problem-solver and a co-planner together with the client, as one who uses her own personality as a therapeutic agent, as one who directly engages the client in occupations as treatment, and as an organizer and leader of task-oriented therapeutic groups" (4).

PRACTICE SITES

Tiffany (5) has identified three levels of mental health services. Primary care or prevention is the first level and is a relatively recent concern of mental health professionals. Through education and counseling, attempts are made to head off serious psychological disturbances. Early intervention for relatively minor disturbances helps to prevent more severe problems from developing. Secondary care is the direct intervention in a psychological dysfunction or disease that has developed. Tertiary care is concerned with maintaining an optimum level of function in chronically ill clients and with providing them the necessary support services to prevent regression or deterioration. Occupational therapists in the past have been involved mainly with secondary and tertiary care. Preventive services are now being given greater emphasis; increasing numbers of occupational therapists will work in preventive programs in the future.

There are multiple settings for occupational therapy practice with psychosocial dysfunctions. Large public institutions for the mentally ill used to be the predominant site for occupational therapy services for this population. These institutions continue to exist but now serve a limited population of chronically disabled clients with severe mental disorders. Specialized institutions have been developed for the treatment of psychotic or severely disturbed children and adolescents, clients with drug and alcohol abuse problems, and court-committed clients. Such institutions are usually residential, with clients remaining in treatment for an extended period of time. Occupational therapy departments in institutional settings tend to be large and may include other activity specialists as well as occupational therapists. Group treatment approaches are common, although individual therapy goals for clients are usually identified.

Acute care hospitals in local communities most often provide the immediate care for psychologically disturbed clients. Many hospitals have a small inpatient psychiatric unit that admits clients experiencing a psychotic episode or a psychological crisis that prevents them from functioning in their customary environment. The average length of stay in these units is short, and the goals of treatment are often limited to evaluation of the problem areas and provision of a therapeutic environment in which clients can reorganize and begin to deal with their immediate problems. Medication may be prescribed and adjusted to clients' needs during their stay on the inpatient unit. Once each client's condition is stabilized, he or she is usually discharged and referred to an outpatient or community-based program if further treatment is indicated. Team members working on psychiatric units of acute care hospitals may include psychiatrists, nurses, social workers, psychologists, and occupational therapists (6).

The largest proportion of treatment services for the mentally ill and psychologically disturbed is available through community mental health centers. These programs have been designed to offer psychiatric care to clients close to their home community and may include outpatient therapy, crisis intervention, group homes, and geriatric programs, specialized services for children and adolescents, family therapy, drug and alcohol abuse programs, and outreach services. Team members include the same professionals found in hospitals but may also include lay workers and members of the community. Barris, Kielhofner, and Watts (4) point out that work in community clinics is quite different from that on an inpatient hospital unit. There is generally less structure in community programs, fewer physical boundaries, and less domination of the treatment process by physicians. Community clinics tend to be egalitarian, with co-workers sharing decision-making responsibilities and taking an active part in program planning. The occupational therapist in a community mental health clinic is more likely to work with clients in a friendly, collaborative relationship rather than a directive one. It is important that the community clinic occupational therapist and therapy assistant have a good working knowledge of community resources and services so that they can refer clients to appropriate related programs. They also need to be aware of local standards and cultural patterns so that clients can be helped to adapt their behavior to fit with community norms and customs. Community-based treatment programs offer great advantages to clients, since they can seek treatment without leaving their homes, their families, or their employment. Treatment can be better adapted to their personal needs and environment, and mental health workers can better judge when to fade out their support as clients are able to assume more control of their lives. Community mental health centers seem to be living up to the high expectations that were held for them and will continue to be the site of most mental health services.

Day hospitals or day-care programs are another site of mental health services and may be part of the overall program of a community mental health center or may be an extended service of a local hospital. Day hospitals are a transitional stage between hospitalization and community living. They offer a full range of treatment services and maintenance programs for chronically ill clients who are at risk for repeated hospitalizations. Occupational therapy is an important part of the program. A balanced program of daily activities may be available to clients, including training in self-care and independent living, work habits and skills, and leisure time activities. The end goal is stabilization of the client's status so that the client can maintain himself or herself, perhaps with some assistance, in the community (7, 8).

In addition to the settings already mentioned, there are other specialized treatment facilities that deal with only one type of psychosocial problem. Drug and alcohol abuse programs are an example, with some being part of a larger institutional setting and others operating as free-standing community agencies. These programs employ a variety of health-related professionals, counselors, psychologists, social workers, and sometimes representatives of the criminal justice system. Many programs employ former addicts as lay workers to assist with the therapeutic program. Group therapies are usually a major part of the treatment effort, and clients often spend an extended period of time in a program. Occupational therapy can provide useful insights into the effects of addiction on occupational performance and can help clients regain performance skills that have been lost or neglected during periods of substance abuse. Constructive use of leisure time is another contribution of occupational therapy to the total treatment program. Prevention is an additional thrust of these programs, and efforts are made to educate the public about substance abuse and the need for early intervention (4).

Home treatment for psychosocial dysfunction has not been frequently used but could become more prominent if it becomes a reimbursable mental health service. Occupational therapists could play a role in such programs, just as they now do in home care for the physically impaired.

A small number of occupational therapists have pioneered work in correctional institutions as part of a general program of rehabilitation for convicted criminals. Occupational therapy concepts and methods could be of great value in such settings, and we may see more OTRs and COTAs employed within the correctional system in the future.

Psychosocial occupational therapy has gone through a long and unsettled transition period as mental health services changed their emphasis and relocated from institutional to community settings. Although occupational therapists working in this practice area have not achieved consensus on a unified theoretical approach, they appear to be moving toward greater agreement. If occupational therapy can demonstrate that it has a unique service role in the treatment of psychosocial disorders, it will continue to be a viable part of mental health programs. The AOTA projects that community programs will be the location of most mental health treatment and that more occupational therapists and therapy assistants will be needed as these programs expand their services. In addition, nursing homes are beginning to identify the need for more occupational therapy personnel to work with residents who show psychosocial disturbances. These two settings are viewed by the AOTA as having the greatest growth potential for the use of psychosocial occupational therapy (1).

CASE STUDY: CHRONIC UNDIFFERENTIATED SCHIZOPHRENIA

Let's look at one of the new community-based programs and see how occupational therapy fits into the total service program. Hillside Hospital is an acute care hospital in a small Northeastern city and runs a psychiatric adult day treatment program as an extension of its inpatient psychiatric services. The program was developed to improve clients' level of functioning in home, work, and community settings; to teach clients adequate coping skills so that they could better deal with the stresses of daily life; and to provide a controlled environment in which these skills could be practiced. The program is staffed by a consulting psychiatrist and social worker, psychiatric nurses, and registered occupational therapists. It is located in a wing of the hospital and is open from 7:30AM to 4:30PM each weekday. Services of the day program include one-to-one counseling, verbal and practice groups aimed at developing or improving a variety of personal and job-related skills, individual and group occupational therapy, medication monitoring, liaison services with clients' referring physicians, and referral to other community agencies when indicated. Funding is through private insurance coverage and state and county sources.

When clients are accepted into the program, they must agree to attend regularly, maintain confidentiality, maintain contact with their referring physician, actively participate in program activities, provide their own transportation, and meet the financial obligations of their treatment. Clients are not permitted to attend if intoxicated by drugs or alcohol. The length of client involvement with the adult day program varies, depending on the client's diagnosis, motivation for change, and ability to follow through on recommendations.

The occupational therapy staff plays an important role in the day treatment program by organizing and supervising task groups that provide shared work experience for clients, by providing sensory integration and movement activities for clients in need of better perceptual and cognitive functioning, by providing training in daily living tasks, and by offering individual and group treatment sessions tailored to a client's particular needs and interests. The occupational therapy staff works with the nursing staff to provide group therapy, assertiveness and parent training, and self-awareness sessions.

Ann represents a typical case seen by the occupational therapy staff at the adult day treatment program. She is a 32-year-old woman who has had no specific job training and is unemployed. She was referred to the program by her psychiatrist at a community mental health center. Ann had been diagnosed as having chronic undifferentiated schizophrenia and has had a long history of psychiatric problems with many long-term hospitalizations. At the initial interview with the occupational therapist, Ann showed poor coping skills. She was inclined to sit and worry about problems, tending to cry hysterically and hyperventilate, rather than take any positive action. Her motivation was poor. She had tried several volunteer positions and sheltered employment but was unable to follow through in any of these jobs. Her communication and social skills were poor. Ann had tried to live in her own apartment but had difficulty coping with the day-to-day challenges of independent living. She had trouble managing her money, often spending money on unnecessary items rather than paying her bills. She had little knowledge of nutrition and had become obese. Her self-confidence was low. At the time of the interview, she was on a combination of three medications prescribed by her physician: an antipsychotic medication, another to minimize side effects caused by the former drug, and a third medication to decrease anxiety.

Ann's social history indicated that she had had a difficult childhood. Because of rebellious behavior, she had spent a lot of time in foster homes and in different school systems. Intellectually Ann was in the low-normal range. Since 1969 she had had multiple hospitalizations. In 1978 she was married but divorced within three months. Ann held brief jobs as a maid and a kitchen worker but was unable to maintain employment because of her poor attitude, lack of motivation, and inability to assume responsibility. Her physical health was generally good, although she had sustained a back injury that prevents her from doing any heavy lifting.

The Framingham Functional Assessment Scale was completed by the treatment team when Ann entered the adult day treatment program and was readministered every three months that she remained in treatment. The results of the initial evaluation showed that Ann had minimal concentration. She needed constant guidance in performing tasks, and her functioning broke down under the slightest stress. She needed assistance to reengage in the task. Her social functioning was severely limited. She rarely initiated contact with others. She expressed discomfort and anxiety when in a group of people and tolerated only limited interactions with staff members. Although she sometimes referred to her own emotional state, she showed little objective understanding of emotions and seemed to be overwhelmed by her own feelings.

Physically, Ann could take care of her own personal needs; however, she had some difficulty with grooming and hygiene skills. Psychologically, she had great difficulty coping with the day-to-day demands of her life. She had few mechanisms available to handle stress and tended to become hysterical when situations arose that she couldn't handle. Ann often displayed physical manifestations when under stress (headache, backache) and tended to deal with problems by expecting others to handle them for her. She felt extremely inadequate, making self-derogatory remarks and becoming easily discouraged. She had limited understanding of the role of diet and exercise in regard to weight loss. She needed assistance with planning and preparing nutritious meals, as well as with shopping for and maintaining her clothing.

When asked about her leisure interests, Ann recalled that she had enjoyed activities like crocheting, knitting, needlepoint, volleyball, and exercise classes in the past. Recently, however, she had not been able to motivate herself to participate in any of them. She reported that she had a few friends but had not contacted them in the past year.

Her cognitive abilities were limited. She had an attention span of approxi-

mately 10 minutes. She was oriented to person and place but was frequently confused as to the date and time of day. She had difficulty in organizing tasks and often moved to the next step of a task without completing the first one. Her awareness of other people was minimal. Her verbalizations were often child-like and whiny. In a group situation she would frequently attempt to dominate, interrupting others in a loud voice and refusing to allow them to take part in decisions. Her conversation in group sessions was usually only with the therapist.

The occupational therapist considered the behaviors that Ann was displaying and identified several areas where intervention seemed to be needed. The resulting treatment plan focused on several problem areas in which occupational therapy could offer assistance. Occupational therapy objectives included helping Ann build greater confidence in her own abilities, teaching her more effective ways of dealing with stress, helping her develop better work skills, encouraging more appropriate group interaction and communication skills, and helping her to improve her physical health.

To assist her in these areas the OTR scheduled her to participate in individual occupational therapy treatment sessions three times a week. During these sessions, Ann and the OTR worked to improve Ann's self-confidence by completing familiar activities together and by gradually introducing new leisure-time activities that Ann could continue at home. Ann was also taught methods of stress reduction and was helped to see that some of her physical symptoms were stress related. The OTR persuaded Ann to attend a relaxation group each week that used progressive relaxation techniques, videos, and music to help group members achieve physical and mental relaxation. Ann was encouraged to use these methods when she felt under stress and to practice them regularly at home. She also began to attend a work skills group twice a week to develop job-related skills and better work habits. Communication and group interaction skills were worked on in a weekly social skills group where Ann learned to present herself more effectively, to use appropriate grooming and hygiene methods, and to be more comfortable in group situations. A weekly exercise class rounded out her schedule, with a home exercise routine organized for her to help her lose weight and improve her physical condition. Ann also participated in a weekly ADL (activities of daily living) group where she learned to plan and prepare nutritious low-calorie meals for herself, budget her money, and take care of her clothing.

Plans were made to review Ann's progress each week with the treatment team. The treatment plan was updated on an ungoing basis and monthly reports were sent to Ann's physician.

Ann participated in the adult day treatment program for approximately one year, attending three days a week. At the end of this period, Ann had established a positive relationship with the occupational therapist and with other staff members. Initially she missed some sessions due to physical complaints, but as time went on her attendance became more consistent. She was able to learn more appropriate methods of stress reduction and can now utilize relaxation techniques and satisfying leisure activities for this purpose. She feels more positive about her achievements and often brings in samples of needlework that she has completed at home in her leisure time. Ann did follow through on her nutritional program and her home exercise routine, losing at total of 20 pounds.

Ann improved her communication abilities and is now able to reach out to the other clients socially, initiate conversation, and maintain eye contact with others. Her verbalizations are more adult and appropriate. Her appearance has markedly improved. She has joined a community recreation program that she attends regularly and has made some new friends. Her involvement in the adult day treatment program has largely been replaced by volunteer work at a child care

center. She works there three days a week for half-days and gets much positive feedback from the staff on her work with the children.

A very satisfactory improvement in behavior and community living skills resulted from Ann's participation in the adult day treatment program. Plans have been made for her to continue her individual session with the OTR once a week for several months. The therapist will continue to offer her support and will assist with problems if necessary. Ann continues to see her psychiatrist at the mental health center periodically for regulation of her medications. She lives alone in a small apartment and is able to care for her own needs with minimal assistance. The long-term goal is to prepare Ann for paid part-time employment in a suitable environment. In view of her progress so far, this appears to be achievable.

DISCUSSION QUESTIONS

1. Although no COTA was employed in this program, are there parts of the occupational therapy treatment program that could have been conducted by a COTA? Discuss the potential contributions of a COTA in this setting.

2. How might the occupational therapist use himself or herself as a therapeutic tool in a program such as that described for Ann?

3. How were treatment activities graded in Ann's program?

4. How did the treatment activities conducted by the occupational therapist ease Ann's ability to fit into community activities?

5. Did the therapist work with Ann in a directive way or in a collaborative way? Why?

6. What personality attributes do you imagine an occupational therapist or therapy assistant would need to work effectively with a client like Ann?

REFERENCES

1. Ad Hoc Commission on Occupational Therapy Manpower: *Occupational Therapy Manpower: A Plan for Progress*. Rockville, MD, American Occupational Therapy Association, 1985, pp 55–59.
2. Smith D: Effects of psychotropic drugs on the occupational therapy process. *Mental Health Special Interest Newsletter*. American Occupational Therapy Association, 4:1, 1981. (Reprinted in *Occupational Therapy in Practice*. AOTA, 1985, pp 93–95.
3. Allen CK: *Cognitive Disabilities: Occupational Therapy Assessment and Management*. Boston, MA, Little, Brown & Co., 1986.
4. Barris R, Kielhofner G, Watts J: *Psychosocial Occupational Therapy: Practice in a Pluralistic Arena*. Laurel, MD, Ramsco, 1984, pp 3–172, 262–280.
5. Tiffany E: Psychiatry and mental health. In Hopkins H, Smith HD (eds): *Willard and Spackman's Occupational Therapy*, ed 6. Philadelphia, JB Lippencott, 1983, pp 267–333.
6. Rider B, Gramblin J: An activities approach to occupational therapy in a short term acute mental health unit. *Mental Health Special Interest Newsletter*. American Occupational Therapy Association, 3:4, 1980. (Reprinted in *Occupational Therapy in Practice*. AOTA, 1985, pp 96–98).
7. Gabriel J, Day treatment. *Mental Health Special Interest Newsletter*. American Occupational Therapy Association, 3:4, 1981. (Reprinted in *Occupational Therapy in Practice*. AOTA, 1985, pp 87–88.
8. Day treatment services. *Mental Health Special Interest Newsletter*. American Occupational Therapy Association, 3:3, 1980. (Reprinted in *Occupational Therapy in Practice*. AOTA 1985, pp 100–101.

SUGGESTED READINGS

Anthony WA. *Principles of Psychiatric Rehabilitation*. Amherst, MA, Human Resource Development Press, 1979.

Briggs AK, Agrin AR (eds): *Crossroads: A Reader for Psychosocial Occupational Therapy*. Rockville, MD, American Occupational Therapy Association, 1981.

Kaplan B: *The Inner World of Mental Illness*. New York, Harper & Row, 1964.

Nathan PE, Harris SL: *Psychopathology and Society*. New York, McGraw-Hill, 1980.

Sylph JS, Ross HE, Kedward HB. Social disability in chronic psychiatric patients. *Am J Psychiatry* 134:1391–1394, 1977.

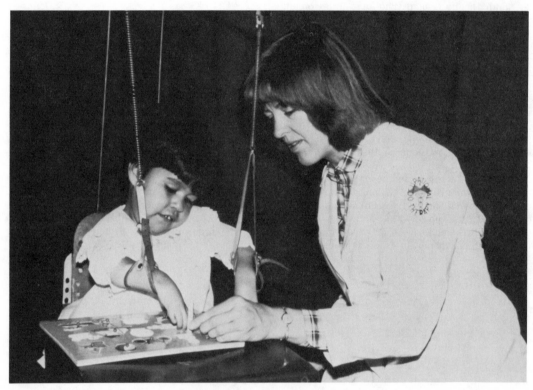

Courtesy AOTA

TWELVE

Practice with Developmental Disabilities

Occupational therapy has a long tradition of involvement with clients who have lifelong disabilities. The early literature in the field had many references to occupational therapy interventions for clients with cerebral palsy, birth defects, and multihandicapping conditions. Many of these lifelong disabilities are now grouped under the general term of *developmental disabilities*. Federal funding, beginning in the 1960s, helped to support the development of new therapeutic programs for this group of disabled people and gave rise to many new opportunities for occupational therapists and therapy assistants to work with this population.

FEDERAL SUPPORT FOR PROGRAMS

In the early 1960s, President Kennedy formed a special panel to investigate the needs of the mentally retarded population. The report of this panel led to the enactment of Public Law 88-164, which provided for the development and construction of research and treatment facilities for the mentally retarded and established a network of university-affiliated facilities to conduct research and educate students who work in the disciplines relevant to mental retardation. During this period, care of the retarded was beginning to shift from large institutional settings to community-based programs. There was renewed concern over the civil rights of retarded persons and an interest in seeking alternatives to institutional living. The Developmental Disabilities Services and Facilities Construction Act of 1970 (P.L. 91-517) broadened the mental retardation law to include a wider range of disabilities, including cerebral palsy and epilepsy. Later, the Developmentally Disabled Assistance and Bill of Rights Act of 1975 (P.L. 94-103) expanded the 1970 law even further to include autism and dyslexia (when related to a neurological condition).

DEFINITION OF DEVELOPMENTAL DISABILITIES

The Developmentally Disabled Assistance and Bill of Rights Act of 1975 provided a broad definition of developmental disabilities that, with minor revisions, remains in general use today. The 1978 extension of the act defined a developmental disability as follows:

A developmental disability is a severe, chronic disability of a person which
a) is attributable to a mental or physical impairment, or a combination of mental and physical impairments;
b) is manifested before the person attains age twenty-two;
c) is likely to continue indefinitely;
d) results in substantial functional limitations in three or more of the following areas of major life activity:
   1) self-care
   2) receptive and expressive language
   3) learning
   4) mobility
   5) self-direction
   6) capacity for independent living, and
   7) economic self-sufficiency; and
e) reflects the person's need for a combination and sequence of special, interdisciplinary, or generic care, treatment, or other services which are individually planned and coordinated (1).

The law intentionally did not list diagnostic categories because its authors wished to avoid labeling clients. Mental retardation had long had a negative stigma attached to it, and it was felt that this new, neutral term would avoid traditional stereotypes associated with the term *mental retardation*. The authors of this act also wished to focus attention not on the causes of these disabilities but on their effects. The limitations in functional performance and adaptive living skills were the areas in need of training and development, and the federally funded programs were aimed at helping these persons develop their optimum potential for living a full and satisfying life. The key element in the definition that distinguishes these disabilities from others is the fact that the disorder must be manifested during the developmental period of the individual's life (before age 22). The rationale for this part of the definition is that major disabilities that have their onset early in life are generally more severe and cause the individual to have problems in many areas of life. These disabilities may give rise to secondary disabilities and usually interfere with the person's ability to acquire basic life skills. For these reasons, developmental disabilities represent a special problem that requires the help of a variety of professionals during different periods of life. Developmental disabilities are chronic in nature, and although functional improvements can and do occur, the condition cannot be cured and will persist for the lifetime of the individual (1).

STATE SERVICES

The Developmental Disabilities Act of 1970 (amended in 1975) established a planning council in each state and required that states draw up a plan for services to their developmentally disabled citizens. Federal funds were allocated to help support a wide range of services: diagnosis, evaluation, treatment, personal care, day and residential care, special living arrangements, training, education, sheltered employment, recreation, counseling, protective and other social and legal services, information and referral, follow-through services, and transportation. These pieces of legislation provided both incentive and funds to support major improvements in the care of developmentally disabled people in the United States. For the first time a network of services was developed specifically to meet their needs. It was increasingly recognized that developmentally disabled clients were not only children but also adults who had their own set of needs and wants: better housing arrangements, vocational training and employment, recreational programs and facilities, and integration into their communities as fully participating citizens. The concept of a continuum of services was proposed, because the needs of the developmentally disabled varied as they moved through their life stages. The need to educate professionals who could function in the multidisciplinary environment was apparent, and a variety of educational programs were developed to train the additional personnel needed. Professionals working with the developmentally disabled also had to act as advocates for their clients in many situations, to ensure that their rights were protected and that their best interests were being served. Developmental disabilities includes an extremely large client group (1975 estimate, at least nine million persons), and these clients have a primary need for occupational therapy services. Job opportunities for OTRs and COTAs have vastly expanded for this clientele and are expected to continue to do so in the next decade (2,3).

MODELS OF SERVICE DELIVERY

At least five different models of practice have been used by professionals who provide service to persons with developmental disabilities. The most traditional is *the medical model*, which views the developmentally disabled person as one who has suffered a physiological insult that has resulted in reduced functional capacity. The medical model has helped to provide information on some of the causes of developmental disability and has contributed to the assessment of impairment but has been unable to provide many "curative" or intervention strategies for some disabilities, such as mental retardation.

The medical model uses the conceptual framework of "illness" and "normality" when looking at developmental disorders, and these concepts are often less useful when dealing with chronic conditions. It has also helped to stigmatize the mentally retarded by labeling them as subnormal and, by implication, incapable of improvements in behavior and functional abilities. Although the medical model continues to have value in its focus on the biomedical components of developmental disability, it does not offer solutions to the broad range of functional limitations seen in this population.

The child development model has also frequently been applied to the education and treatment of the developmentally disabled. This model assumes that the physical, social, and emotional development of the person goes through a series of recognizable stages. Failure to achieve certain developmental milestones is viewed as preventing or interfering with the development of later, more advanced skills. This model has made contributions through its focus on the progression of the individual in his or her own developmental stages and provides a realistic frame of reference when looking at the functional abilities of the disabled person. It may have contributed, however, to the treatment of older disabled individuals as children. Normal adult states of development were not emphasized to the extent that childhood stages were, and this resulted in a lack of awareness of adult needs and goals. Remedial approaches using this model tend to focus on helping the individual master basic developmental skills. Some critics feel that normal development is not an appropriate model for those with developmental disabilities and suggest that it is preferable to teach skills to the developmentally disabled that are adapted to their limitations and to their specific natural environment.

Another model in current use may be

described as *the social-ecological model.* This model is rather recent and is not in wide use but is finding growing acceptance. It looks at disabled individuals in relation to their "social ecology" and takes into account their habits, modes of life, and relationship to their surroundings. The principle of normalization is an important concept in this model. The idea of providing a life-style for the disabled person that is similar to that of the normal population is proposed, getting clients out of the institutional environments and into less restrictive environments. This model focuses more on the needs of the developmentally disabled for a normal life-style than on the nature of the disability. Intervention may be directed at changes in the environment, offering specialized facilities, the use of educational equipment, and training materials. The model is less well defined than some of the others, however, and can be misinterpreted and inappropriately applied. Its appeal lies chiefly with its emphasis on the individual in the context of his or her social environment, and concepts that arose from this model (normalization, deinstitutionalization) have been the subject of much discussion.

The behavioral model has been accepted as a dominant influence in programs for the mentally retarded. This model, which is based on the concepts of Skinner and other behavioral psychologists, is supported by two decades of research and clinical application. According to this model, human behavior is learned through well-established learning principles. The behavioral model holds that abnormal or deviant behavior can be changed through the systematic application of basic learning principles. Methods include the use of classical and operant conditioning, involving reinforcement and extinction procedures, shaping techniques, modeling, and precision-teaching

methods. This model has proven to be successful in teaching new skills to the retarded and to other developmentally disabled clients. Because this approach focuses on behavior rather than on the diagnosis or disability, it avoids labeling individuals and does not force them into an "illness" category. It has been criticized because some of its adherents seen unable to consider alternatives and because ethical and moral issues can be raised over its application in some situations. It also tends to ignore intrinsic motivation and the importance of self-directed capability in the individual. This model is in wide use, however, and continues to play a role in the treatment of many developmental disabilities.

The psychoeducational model is a synthesis of some of the models already mentioned. This model also focuses on learning and is based on first assessing the individual's skill deficits and then setting target goals to be achieved. A course of programmed instruction is designed to lead the individual systematically toward goal achievement, with the end goal being increased competence. This model is often applied to groups rather than to individuals and relies on systematic training programs that focus on highly specific skills. There is no disease orientation in this model. Instead an educational orientation is used, with prescriptive teaching as the method to be applied. The model has the potential for wide application by a range of professional disciplines and can be used for prevention and early intervention when problems are anticipated (4).

The five models described are currently in use; the choice of practice model depends on the philosophy of the staff and the program. Occupational therapy personnel working in developmental disabilities need to be familiar with all of the models to be prepared for broadly based practice in this specialty area.

KEY CONCEPTS OF PRACTICE

An important concept for the occupational therapist working in developmental disabilities is that of habilitation. In working with the physically handicapped, we have discussed *rehabilitation*, by which we usually mean the relearning or restoration of skills and functions that have been lost or impaired because of illness or injury. Clients who have a developmental disability, however, have never developed some of the basic skills and abilities that are needed to function in society. Their need is for *habilitation*: the development and acquisition of abilities that were not previously present and that may need to be learned "from scratch." This fundamental difference characterizes practice in the specialty area of developmental disabilities. One cannot build on a client's memory of how it felt to move normally when he or she has never experienced normal movement. The therapist must build in to the treatment program many opportunities for clients to feel and experience these "normal" patterns of development so that they can learn to eventually achieve them more independently. Mentally retarded clients who have not had adequate opportunities to learn how to use their senses to gather information and explore the environment must be given structured experiences that will encourage them to develop these abilities. The basic skills must be built rather than rebuilt, and the OTR and COTA working in this area must have a good knowledge of normal growth and development in order to provide optimum habilitation experiences for developmentally disabled clients.

The principle of normalization was mentioned when the social-ecological model of practice was discussed. This concept is based on the idea that the quality of life increases as access to culturally typical activities and settings increases. A closely related concept is that of deinstitutionalization, which holds that the mentally retarded should be able to live and work in the least restrictive environment compatible with their functional limitations. These two ideas have been influential in promoting the integration of the mentally retarded into the mainstream of society. Although both concepts continue to be controversial, most professionals agree that they are desirable goals. Programming has moved systematically in the directions suggested by these two concepts. In 1967 the mentally retarded population in public institutions in the United States had reached an all-time high of nearly 200,000. By 1984, however, that figure had fallen 55% to about 110,000. Deinstitutionalization for mentally retarded persons began 12 years later than for the mentally ill and proceeded more gradually. As a result, there were fewer failures in the transition. Even so, there have been deficiencies in addressing the needs of diverse groups within the mentally retarded population. Many retarded individuals who were discharged from institutional settings were inappropriately placed in nursing homes that were ill-equipped to offer them the services they needed.

Landesman and Butterfield (5) identified three things that are critical to successful deinstitutionalization: 1) alternative community care and training programs, 2) predischarge preparation of residents for community living, 3) a community environment able to protect the rights of the retarded and sensitive to their needs.

Follow-up studies of residents discharged from institutional settings suggest that even the most severely and profoundly retarded individuals can progress in community settings if they are given adequate support systems. Continued study of the results of deinstitutionalization is necessary, but the preliminary findings tend to support the general idea that retarded individuals can live and function adequately in community-based programs. There will be some individuals who cannot, and institutional care may need to continue as an alternative source of care for such clients. A diversity of programs and living arrangements may be the best arrangement, since the needs of the developmentally disabled are so varied (5).

CONTINUING SERVICE NEEDS

One group that has not been adequately considered in planning is that of the aging developmentally disabled. In 1985 this population was estimated to include at least 200,000 persons, many of whom live in long-term care settings. Although only about 5% of the overall elderly population are institutionalized, that percentage rises much higher for aging developmentally disabled persons. People with mental retardation and other developmental disabilities are living longer than they once did, and states need to plan adequate care for this group. In 1985 a survey conducted by Janicki, Ackerman, and Jacobson (6) found that only 34% of state agencies for the aging had a state plan for the care of aging developmentally diabled clients. State developmental disabilities plans usually did not address the needs of the aging developmentally disabled population, and those that did used varying cutoff ages for defining this population. A more unified approach is needed, with collaboration between state agencies dealing with the elderly and those dealing with the developmentally disabled to provide adequate plans for the care of this group.

Attempts are being made to broaden the range of community care alternatives available to the developmentally disabled and to secure funding to pay the costs of such programs. In 1983 Senator John Chaffee introduced Senate Bill 2053, the Community and Family Living Amendments Act of 1983. This bill was intended to extend Medicaid funding (Title 19) to cover home and community care settings as well as institutional care. Although the bill has not been passed at this writing, it offers the kind of fiscal support that is needed if community care is to be a realistic alternative to institutionalization (7). The Health Care Financing Administration of the United States Department of Health and Human Services has issued guidelines for the appropriate placement of mentally retarded individuals in care settings and suggests that facilities should be selected based on whether the care they provide is developmental or medical. Developmental needs include a broad range of skills for which training should be provided, such as daily living skills, communication skills, and problem-solving skills. Few skilled nursing facilities or intermediate care facilities offer developmental training. Their report estimates that up to 10% of the residents of those institutions are mentally retarded individuals (8).

IS DEVELOPMENTAL DISABILITIES A SPECIALTY AREA?

One of the issues facing occupational therapists and COTAs working with developmental disabilities is whether they should practice as a generalist or as a specialist. Because developmental disabilities includes such a variety of conditions and functional deficiencies, some therapists believe that preparation as a generalist is appropriate. A broad knowledge of human growth and development, an understanding of a variety of chronic disabling conditions, and a repertoire of theoretical approaches to the functional limitations seen in these conditions may be needed to enable the OTR or COTA to help developmentally disabled clients reach their maximum potential. Other therapists feel that developmental disabilities is a true specialty area. They point out that one develops specialized knowledge about the problems of clients in a specific diagnostic group, such as cerebral palsy, mental retardation, or autism. Some therapists also tend to specialize in a specific age range, focusing on the needs of infants or teenagers. Here too, specialized knowledge about these stages of growth and development is applied to the limitations of the developmentally disabled client (9). In a small-scale survey conducted by the AOTA Developmental Disabilities Special Interest Section in 1983, respondents most frequently considered themselves generalists and believed that they were most effective using this approach. Respondents reported serving clients from ages 3 to 94 years of age, and all were seeing some adult clients in their practice. Respondents agreed that the greatest unmet need among their client groups was for more emphasis on the needs of the adult developmentally disabled population. More appropriate evaluation methods, ideas for treatment activities and equipment, and methods for improving independent living skills in the adult client were felt to be needed. Respondents overwhelmingly agreed that OT education should place more emphasis on developmental disabilities throughout the life span and suggested an increased emphasis on psychosocial issues for the developmentally disabled group (10).

PRACTICE SITES

Today OTRs and COTAs work in a variety of programs that deal with developmental disabilities. These programs include infant intervention programs (often seeing children from 0 to 3 years of age), family support and home care programs (where the OTR or COTA teaches the family how to promote optimum growth and development of the child), public and private school programs, sheltered workshops and other vocationally oriented programs, community living facilities, institutional care programs, and medically based programs (skilled nursing facilities, intermediate care facilities). A more recently developed type of facility is the intermediate care facility for the mentally retarded. Such programs provide active treatment and developmental training specific to the needs of the mentally retarded. In recent years there has been a renewed interest in work-related programs for this client group, and occupational therapists are again recognizing their responsibilities for contributing to the vocational rehabilitation process (11). Emshoff (12) has described an adapted vocational program for severely handicapped adults in which therapeutic activities are combined with job training. Gradually work skills are developed, and clients can also become more independent in daily living skills. Such adapted vocational programs are an important addition to the range of services provided for developmentally disabled clients. Although many will never be economically independent, pride in achievement and increased self-esteem are fostered through workshop programs.

TECHNICAL AIDS

Along with other groups of handicapped individuals, developmentally disabled clients have benefited from modern advances in technology. The use of technical aids has expanded the range of therapeutic activities available to the occupational therapist and has provided clients with job-related skills. The use of augmentative communication systems, environmental control units, and mobility systems have enabled clients to more easily communicate with others, control their immediate environment, and improve motor performance. Microcomputers, with adapted input and output devices, allow the severely handicapped individual to tap into the potentials of the computer for many practical purposes. The science of technology for the handicapped is in its infancy and has enormous potential. Special software packages are being developed to meet specific needs. Basic perceptual concepts (matching, sound discrimination, recognition of rhythms, numbers, and letters and problem-solving skills) are examples of programs designed for training. Occupational therapists of the future may find themselves taking required classes in applications of technology in rehabilitation (13).

ATTRIBUTES NEEDED FOR WORK WITH THE DEVELOPMENTALLY DISABLED

The OTR and COTA working with developmentally disabled clients need more than an average amount of patience and perseverance. Gains tend to be made in small increments and over relatively long periods of time. One has to also work to maintain the gains that have been achieved. Special senstivity to the needs of client's families is important, since families often share a sense of guilt and responsibility for a developmental disability. Family counseling and the use of family support groups are often needed to help families come to terms with their situation. Another attribute especially needed for work with this population is flexibility. The OTR and COTA must be prepared to revise goals when needed or to seek alternative means of accomplishing a goal. The course of most training programs is not a smooth, upward rising line but rather a series of up and down lines charting a gen-

erally upward trend. Small gains should be rewarded and then built on to achieve greater ones. Coaching is an important role for the OTR or COTA working with this disability group.

The OTR and COTA need good team skills, because developmental disabilities represent complex conditions that require a multidisciplinary approach for effective intervention. The OTR and COTA are likely to be working with physicians, nurses, psychologists, educators, physical therapists, social workers, workshop personnel, and vocational rehabilitation workers. The OTR or COTA must clearly outline what contributions they can make to the total programming for developmentally disabled clients. Often the OTR is viewed as an equipment specialist and is consulted when the client has special needs for custom equipment. Skill training in independent living is another major focus of occupational therapy personnel and is often the core of a training program.

Along with other team members, the OTR and COTA should be prepared to fulfill an advocacy role for their developmentally disabled clients. Safeguarding client's and families rights and ensuring that adequate facilities and programming are available to meet client's needs are responsibilities that must be taken seriously. Lobbying and testifying for legislation to benefit this client population is increasingly necessary in an era of cost-cutting and tight fiscal control. The OTR and COTA also share in the general responsibility to help the families of developmentally disabled clients plan realistically for the future. Many families worry about what will happen to children when they themselves can no longer care for them. Discussing alternative living arrangements with clients and their families can help them to make appropriate choices for the continued care of their family member.

CASE STUDY: A MULTIPLY HANDICAPPED CHILD

The case of Mack represents the kind of problems typically seen in a developmentally disabled person who is severely limited. Mack is a 9-year-old boy who is currently enrolled in a residential school and treatment center for multihandicapped children. Belle Harbor School is a private residential facility that serves children from age 0 to 21 years. It provides a home-based infant development program, a group treatment program for disabled infants and their families, a half-day preschool program and a school program. The educational programs offered conform to state and federal regulations governing the education of handicapped children, and the physical and occupational therapists on the staff work closely with members of the education staff.

Mack was a normal, healthy infant until the age of 19 months when he was involved in an automobile accident. He was not in a car seat restraint and was thrown from the vehicle. Immediately after the accident he was rushed to a hospital and stopped breathing en route. He suffered multiple cuts, fractures, and bruises to the head, particularly the right side of the skull. He underwent surgical debridement of the skin and a subtotal craniectomy. A CT scan revealed a subdural hemotoma, which was removed. Mack remained in an unresponsive state, and two months later a feeding gastrostomy was performed. After the craniectomy, Mack showed some response to light touch, verbal stimuli, and colored objects. Other problems that were evident were chronic infection of the right inner ear, a seizure disorder, spastic quadriplegia, right eye blindness, and partial right ear hearing loss. Retardation was believed to be in the profound range.

Three months after the accident, Mark entered a rehabilitation hospital where he remained for six weeks. Then followed a period of therapy at home. At the age of two years, he began attending the preschool program at Belle Harbor School for half days. When a sibling was born, Mack's parents placed him in residential care at the school. He now lives in a group home at Belle Harbor School and attends school full-time in a class for the multihandicapped.

Mack continued to have several physical impairment. His movement was limited to primitive reflex responses. There was overall muscle spasticity (tightness) that was greater on the right side. He had facial weakness on the lower right side and diminished right lip closure. After a time he no longer needed the gastrostomy tube for feeding and could eat soft foods. External jaw control was needed for cup drinking. His overall level of functioning was estimated at 7–8 months of age and his level of retardation was later thought to be in the severe to profound range (an decrease from the original estimate).

When assessed by the occupational therapist, Mack was found to be dependent in all areas of self-care. He could assist minimally in feeding by helping bring a spoon to his mouth. In dressing, he was almost totally dependent. He was unable to walk and required an adapted wheelchair with special supports to keep him properly positioned. Mack communicated his basic needs by crying, vocalizing, use of body language, and facial expressions. He was unable to manipulate objects, except for batting at objects with his left hand.

When performance components were analyzed, Mack was observed to be more severely limited on his right side. He was functioning at the brain stem level of reflex development and was dominated by primitive postural reflexes that controlled his movement. He could not perform isolated movements but moved in total body patterns. Total body extension was the dominant pattern seen, with his head, neck, and back arched backward. Another result of the accident was that Mack was blind and had a moderate hearing loss on the right side. He got most of his information about the external environment through touch and hearing. He enjoyed movement sensations such as rocking, swinging, and riding on the bus.

According to the psychological evaluation, Mack had a tested IQ of about 25. He was functioning in the severe-to-profound range of mental retardation. He was able to anticipate familiar events and to discriminate between familiar people. He had some awareness of bowel and bladder function, since he cried when soiled or wet. Mack enjoyed physical contact with his adult caretakers and peers. He was attentive toward familiar voices and would become quiet and turn toward a recognized voice. His grandparents became his only family contacts, and he occasionally went on overnight visits to their home. He was involved in recreational activities at his group home and particularly enjoyed swimming, rocking or swinging, and roughhousing with staff members. When content, Mack would lie quietly in a relaxed position.

Because of the severity of his handicaps, Mack required a number of pieces of adapted equipment. He now uses an adapted wheelchair for positioning and transportation that is equipped with trunk supports, a head support, adductor pads, footrests, and a tray. He uses a flexion side-lying device and a corner chair for positioning in his classroom. A supine stander is used both in school and at home to support him in an upright position. Mack wears ankle-foot or thoses (splints) on both feet to reduce muscle tone and to prevent contractures. He also uses a resting pan splint on his right hand because the hand is usually held in a fisted position. A built-up handled spoon is used to assist in hand-over-hand feeding, and various toys have been adapted so that they can be operated by only gross hand movement.

To prevent further limitations, range of motion exercises are performed three times a day. Various pieces of adapted equipment and positioning devices are used to inhibit Mack's high muscle tone and to position him properly. Relaxation methods are also used to reduce muscle tone. Other preventive measures include ongoing orthopedic consultation, nursing care, and nutritional and dietary monitoring.

The overall goals for Mack's school program are included in an Individual Education Plan that is written annually and revised three times during the year. The occupational therapy treatment plan is part of the Individual Education Plan and contains several objectives for this year. They include increasing his ability to communicate through vocalizing or facial expression, increasing his responses to external stimuli, maintaining the present range of motion in all of Mack's joints, increasing his tolerance for standing in the supine stander, improving his ability to drink liquids, and increasing his ability to feed himself finger foods.

To help Mack achieve the treatment objectives, a daily session with the COTA has been scheduled. She is responsible for carrying out activities recommended by the OTR for each objective listed. Behavior modification methods are being used to elicit greater communication, and a variety of sensory stimuli are presented to elicit responses from Mack. The COTA ranges all of Mack's joints daily so that their mobility will be maintained and positions Mack in the supine stander for increasing periods of time during the therapy sessions. The OTR works with the classroom aide who feeds Mack his meals so that consistent feeding and positioning methods are used, thus improving his ability to drink liquids and finger-feed. The COTA reports her results weekly to the OTR so that modifications in the program can be made if needed.

In addition to supervising individual therapy, the OTR consults with classroom teachers and aides to ensure consistent programming and carryover. She also monitors orthopedic and equipment needs. In consulting with the classroom staff, she instructs them on the use of equipment, positioning and handling techniques, lifting and carrying techniques, and methods for carrying out the occupational therapy objectives. She also frequently consults with Mack's parents and other related health professionals.

Mack's Individual Education Plan is reviewed monthly, and a full annual review is conducted by the entire treatment team. Progress is reviewed quarterly in the residence program. Since Mack's admission to the residential school program, he has shown improvement in head control, increased vocalizations, increased environmental awareness, successful prevention of deformities, and increased body awareness. Although the current objectives of his program are very basic, they may eventually lead to less total dependence in postural and movement abilities and the ability to assist with some self-care tasks. Occupational therapy in this case is concerned with avoiding further limitations, maintaining existing levels of ability, and building some basic physical and cognitive skills. Improving the quality of Mack's life is another consideration, because his handicaps will remain throughout his lifetime. Plans for Mack's future placement are not known, but he will continue to need supportive services all his life.

DISCUSSION QUESTIONS

1. More severely developmentally disabled individuals are surviving today because of medical advances and improvements in care. Their needs for a continuum of care throughout life place a heavy financial and social burden on society. Is it ethical to discontinue life support for multiply handicapped individuals if they or their families wish it? Who should make this decision?

2. As this chapter showed, the trend is toward services being located in the community rather than in institutional settings for developmentally disabled clients. Do you think Mack could be adequately cared for by community programs? If so, what kind of support ser-

vices would he be likely to require during his lifetime?

3. Is improving quality of life for a severely handicapped individual a realistic goal for occupational therapists and others involved in treatment programs for the developmentally disabled. Will insurance companies and social security coverage pay for such programs?

4. Take a look at your state's developmental disabilities plan. What priorities does it set for the care of developmentally disabled individuals? What services are available? Do they provide for a continuum of care throughout the lifetime of a client?

5. What facilities are available in your area for the aging developmentally disabled person? Are nursing home personnel given additional training for dealing with this population? Are there special housing facilities available?

6. Have you had any personal experiences with developmentally disabled individuals? Discuss these with your classmates. What are your feelings and reactions when trying to communicate and relate to a severely handicapped person?

7. Largely in response to the demands of families for improved services, the federal government has established more adequate facilities and services than existed prior to the 1960s. In the light of increasing cost-containment efforts in medical care, can we continue to afford the amounts we are spending on programs for the developmentally disabled? Should the federal government continue its involvement in this aspect of health care?

REFERENCES

1. Summers J: The definition of developmental disabilities: a concept in transition. *Ment Retard* 19:259–265, 1981.

2. Moersch M: Developmental disabilities. *AJOT* 33:93–99, 1978.
3. Hightower-Van Damm M: Nationally speaking: developmental disabilities act: an historic perspective. Part I. *AJOT* 33:355–359, 1979.
4. Baldwin S: Models of service delivery: an assessment of some applications and implications for people who are mentally retarded. *Ment Retard* 23:6–12, 1985.
5. Landesman S, Butterfield E: Normalization and deinstitutionalization of mentally retarded individuals: controversy and facts *Am Psychol* In press.
6. Janicki M, Ackerman L, Jacobson J: State developmental disabilities/aging plans and planning for an older developmentally disabled population. *Ment Retard* 23:297–301, 1985.
7. Bates M: S-2053: shifting the D D funding focus. In *The Blueprint*. Madison, WI, Wisconsin Council on Developmental Diabilities, 1984, p 1–3.
8. Steck J: *PT21, Chicago Regional State Letter No. 2-85: Clarification of Developmental Needs as Related to Mentally Retarded Individuals.* Region V, Health Care Financing Administration, US Departmentof Health and Social Services, 1985.
9. American Occupational Therapy Association. Developmental disabilities: implications the confusion in their definition may have for O.T. practice. *Developmental Disabilities Special Interest Section Newsletter* 5(2):3, 1982.
10. American Occupational Therapy Association. Readers' response to "developmental disabili-

ties: implications. . ." *Developmental Disabilities Special Interest Section Newsletter* 6(2):3, 1983.
11. Creighton C: Work-related programs: an overview. *Developmental Disabilities Special Interest Section Newsletter* 8(1):1–2, 1985.
12. Emshoff M: Adapted vocational program for severely handicapped adults. *Developmental Disabilities Special Interest Section Newsletter* 8(1): 3–4, 1985.
13. Gordon R: Use of technical aids in occupational therapy treatment. *Developmental Disabilities Special Interest Section Newsletter* 7(1):1–4, 1984.

SUGGESTED READINGS

Amary IB: *The Rights of the Mentally Retarded-Developmentally Disabled to Treatment and Education.* Springfield, IL, Charles C Thomas, 1980.
Cohen H: Trends in service delivery and treatment of the mentally retarded. *Pediatr Ann* 11:458–469, 1982.
Gibson D, Brown RI: *Managing the Severely Retarded.* Springfield, IL, Charles C Thomas, 1976.
Koch R, Koch KJ: *Understanding the Mentally Retarded Child.* New York, Random House, 1974.
Schulman ED: *Focus on the Retarded Adult: Programs and Services.* St. Louis, CV Mosby, 1980.

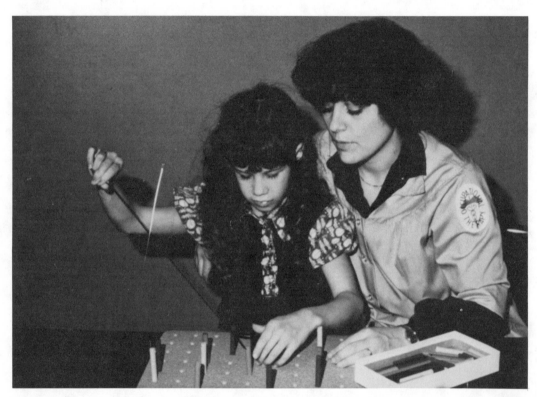

THIRTEEN

Practice in Public Schools

One of the most dramatic changes in occupational therapy practice in recent years has been the rapid growth of services in public and private schools. The 1985 AOTA Manpower Report showed that schools are now the second most common employment setting for OTRs and the third for COTAs (1). Occupational therapists had long worked in schools for handicapped children, but the impetus for increased services in schools came from two pieces of federal legislation. The Education of All Handicapped Children Act of 1975 (Public Law 94-142) and Section 504 of the Rehabilitation Act of 1973 permanently changed the kind of education and services available to handicapped children in the United States.

PROVISIONS OF LEGISLATION

By the early 1970s some states had already passed legislation requiring free public education for all handicapped children, but many states still refused to accept some types of handicapped children in special education classrooms. Those with the most severe handicaps were frequently excluded. In an effort to establish a uni-form national standard, Public Law 94-142 guaranteed a free public education to all children, regardless of type or severity of handicap, and required that the effectiveness of educational programs for handicapped children be monitored. Among the provisions of this law was the inclusion of occupational therapy as one of the related services that might be required to enable a handicapped child to benefit from special education. Occupational therapy was described as "services directed at improving, developing, or restoring functions impaired or lost through illness, injury, or deprivation; improving ability to perform tasks for independent functioning when functions are impaired or lost; and preventing, through early intervention, initial or further impairment or loss of function" (2). The legislation applied to children from 3 to 21 years of age, although states were only required to provide special education to children from 3 to 5 years and from 18 to 21 years if educational programs were offered to nonhandicapped children in the same age groups. [In 1986 amendments to the law were added that required all states to provide education and related services to children from 3 to 5 years if receiving federal funds (3). The term *handicapped children* referred to those who were mentally retarded, hard of hearing, deaf, speech impaired, visually handicapped, seriously emotionally disturbed, orthopedically impaired, deaf-blind, multihandicapped, or who had specific learning disabilities or other health impairments. The legislation specifically protected the rights of children and their parents, and parental approval and consent was required for implementation of a school's educational plan for a child (2). This legislation revolutionized the way services were provided to handicapped children and made the school the major site of service delivery. Occupational therapy, along with other related services, was integrated into the educational program for handicapped children and became a part of their total educational experience.

Another law, Section 504 of the Rehabilitation Act of 1973, prohibited discrimination against handicapped persons in any programs that received federal funds and mandated that handicapped children be educated in the least restrictive environment possible for each individual. This meant that handicapped children did not all need to remain in segregated classrooms. Those who could participate in regular educational activities for all or some instruction were to be mainstreamed into the regular educational program. Schools were required to provide learning environments that were accessible to handicapped students and that contained facilities for instruction that were equal to those provided for "normal" children (4).

As a related service, occupational therapy can only be provided to children who have been identified as handicapped under the provisions of Public Law 94-142 and who are in need of special education. Thus occupational therapy programs are ancillary to a child's educational program and are intended to help the child develop the skills that are necessary for academic learning and vocational training. The occupational therapist or therapy assistant employed in a school works as a member of an interdisciplinary educational team and must learn to communicate and work collaboratively with teachers, school administrators, psychologists, speech and language therapists, physical therapists, counselors, and classroom aides.

MEDICAL MODEL VERSUS EDUCATIONAL MODEL

Stephens (5) and Ottenbacher (6) have pointed out that occupational therapy personnel are usually educated in the medical model. This may make for some conflicts and misunderstandings when they practice within the educational system, because the models of practice are quite different. The medical model focuses on identification of disease or dysfunction and develops strategies to intervene in the disease process or to reduce dysfunction. The educational model is concerned with normal growth and development and with helping children achieve mastery of the skills needed to function in society. Teachers and therapists may view the needs of a child differently because of these variations in philosophy and goals. Table 13.1 illustrates some of the differences between educational and medical settings (5). Ottenbacher believes that these differences in philosophy and practice can be minimized if therapists and educators can put aside their biases and differences in perspective. He suggests that therapists merge their goals with those of educators and develop cooperative and mutually supportive relationships with them. Because occupational therapy has found the medical model limiting, the educational model may offer additional opportunities for the occupational therapist to become fully involved in the daily needs of handicapped students (6).

Table 13.1.
Comparison of Medical and Educational Systems[a]

	Hospital	School
Function	Saving lives, caring for the sick, curing or healing the injured	Instruction and development, preparation of life
Type of system	Relatively closed; must have credentials to participate; restricted areas; may be located at a distance from consumer; must pay fee or make appointment to enter	Relatively open; public has general knowledge and experience; building open to all; part of community; records accessible; parents and others urged to participate
Contact with system	Intermittent; contact when problem arises; consumer chooses when and where to enter system	Constant; continues through age 16 + ; admittance and attendance required by law
Barriers to consumer provider interaction	Medical mystique; lack of understanding of terminology, clothing (nametags, uniforms, patient's gowns); inaccessible records; accessible only through receptionist or answering service	Teachers' lounge; teachers' dining area
Delivery of services	Cooperative team headed by physician; consumer usually not part of team	Individual professionals or collaborative and consensual decision making by team; consumer (parent) is team member
Administration	Appointed board members (prestigious citizens); board meetings usually closed with little consumer input	Board members elected by public (members of community); board meetings open with frequent consumer input
Funding	Private pay; insurance; federal funds; grants; taxes; fee for service; salaries usually not public	Property taxes, state and federal funds; indirect pay for service; salaries public knowledge

[a]Reproduced by permission from Clark P, Allen A: *Occupational Therapy for Children*. St. Louis, 1985, The C. V. Mosby Co., p. 474.

OCCUPATIONAL THERAPY PROCESS IN SCHOOLS

The occupational therapy process follows many of the same steps in school settings that it does in medical settings. The differences center around specific procedures that are mandated by Public Law 94-142. Children are not eligible for occupational therapy or other related services unless they have been judged to need special education. The assessment of a child's educational needs is the first step in service delivery in schools. The occupational therapist may or may not be a part of the initial referral/assessment process.

According to Rourk and her colleagues (7), two types of screening occur in the educational setting. The first is type 1 screening, in which high-risk children are identified who may need special education. An example of type 1 screening is the routine prekindergarten assessment that is conducted to determine readiness for entry into kindergarten. A child who is found to have visual problems, motor impairment, or a hearing loss during this initial screening is referred for a more complete assessment. The in-depth assessment is type 2 screening and is conducted by a multidisciplinary team. The occupational therapist and other related service personnel may be asked to evaluate the child and contribute data to this more detailed assessment. The child's family may also be asked to contribute information. When all of the relevant data have been collected, the multidisciplinary team meets to analyze findings and determine the child's total educational needs. If the child has a need for special education, the team prepares an individualized educational program (IEP), which outlines the child's present level of function, sets annual goals and short-term objectives, identifies the special education and related services that need to be provided, establishes the date for starting service, estimates how long services are expected to continue, and sets the criteria for measuring the achievement of goals and objectives. The IEP becomes the blueprint for the child's educational program for the school year. If occupational therapy is recommended as a related service, the child is referred to the OTR attached to the school program. A physician's referral for occupational therapy services in schools is needed in some states, and the therapist is responsible for following whatever referral procedures are required by the state and by local education agencies.

An occupational therapy intervention plan is then developed, but the objectives in this plan must relate to the overall IEP objectives. The occupational therapy plan includes short-term objectives, strategies to be used to achieve the objectives, relevant treatment concepts, a statement of how frequently the child will be treated and for how long, and a statement of the predicted outcome. The COTA may assist in developing the intervention plan. The plan is then initiated and results are regularly assessed. Implementation is the responsibility of the OTR, but some intervention activities may be delegated to the COTA, the classroom teacher or aide, the family, or a combination of these individuals. Changes that are seen in the child's abilities must be documented objectively. Each child's IEP is reviewed annually, and a comprehensive assessment by the multidisciplinary team is required at least every three years.

MODES OF SERVICE DELIVERY

Occupational therapists and therapy assistants work in school settings in three major ways. 1) In *direct service delivery*, therapists or assistants carry out occupational therapy interventions with children on a regular basis. Children may receive occupational therapy either individually or in small groups. Some problems may require one-to-one intervention and this is built into the child's daily or weekly schedule. Other therapy interventions may be scheduled in small groups to work on similar objectives. This method has the advantage of saving time for the OTR or COTA and is comparable to groupings used for classroom instruction.

2) The OTR may *monitor* therapy programs being carried out by others. In this type of service delivery the OTR directly supervises nonoccupational therapy personnel who implement all or part of the therapy program. The therapist is responsible for teaching correct procedures to the assistants, maintaining regular contact with the assistants to ensure proper implementation of the program, and reassessing to determine whether adequate progress is being made or whether adjustments are needed in the program.

3) Through *consultation* the OTR may offer services to classroom teachers, families, and colleagues in the school setting. The occupational therapist may be able to offer expertise to the school system as a whole when new programs are being planned or system-wide changes are being considered.

UNIQUE FEATURES OF SCHOOL PRACTICE

Caseloads (the number of clients seen by an individual therapist or therapy assistant) vary considerably in school settings, depending on factors such as the type of service delivery pattern that is being used, the type and severity of students' handicapping conditions, and the amount of support staff available. Many occupational therapists serve more than one school and function on an itinerant basis, traveling from school to school. In this situation the geographic area to be covered and the amount of travel time needed must also be considered in determining caseload.

In school practice some times of the school year are more demanding than others. At the beginning of the year, more time is spent in IEP meetings, in assessing the needs of children, and in initial documentation. At the close of the year, time is needed for annual reassessment of student IEPs and for making placement plans for the following year. Paperwork is a necessary evil in school practice, just as in medical settings, although it takes different forms. Therapists may also need to set aside time for consultation with families, home visits, and team meetings.

The OTR and COTA may conduct occupational therapy treatment activities in self-contained clinic areas or they may implement their therapeutic programs in the child's classroom. Although the site of therapy may vary from one school to another, the occupational therapist is frequently called on to advise classroom teachers and families about special equipment that may be needed to position the child optimally and to help the child perform academic work. Adapted equipment needs are assessed along with the rest of the child's needs and special equipment is ordered or constructed as required.

Unlike medical settings, occupational therapy personnel who work in schools usually do not have a departmental structure in which to operate. Because they are part of the total educational program, they are individually assigned to schools or classroom units and are supervised by a school administrator. In some situations this can make therapists feel professionally isolated from their peers, and it is important that therapists develop a system of colleague communication and support to prevent loss of professional identity and peer interaction. Some states require school occupational therapy personnel to hold teacher certification or cert-

ification as a school therapist in addition to their professional certification or licensure.

OTR AND COTA ROLES

The American Occupational Therapy Association has identified the following roles of occupational therapists in school settings (8):

---

1. Evaluating students with suspected educational handicaps to specify the need for and goals of an occupational therapy intervention program;
2. Participating in educational program planning for individual students to coordinate occupational therapy goals and program plans with the total educational program;
3. Implementing an intervention program to facilitate an individual's optimum functioning and enhance the student's ability to learn and develop;
4. Consulting with school personnel and parents regarding services provided by occupational therapy; and
5. Managing and supervising school-based occupational therapy programs.

In school-based occupational therapy programs, COTAs are an important part of the team. In many cases they provide the day-to-day implementation of the intervention plan developed by the OTR, releasing the OTR for more involvement in consultation, program planning, and assessment of student needs. Walker (9) has provided an example of how the service roles were divided in an Oregon school system. In this program the OTR was responsible for developing the policies and procedures for service delivery, determining student eligibility for occupational therapy services, communicating with physicians, writing reports, designing adapted equipment, determining the need for changes in student programs, and supervising COTAs. The COTAs' responsibilities included maintaining an inventory of supplies and equipment, fabricating pieces of adapted equipment, ordering supplies, recording services performed, and providing guides for recreational and community resources. In this school program the COTAs trained students in activities of daily living and conducted treatment activities to improve motor functions and sensory integration.

A role that is gaining acceptance with school occupational therapists is that of increasing involvement in vocational education for handicapped students. Creighton (10) notes that the occupational therapist's skill in task analysis is an ideal qualification for analyzing the vocational tasks for which handicapped workers will be trained. The OTR is particularly well-equipped to assess a handicapped student's physical skills and job-related behaviors and help to match students with suitable job placements. The occupational therapist, says Creighton, may be the only member of the educational team who understands the principles and methods of adapting equipment and simplifying work tasks. These skills are directly relevant to vocational training. Creighton suggests that school occupational therapists become more active in vocational education, where they can put these skills to use with handicapped students who are in vocational education programs.

RURAL-URBAN DIFFERENCES

Regan (11) has described some of the differences between rural school systems and those in urban areas. She notes that rural communities are often more conservative and hold more traditional values toward schools and educational services. These communities may be less likely to see the need for an array of related services for handicapped children in local schools

and may need to be educated as to the value of such services. Regan suggests that occupational therapists and other health care workers immerse themselves in the local community and take the time to learn about its standards and values before implementing a new program. These efforts may help to gain community support and acceptance for programs that initially may be viewed as unnecessary.

EMPLOYMENT PATTERNS

Employment patterns are somewhat different in school systems than in traditional medical settings. School therapists are usually employed on the basis of an annual contract with the school system. Employment may be on a 9- or 10-month basis rather than for a full 12-months. Salaries for school-employed therapists tend to be comparable to those of beginning teachers in the school system. In many school districts, teachers and other educational personnel are unionized, and salary, working conditions, and fringe benefits are settled through collective bargaining. Salary increases may depend on earning additional college credits and years of experience as well as satisfactory job performance. An educational administrator rather than a supervising OTR evaluates the job performance of OTRs and COTAs. There is often no direct method by which an OTR or COTA may be promoted to higher responsibilities within the school setting. Administrative functions are usually carried out by persons with an education background, and it is rare to find an occupational therapist in an administrative position in a school system.

FUTURE TRENDS

Schools will continue to be a prime employer of OTRs and COTAs. In 1985 more than four million handicapped children were served under the programs mandated by Public Law 94-142 and its amendments. Today 93% of all children with disabilities receive special education and related services (12). More school-based practitioners will be needed, because the school population is again increasing and a corresponding increase in the number of handicapped children is anticipated (1). The school setting offers a multitude of opportunities to the OTR and the COTA to directly contribute to the education and development of handicapped children. This practice area is the most rapidly growing area in occupational therapy, and schools may become the most common employment site for occupational therapy personnel in the future.

CASE STUDY: CEREBRAL PALSY

To illustrate what occupational therapy contributes in public school programs, let's consider the case of Erin. Erin is 4 years 7 months of age and is enrolled in a preschool program for hearing-impaired children. Her diagnosis is cerebral palsy, athetoid type, and is moderate to severe in degree. She has a 50% hearing loss in both ears that is corrected to 30% with hearing aids. Erin has an extensive history of medical problems.

She was born prematurely at 32–34 weeks gestation and weighed only 3 pounds 4 ounces. At birth she was found to have severe hyaline membrane disease, a respiratory disorder in which there is inadequate development of the lungs. Erin had also suffered a ventricular hemorrhage that resulted in hydrocephalus; a mechanical shunt was installed to ensure circulation of cerebrospinal fluid. Erin's history also includes episodes of pneumonia, spinal meningitis, and a number of chronic ear infections. Despite these problems, Erin appears to have normal intelligence and is an outgoing, well-adjusted child.

In Erin's state, children are eligible for special education services at the age of 3

years. Erin entered the preschool program at that age and will continue to be eligible for school services until the age of 21. Her current educational program focuses on language development, learning total communication (the use of both signed language and speech), and the development of self-help skills.

When initial screening showed that Erin was likely to need special education services, she was referred for a type 2 screening by a multidisciplinary team. Her problem areas were identified, and the team developed an individualized educational program that established annual goals and short-term objectives. Among the related services that were recommended for Erin were physical and occupational therapy. Because Erin lives in a state that requires a physician's referral for both services, this was obtained and must be renewed annually for services to be continued.

The assessment conducted by the multidisciplinary team revealed several areas of dysfunction that occupational therapy could address. Erin had fluctuating muscle tone, causing her movement patterns to be uncoordinated and unreliable. She tended to appear floppy, with overly flexible joints. When she reached for a toy she had difficulty holding her head and trunk steady to allow her to reach accurately and smoothly. Sometimes her muscles tightened, contributing to her incoordination. She had excessive range of motion in her elbows, wrists, and fingers. Coordination was a major problem for Erin. The more demanding a fine-motor task was, the more difficult it was for her to perform. For example, she could manage to get her coat on but could not manipulate buttons or use a zipper.

Erin was strongly motivated to master developmental tasks. Her normal level of intelligence promoted a strong desire for independence, and she had been known to give helpful adults a swat when they offered to help her with a task she would prefer to do alone. She fell frequently while walking, but this did not discourage her. The OTR made knee pads for her to wear to protect her sensitive joints. Erin enjoyed her preschool program and tried hard to keep up with the other children. Although all were hearing-impaired, none had movement problems as severe as Erin's.

Erin's family was warm and supportive and offered her many opportunities for independence in her daily routine. They gave her extra time to dress in the morning and overlooked spills at the dining table so that her independence in everyday tasks would be encouraged.

The occupational therapy intervention plan for Erin focused on helping her to develop self-care skills, on providing environmental adaptations to enable her to function at school and at home, and on improving her physical stability while working toward coordinated movement. The following short-term occupational therapy objectives addressed tasks that Erin needed to be able to do at home and at school:

1. Erin will be able to hold her head steady in a midline position while reaching for objects on her desk in two out of three attempts.
2. Erin will be able to put on her shoes independently and close the Velcro fasteners within a 10-minute period 80% of the time.
3. During counting activities in her classroom, Erin will be able to grasp half-inch thick plastic "coins" and place five "coins" in a slotted bank in four out of five trials.
4. Erin will be able to use the toilet independently at school 100% of the time with the aid of grab bars on each side of the toilet stall.
5. Erin will be able to perform the finger movements needed for at least five basic signs to indicate her needs in the classroom.

A COTA was assigned to see Erin for daily occupational therapy sessions. The OTR conferred with Erin's classroom teacher and parents to discuss therapy objectives and suggest related activities that could be carried out in the classroom and at home. During the daily treatment sessions the COTA used a variety of activities (most of them in the form of play) to help Erin achieve her objectives. A therapy session might involve a game of "push me over, push you over" or "ride the wild therapy horse" (a suspended bolster) to help Erin develop better ability to stablize her neck and truck during movement. Sometimes the COTA and Erin would play "hanging out the wash," with Erin hanging weights on a line with clothespins, or have "turtle races" down the hall. (The "turtle" is a riding toy powered by arm movement, which required Erin to contract her shoulders and rotate her trunk to make it go.) On other days the COTA and Erin played dress-up games to work on dressing skills. Sometimes Erin was allowed to make a Cheerios necklace that she could later eat as a reward for good work. In all of these activities, the goal was to help Erin develop adequate body stability so she could move more easily from a fixed position. Later the emphasis would move to better fine-motor coordination.

While the COTA worked directly with Erin, the OTR recommended the following environmental adaptations that would make classroom participation easier for Erin:

1. Installation of plastic pipe grab bars in the toilet stall so that Erin would have enough stability to safely use the toilet by herself.
2. Use of a cut-out table with raised edges. This allowed Erin to rest her arms on the table while using her hands and prevented objects from falling off the table when knocked about by Erin's flailing arms.
3. Use of a prone stander for some classroom activities and in therapy sessions. This piece of equipment allowed Erin to stand in a supported position and helped her develop stability around her weight-bearing joints.
4. Use of a well-fitting and supportive

chair with a footrest during classroom activities. This provided better stability for Erin while seated and allowed her to participate more easily in tabletop activities.

Erin has been seen in occupational therapy for two years and has carried over her therapy activities in the classroom and at home. She has made considerable gains in several areas of function. The most notable has been her increasing independence in self-care and her developing communication skills. Her use of signing and the number and quality of signs used has increased considerably. Self-help and fine-motor tasks are now achieved in less time and with greater ease. Her improved body stability is reflected in improved gait while walking and in an overall improvement in posture and movement skills.

The occupational therapy program directly contributed to Erin's performance in the classroom and at home. Because her teachers and parents assisted with the therapeutic program gains occurred faster and with greater consistency than if Erin had only been seen by the COTA. Although long-term predictions cannot be made, her therapist and teachers expect that Erin will be able to master most educational tasks and should be able to lead a productive adult life.

DISCUSSION QUESTIONS

1. How does your local school district provide occupational therapy services to children such as Erin? At what ages are children eligible for services?

2. Discuss some of the differences in occupational therapy roles and functions in medical settings and in schools. Are different outcomes emphasized in the two settings?

3. Does your state require any special certification for OTRs and COTAs who work in public schools? If so, what are the requirements for certification?

4. What kinds of programs are available in your area for handicapped persons beyond the age of school eligibility who have a need for further training or sheltered work?

5. Discuss the concept of mainstreaming for handicapped children. What are some of the advantages and disadvantages of this approach?

REFERENCES

1. Ad Hoc Commission on Occupational Therapy Manpower: *Occupational Therapy Manpower: A Plan for Progress.* Rockville, MD, American Occupational Therapy Association, 1985, pp 6–7, 55–59.
2. Government and Legal Affairs Division. American Occupational Therapy Association. Final regulations, PL 94-142, Education of All Handicapped Children Act. *Federal Report* 77-5:3–17, 1977.
3. DeBello L: New law provides occupational therapy for preschoolers. *Occup Ther News* 40(12): 6, 1986.
4. Nondiscrimination on basis of handicap: programs and activities receiving or benefiting from federal financial assistance. *Federal Regulations* 42:86, 1977.
5. Stephens L: Occupational therapy in the school system. In Clark P, Allen A (eds): *Occupational Therapy for Children.* St. Louis, CV Mosby, 1985, pp. 471–489.
6. Ottenbacher K: Occupational therapy and special education: some issues and concerns related to Public Law 94–142. *AJOT* 36:81–84, 1982.
7. Rourk J, Andrews J, Dunn W, Stephens L, Wendt G: *Guidelines for Occupational Therapy Services in Schools.* Rockville, MD, American Occupational Therapy Association, 1986, pp. 12–23.
8. Gilfoyle E: The role of occupational therapy as an education-related service. *AJOT* 35:811, 1981.
9. Walker N: COTA and OTR treatment team in schools. *Occup Ther News* 38(10):6, 1984.
10. Creighton C: The school therapist and vocational education. *AJOT* 33:373–375, 1979.
11. Reagan N: Implementation of occupational therapy services in rural school systems. *AJOT* 365:85–89, 1982.

12. Tenth anniversary of handicapped children education act recognized. *Occup Ther News* 40(4): 1–2, 1986.

SUGGESTED READINGS

Ayres A: *Sensory Integration and the Child.* Los Angeles, CA, Western Pyschological Services, 1979.

Banus B, Kent C, Norton Y, Sukiennicki D, Becker M: *The Developmental Therapist*, ed 2. Thorofare, NJ, Slack, 1979.

Clark P, Allen A: *Occupational Therapy for Children.* St. Louis, MO, CV Mosby, 1985.

Cruikshank W (ed): *Cerebral Palsy: Its Individual and Community Problems*, ed 2. Syracuse, NY, Syracuse University Press, 1966.

Gilfoyle E, Grady A, Moore J: *Children Adapt.* Thorofare, NJ, Slack, 1982.

Reilly M (ed): *Play as Exploratory Learning.* Beverley Hills, CA, Sage Publications, 1974

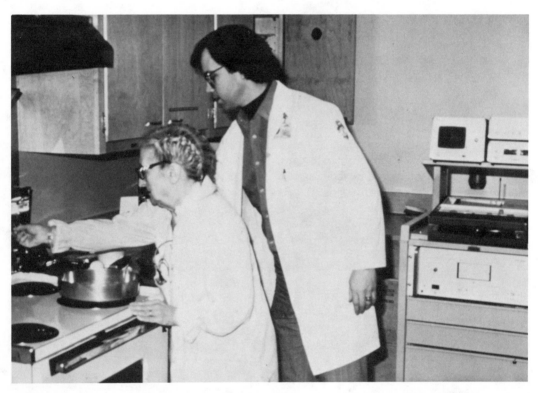

Courtesy AOTA

FOURTEEN

Practice with Elderly Populations

Old age is not a disease, but older people in our society are often viewed in terms of diminished physical capacity, mental competency, and status. The general public tends to have some fixed beliefs about aging that often influence public policies relating to care of the elderly. How accurate are your ideas about the elderly population of the United States? Take the following quiz to find out.

T F 1. The human body begins to physically deteriorate at an average age of 62 years.

T F 2. For most older people, old age is a period of tranquility and satisfaction.

T F 3. The current figure of 2.6 million people over the age of 65 in the United States is expected to remain relatively stable over the next 25 years.

T F 4. Florida has the largest population of people over the age of 65 of any state in the union.

T F 5. Twenty-five percent of the over-65 population live in institutional settings.

T F 6. Old people are unable to change or learn new things.

T F 7. Old people are unproductive and a burden on society.

T F 8. Most people over the age of 80 are senile.

T F 9. Old people prefer to live with others of their own age so that they can have peace and quiet.

T F 10. Most older people have adequate financial resources to provide for themselves in their old age.

If you marked all of the above statements false, you have a better than average awareness of aging and the elderly population. Each statement in the quiz represents a common myth about aging. Now let's look at the facts.

WHO ARE THE ELDERLY?

Medical science shows no evidence that physical decline is directly related to chronological age. People age at different rates. Major illnesses or injuries can severely damage the body at any age. The aging process is individual, although conditions such as poverty and life-style can influence one's physical and mental health (1).

Although old age is idealized as a period of peace and contentment, it is a highly stressful time of life for many people. Loss of family and close friends, financial crises, and the cumulative effects of chronic diseases can cause great anxiety in elderly people. Our image of the happy cookie-baking grandma and the contented grandpa in his rocking chair is largely mythical (1,2).

The population of people over the age of 65 is rapidly increasing in the United States. The number of people in this age group doubled from 1950 to 1980, and government agencies estimate that by the year 2030 there will be 55 million people in this age range. In addition, the population of "old" old people (those over 80 years of age) will have increased 900% by the end of the century. This does not mean that the average life expectancy at birth has increased. It remains at about 67 years for males and 74 years for females. There is an increased number of elderly persons because of improved nutrition and better medical care. In most societies women outlive men. In the United States in 1980 there were about 147 women aged 65 and older for every 100 men in the same age range. There will be a need for more personnel to staff services and facilities for the over-65 population in the future (2–5).

Although Sunbelt states are popular locations for retired people to live, sizable concentrations of retirees live in the Midwest and in upper New England. New York State has the largest over-65 population. Many older people are willing to accept cold winters and greater population densities rather than leave their families and friends for a more congenial climate in their last years. The large majority of older people continue to live in their own homes. Only 5% of the over-65 population are institutionalized, and 20% of this group are aged 85 or older. Nursing home care is usually necessary because of two factors: 1) chronic disease that substantially impairs function and 2) lack of community support services that would enable the elderly person to remain at home. Most older people, however, are able to live at home with a spouse, family, or friends. About 80% remain independent in all daily living activities; approximately 15% have some degree of physical or mental impairment (1,2,5).

The myth that older people are set in their ways and unable to adapt to new demands has not been confirmed by research. Studies show that the ability to adapt to changing situations is more closely related to the adult personality or character than to the aging process. Some older people may become more conservative in their views, but this is often related to the socioeconomic pressures that they are under. It is difficult to vote for a new swimming pool in the local school when one is on a fixed income and is already having trouble paying one's property taxes. The ability to learn and be creative is present in the aged, just as it is in other age groups. Those people who were creative in their youth usually remain so in old age. Older people tend to maintain their interests and even expand them given opportunities to do so (1).

Rather than being unproductive members of society, many older people make substantial contributions to their communities. Approximately 14% of the over-65 population is still employed in the work force. Butler and Lewis (1) state that of the total population of older people, 33% of their income comes from employment, 45% from pensions that they earned during their working years, and 15% from savings. Only 5% of their total collective income is derived from public assistance programs. Many of those who retire from paid employment after age 65 take an active role in volunteer programs and contribute time and energy to community activities. As a whole, the elderly population continues to be productive and makes solid contributions to society. (Local and regional agencies could, however, learn to use the talents of the elderly population more effectively.) About 14% of all older people live below the poverty level. This is particularly true for women and minority groups (1,3).

The conditions formerly referred to as "senility" are now considered to be various types of organic brain disorders. Fifteen percent of people in the 65–75 age group and 25% of those 75 years and older show disturbances that are due to organic brain disorders. Organic brain syndromes may be either acute (reversible) or chronic. The two most common diagnoses are chronic brain syndrome and cerebral arteriosclerosis. Some of the mental confusion and disorganization seen in elderly persons may be influenced by medication, disorienting environmental conditions, and physical disorders. Organic brain syndromes are not common conditions, however, and they occur in only a small proportion of elderly people (1).

Although some retired people choose to live in retirement communities, many others prefer to remain in their own neighborhoods and enjoy being part of the mainstream of their community life. Often, however, when one spouse dies the surviving spouse may be unable to afford to maintain the family home and may be forced to move to age-segregated housing. In 1986 real estate developers conducted surveys to determine what type of housing was preferred by elderly people who could afford a choice of housing options. They found that the majority wished to remain in their own homes, adding improvements to accommodate physical limitations if needed. The greatest demand for retire-

ment housing was in midwest and east coast communities where large populations of older people had family and friends. Because some elderly people are poor they may be forced to live in substandard housing (1,2,6).

People who have been poor all their lives are likely to become even poorer in their old age, and many who have held their own financially until retirement become poor in the postretirement years. The money that is available must go for the essentials of living: food, shelter, and medical expenses. Contrary to popular opinion, Medicare does not cover all the costs of medical care to the elderly. Only about 42% of the health expenses of older people are paid for by Medicare. The rest must be paid by private insurance or personal income. Hearing aids, glasses, dental care, and many other health care items are not covered under Medicare reimbursement. The financing of long-term medical care for older people is a critical issue in health care today that has not been resolved (1,4,5).

BODIES OF KNOWLEDGE IN GERONTOLOGY

The postretirement period of life is a phase of human development, and like other developmental periods it has its own developmental tasks. Occupational therapists and therapy assistants who work with the elderly must be familiar with theories of development that help to explain the maturational process and how individuals adapt to changing life circumstances. Piaget's theory of cognitive development, Erikson's theory of psychosocial development, Kohlberg's theory of moral development, and Maslow's theory of a hierarchy of human needs have contributed to our understanding of adult development and aging. A second body of knowledge that is critical to personnel who work with older people is a set of theories that helps explain the aging process. Many theories have been proposed to help explain the physical and psychological changes that occur during aging. Biological theories attempt to show how aging occurs on the cellular level. Psychological theories help to explain behavioral changes in older individuals. Practitioners working with elderly populations must have a working knowledge of these theoretical constructs to understand their clients' behaviors and abilities (2).

GOALS OF OCCUPATIONAL THERAPY WITH THE ELDERLY

Because the older person is likely to have multiple physical or psychological disorders, it is particularly important that a holistic approach be taken in treatment. The gerontic occupational therapist must be able to deal with independent living needs, physical limitations, cognitive changes, and psychological adjustment. The three diseases that are seen most frequently in the elderly are 1) cerebral vascular disease, 2) arthritis, and 3) Parkinson's disease. These conditions are chronic, and, in the case of Parkinson's disease, progressive. The occupational therapist and therapy assistant will need to carefully assess the elderly client's status in all three functional areas. Care must be taken to consider any secondary conditions that may affect the client's total function; prevention of further disability is an additional consideration. Just as with other age groups, the therapist or therapy assistant should encourage the client to help with the identification of personal goals and priorities so that the treatment program can be individually tailored to the client's needs.

In the elderly client, many of the goals of therapy center on improving cognitive awareness and psychological adjustment.

For clients who have been institutionalized for a period of time, mental confusion and disorientation may be a problem. Therapeutic programs that help the client maintain contact with reality are often helpful. *Reality orientation* provides a structured method of improving cognitive awareness in clients. *Remotivation groups* are aimed at helping clients become more interested in their immediate surroundings and in encouraging them to share their past experiences. *Life review groups* offer opportunities for elderly clients to reminisce about their life, review unresolved conflicts, and integrate their experiences into an acceptance of their life as it draws to a close.

Physical needs are another focus of occupational therapy intervention. Physical fitness is a concern of people of all ages, and the elderly, although subject to some physical limitations, can continue to benefit from mild exercise. *Exercise groups* help clients to maintain joint range of motion and general flexibility as well as provide some social stimulation. Clients who have major physical dysfunctions may need a rehabilitation program to restore as much function as possible and to help compensate for physical limitations. Most older clients will show some degree of sensory loss. Low vision may necessitate the use of magnifiers for reading, large-print reading materials, special lighting, and other environmental adaptations. Hearing loss may prevent some elderly clients from participating fully in social activities and may contribute to the development of paranoid behavior, depression, and social isolation. Telephone amplifiers, use of a hearing aid if feasible, and use of special methods when communicating with hard-of-hearing clients may make it possible to communicate more effectively. Programs of sensory stimulation are sometimes used with elderly clients to maintain their perceptual skills and increase their awareness of internal and external sensory cues. Some elderly persons may be aphasic (language-impaired) as a result of a stroke. These clients will have difficulty understanding spoken or written language and may also have trouble expressing themselves. A multidisciplinary treatment approach can be designed to help clients relearn appropriate language patterns and develop functional communication with those around them.

Daily living skills are an important area of occupational therapy intervention. The occupational therapist or therapy assistant is the most relevant member of the treatment team to assist the elderly client who is having trouble performing the ordinary tasks of daily life. Occupational therapy treatment in this realm may include teaching grooming and dressing techniques, working on feeding skills, teaching the client to transfer safely from wheelchair to toilet or chair, working on bathing and daily hygiene needs, helping the client to master cooking and meal planning, teaching work simplification techniques to relieve stress on joints and to avoid fatigue, and helping the client to develop or maintain avocational interests (2).

PRACTICE SITES

When we think of care of the elderly our first thought is usually of nursing homes. Although only a small proportion of older people need skilled nursing care, there will always be some who require the comprehensive services and protective environment of a skilled nursing facility. Ellis (5) predicts that the need for such facilities will increase as more and more Americans live to advanced ages. The long-term residential care facility is the most restrictive living environment for the elderly, but it can provide programs designed to meet the elderly client's needs for personal safety, healthy nutrition,

environmental comfort and security, and curative or palliative treatment. Ellis proposes greater use of work-oriented activities for nursing home residents and an increased focus on maximum use of residents' abilities in work, leisure, and self-care tasks. Frequently COTAs are employed in long-term care facilities as activity directors. Activity programs help to promote and maintain the physical and psychological health of residents and offer social opportunities for groups of clients. Rehabilitative services can be provided through the addition of a registered occupational therapist. The OTR often provides services to skilled nursing facilities on a contract (private practice) basis and is called in when a resident is found to need occupational therapy treatment services (7).

More and more, occupational therapy services to the elderly are being provided through community agencies rather than in institutional settings. Such programs include day hospitals, adult day-care centers, community mental health centers, programs to prevent institutionalization, visiting nurse services, and home health agencies. The focus of these programs varies with their clientele, the nature and severity of a client's functional limitations, and program funding. Some programs have a strong preventive focus. Cantor (8) described one program in which occupational therapists served as consultants in retirement planning. Using an activities analysis approach, the program provided a structured method for individuals to examine their use of time and helped them develop strategies for changing parts of their activity pattern in ways that would be more satisfying during the retirement years.

Kirchman and her associates (9) developed a program that offered a support system to older people who wanted to remain in their own communities. This program used avocational and recreational activities, an exercise program, and an educational component to achieve its goals. The senior citizens who participated showed significant increases in socialization, general affect, and life satisfaction. This type of program can be of value to the well elderly in improving their overall quality of life and by offering needed emotional support and opportunities for social interaction with others.

Another focus of occupational therapy intervention for elderly clients is assisting with vocational rehabilitation. Kemp and Kleinplatz (10) pointed out in 1985 that vocational rehabilitation is often ignored for older workers because they are believed to have few active years of employment ahead of them. The chances of becoming disabled are greater in later life than in young adulthood; however, work continues to be a meaningful source of satisfaction for older people. Age should not be the criterion for whether a worker receives vocational rehabilitation. Kemp and Kleinplatz urge that occupational therapists apply their knowledge of gerontology and work evaluation to the problems of disabled older workers.

Adult day centers are becoming more common as the needs of the aging receive more attention. Such programs are usually intended for people who are unable to participate in community senior citizens groups but who do not require around-the-clock care in a skilled nursing facility. These programs are typically aimed at health maintenance, treatment of existing medical conditions, rehabilitative services, and preventing institutionalization. Clients come to the centers during the day and receive a package of services designed to meet their individual needs. Some day centers offer specific programs for clients with certain conditions, such as Alzheimer's disease, and others provide respite services so that families can take an occasional break from care of an elderly family member. Occupational therapy involvement in day-care programs ranges from consultation to full-time administration of centers. Adult day care is a growing market for occupational therapy services and provides an appropriate site for gerontological practice (11).

Still another type of program in which occupational therapists are employed are hospice programs for terminally ill clients and their families. Hospice is a concept rather than a place, but hospice programs have been based in hospitals, nursing homes, clinics, and home health agencies. These programs utilize an interdisciplinary team to provide medical relief of pain for terminally ill clients and supportive services for clients and their families. The role of the occupational therapist may vary from simply establishing rapport and listening to clients express their feelings to the development of supportive programs of therapeutic activities and adaptive daily living skills. The goal is to make the final days of each client comfortable and meaningful and to aid families in dealing with the stress of a terminal illness (12). The hospice concept is compatible with occupational therapy philosophy, and it is expected that the occupational therapy role in hospice care will grow and develop in the future.

GENERAL TRENDS

As the population of elderly people increases there will be an increased demand for services. Francese (4) estimates that at least 6000 new nursing homes will be needed by the year 2000, as well as a whole range of community services to support elderly people who are able to remain at home. More doctors, dentists, and allied health professionals with specialty training in geriatrics will be needed to serve the health needs of this population. Ellis (5) predicts a need for 900% more occupational therapists to serve the elderly. The American Occupational Therapy Association confirms a need for more OTRs to work in this practice specialty but expects that the number of COTAs working in gerontology will remain relatively stable. Larger numbers of COTAs are presently employed in gerontology, and more COTAs belonged to the AOTA Special Interest Section in Gerontology in 1985 than any other special interest section (13,14).

Winston (3) has identified the major needs of the elderly in future years to be income security, access to adequate health care, services to facilitate home maintenance and continued living in one's own home, and transportation. Butler and Lewis (1) cite a need for retirement counseling and propose postretirement seminars to help people adjust to the changes that retirement imposes. Mental illness tends to increase in old age, and Butler and Lewis stress the need for adequate diagnosis and care of mental as well as physical disorders in the elderly. Finally, new life-styles may develop for elderly persons. Butler and Lewis suggest that the extended family may need to be reinvented to prevent the social isolation and loneliness that is all too common among older people. Society must also apply advanced technology to the needs of the elderly and give attention to improving the quality as well as the quantity of life for this population (1,4).

TRENDS IN GERIATRIC HEALTH CARE

Occupational therapy in gerontology is an expanding area of practice. In 1985 Hasselkus (15) identified several trends in service delivery to the elderly that were likely to affect occupational therapy services.

1. Rehabilitation services are more frequently being offered to elderly clients. Because of the prospective payment system used by Medicare, many nursing homes have become community rehabilitation centers, because hospital care is limited to the acute phase of illness. Thus more and more of the rehabilitation services are likely to take place in skilled nursing facilities.
2. Functional status rather than diagnosis is becoming the measure of health for older people. Because occupational therapy is based on the concept of function, it should have important contributions to make in the assessment of functional status and care of the elderly.
3. There appears to be a growing recognition on the part of health professionals that active client participation is necessary for successful preventive and health maintenance programs.
4. There is increased attention to the role of the family in helping elderly people remain in the community or adapt to institutional care.
5. Community care options are increasing, and nursing homes, in their new rehabilitative role, are becoming temporary sites for care in many cases rather than permanent placements. Greater community control of health-related services for the elderly is likely.

Because of these and other changes, Hasselkus suggests that the medical model is less useful than the functional model for occupational therapists and therapy assistants who work with the elderly. She urged OTRs and COTAs to assume a leadership role in the evolving community services for older people. Rogers (14) notes that the success of occupational therapy in gerontology will depend on the inclusion of occupational therapy services in legislation. Strategies must be developed to include occupational therapy services not only for the impaired but also for the well but frail elderly.

CASE STUDY: BILATERAL HIP FRACTURES, ARTHRITIS

The following case example illustrates the multiple problems that may require occupational therapy intervention in an elderly client.

Katherine is a 75-year-old retired woman. She was admitted to a local hospital after a fall in her home in which she fractured her left hip. Gastrointestinal bleeding was also present. She had a central fracture dislocation of the left hip and while in the hospital sustained a fracture of the right hip as well. Surgery was done first on the right hip, with a total hip arthroplasty being performed. Later she underwent a left total hip arthroplasty. After a period of recovery she was discharged from the hospital to a skilled nursing facility in her community for continued rehabilitation. Her physician anticipated that a three-month intensive program of rehabilitation would be needed before she would be able to return to her apartment and live independently.

Upon admission to the nursing home she was found to have severe rheumatoid arthritis in addition to her other disabilities. She was on a variety of medications, and precautions were necessary to prevent dislocation of both artificial hip joints. Her endurance was poor. Movement needed to be gentle because of her severe arthritis.

When first seen by occupational therapy, Katherine was able to perform personal hygiene and grooming activities (except for bathing) and could dress and undress the upper half of her body. Areas of dependency included bathing, applying lower extremity clothing, and functional mobility, including transfers, bed mobility, and ambulation. Katherine could feed herself independently, but her arthritis made it difficult for her to grasp standard eating utensils. Before her hospitalization she had been living alone in a one-bedroom apartment and was accustomed to preparing her own meals and managing her household activities independently.

Katherine's ability to use her hands and arms was extremely limited because of chronic rheumatoid arthritis. Her upper extremity strength was graded poor to fair and her endurance, both in general and for specific upper extremity activity, was poor. She quickly became short of breath and needed to rest frequently. She had only half of the normal range of motion in her shoulders, and several of her finger joints had been fused to give her better stability. She could grossly manipulate objects but had poor fine-motor skill. Katherine complained of pain during movement and required assistance to get to a standing position from her wheelchair. In physical therapy she was able to use a walker and hoped eventually to be able to walk with crutches.

Katherine was aware of energy-conservation techniques and the need to protect her joints from further damage. She had also learned to use appropriate body mechanics and had incorporated these principles into her daily living activities. For example, to conserve her limited energy she sat on a stool when working in the kitchen and knew how to open containers in a way that would not cause further damage to her joints.

Katherine was alert and oriented. She had good short- and long-term memory and could concentrate for extended periods of time. She was highly motivated to regain the independent function that would allow her to return to her home. After initial assessment had been completed, the occupational therapist devised a treatment plan that included the following objectives.

1. Client will demonstrate the use of hip safety precautions during bathing and dressing activities.

2. Client will perform lower extremity self-care activities (bathing of lower body, donning slacks, stockings, and shoes) independently with the use of assistive equipment.
3. Client will feed herself independently using adaptive equipment.
4. Client will maintain her present upper extremity range of motion, strength, and coordination.
5. Client will increase her overall endurance for activity by tolerating 30-minute treatment sessions.
6. Client will perform all homemaking activities necessary to live at home independently.

A treatment schedule was established in which Katherine attended occupational therapy sessions twice a day, with her performance to be reassessed weekly. Once the treatment plan was developed, a COTA was assigned to help Katherine carry out her treatment activities. The following activities were utilized.

1. Information and instruction in hip safety precautions was provided.
2. The use of lower extremity assistive equipment for dressing was demonstrated, and practice in the use of the equipment in daily self-care training sessions was provided.
3. A variety of large-handled eating utensils were provided and the ones that worked best for her were selected.
4. Exercises and activities were introduced in the occupational therapy clinic to maintain upper extremity range of motion, strength, and coordination. For example, a macramé project was positioned on an inclined surface to incorporate maximum joint range in the activity.
5. Treatment time in the clinic was gradually increased until Katherine could spend an entire 30-minute period in activity.
6. Practice in meal preparation and other homemaking activities was provided so that the COTA could assess potential problems and suggest solutions.

After one month of treatment, Katherine was regularly following the hip safety precautions to prevent dislocation of her artificial hip joints. She was attempting to use long-handled equipment to put on slacks, stockings, and shoes but had difficulty handling the equipment because of her arthritis. She was more successful with using the large-handled eating utensils. She was able to tolerate the 30-minute treatment sessions but did become fatigued and still needed to rest frequently. She maintained her upper extremity range of motion, strength, and coordination.

Plans were made for a home visit by the occupational therapist to assess Katherine's apartment for accessibility and safety. The physical therapist taught Katherine to ambulate with crutches, and she was able to use them for short distances. Because her apartment had six steps, the physical therapist assumed responsibility for teaching Katherine how to ascend and descend stairs. The nursing staff continued to monitor Katherine's medical needs and served as the liaison with her physician. The social worker communicated with the occupational and physical therapist concerning Katherine's progress and made plans for her discharge.

OUTCOMES OF TREATMENT

Katherine was able to master all needed self-care skills with the use of adapted equipment. She followed her hip safety precautions and knew that she must continue to follow them for three months after the surgery. Because Katherine continued to be easily fatigued, further energy conservation measures and work simplification techniques were discussed with her.

The OTR's visit to her apartment revealed the need for some additional bathroom equipment. A raised toilet seat and toilet rails were installed, as well as grab bars on the walls. A tub bench was provided to allow Katherine to bathe while sitting. Katherine learned to ascend and descend the stairs safely, to move throughout her apartment, to get in and out of bed and off and on chairs, and to handle some meal preparation. Until she felt capable of preparing all of her meals, the social worker arranged for her to have one meal delivered each day by a community meal service. Family members agreed to assist her with shopping, laundry, and housekeeping until she was able to resume these tasks herself. Katherine was pleased to return to her home and was confident that she would eventually be able to resume most of her activities.

DISCUSSION QUESTIONS

1. Did you have a close relationship with a grandparent or elderly friend or neighbor? If so, did this relationship influence your attitudes about aging and elderly people? How?

2. Are there special qualities that are needed to work effectively with older clients? What are they?

3. Do you think that families are carrying their fair share of caring for the elderly? What happens within a family when an elderly relative needs constant care and attention?

4. Have you visited a nursing home in your community? What kinds of programs does it offer to its residents? How much does it cost to live there? Is occupational therapy provided?

5. Did Katherine's occupational therapy treatment plan differ in any significant way from that that might have been prepared for a younger client?

6. Does your state have a Commission on Aging? What services does it provide to elderly citizens?

7. Discuss the relative quality of life available in different kinds of living situations for the elderly. Consider institutional settings, retirement communities, low-income housing, and remaining in one's own home. What type of living situation would you prefer as an older person?

8. In working with elderly or terminally ill clients one must accept death as an everyday reality. Examine your personal feelings and beliefs about death and dying. Do you think it is of value to work with clients who are not likely to improve?

REFERENCES

1. Butler R, Lewis M: *Aging and Mental Health: Positive Psychosocial Approaches*, ed 2. St. Louis, MO, CV Mosby, 1977, pp 3–33, 211–235, 307–317.
2. Lewis S: *The Mature Years: A Geriatric Occupational Therapy Text*. Thorofare, NJ, Slack, 1979, pp 7–171.
3. Winston E: An older population: meeting major needs through occupational therapy. *AJOT* 35:635–637, 1981.
4. Francese P: Elderly may be biggest growth industry. American Demographics, 1984.
5. Ellis N: The challenge of nursing home care. *AJOT* 40:7–11, 1986.
6. Swallow W: Developers find elderly want to stay in own homes. *The Capital Times*, 15 June 1986.
7. *Long Term Care/Nursing Homes*. Rockville, MD, American Occupational Therapy Association, 1985, pp 1–86.
8. Cantor S: Occupational therapists as members of pre-retirement resource teams. *AJOT* 35:638–643, 1981.
9. Kirchman M, Reichenbach V, Giambalva B: Preventive activities and services for the well elderly. *AJOT* 36:236–242, 1982.
10. Kemp B, Kleinplatz F: Vocational rehabilitation of the older worker. *AJOT* 39:322–326, 1985.
11. Ellis N (ed): Special issue on adult day care. *Gerontology Special Interest Section Newsletter* 8:1–5, 1985.
12. *Hospice/Death and Dying*. Rockville, MD, American Occupational Therapy Association, 1985, pp 1–56.
13. Ad Hoc Commission on Occupational Therapy Manpower. *Occupational Therapy Manpower: A Plan for Progress*. Rockville, MD, American Occupational Therapy Association, 1985, pp 57–59.
14. Rogers J: The issue—gerontic occupational therapy. *AJOT* 35:663–666, 1981.

15. Hasselkus B: Changing trends in geriatric health care. *Gerontology Special Interest Section Newsletter* 8:1–3, 1985.

SUGGESTED READINGS

Crepeau E: *Activity Programming for the Elderly.* Boston, Little, Brown & Co, 1986.

Curtin S: *Nobody Ever Died of Old Age.* Boston, Little, Brown & Co, 1973.

Maclay E: *Green Winter: Celebrations of Old Age.* Reader's Digest Press, 1977.

Maguire G: *Care of the Elderly: A Health Team Approach.* Boston, Little, Brown & Co, 1985.

Strauss A, Glaser B: *Chronic Illness and the Quality of Life.* St. Louis, MO, CV Mosby, 1975.

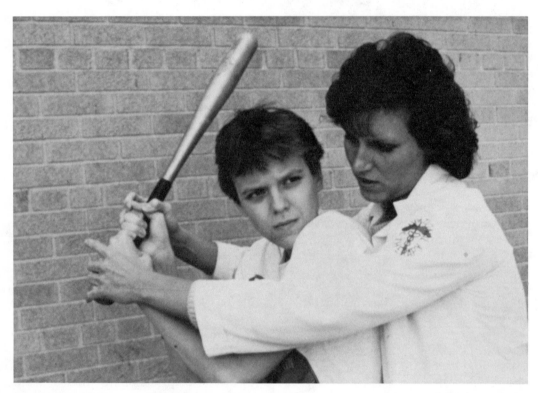

Courtesy AOTA

FIFTEEN

Practice in Community-Based Programs

The movement of occupational therapy services from traditional institutional settings into the community has been one of the biggest changes in the field in the last decade. As the Medicare prospective payment system began to take hold there was a rapid increase in the number of community-based occupational therapy programs that were intended to provide care to persons needing continued therapy after discharge from acute care hospitals and those who needed help to continue to live independently in their homes. According to the 1985 AOTA Manpower Report, there was a 4-fold increase in the number of OTRs working in home health agencies and a 2½-fold increase in the number of therapists in private practice over a nine-year period. Data from the 1986 AOTA Member Data Survey confirmed these increases and showed steady growth in OTR and COTA employment in a variety of community settings (Table 15.1). This survey emphasized that more and more occupational therapy treatment was taking place in community settings as a result of greater community orientation in mental health programs, decreased long-

term care in hospitals, and the development of school system practice (1).

The phenomenal growth of home health agencies supported this trend. Medicare-certified home health agencies were growing nationally at a rate of 100 new agencies every two months, according to 1985 figures of the Health Care Financing Administration. Almost half of the existing home health agencies in 1984 offered occupational therapy services. That was more than double the percentage that provided such services in 1973 (2). The "graying" of America has also contributed to the need for community-based health services.

The concept of home and community-based care is not a new one in occupational therapy. Since the 1920s, occupational therapy services have been available through visiting nurse associations, public health programs, and community- and hospital-based home care agencies. A relatively small proportion of occupational therapy personnel were employed in these programs. By the mid-1970s, however, social and economic changes in the United States were creating

Table 15.1.
Community Employment Settings of OTRs and COTAs in Percentages[a]

Setting	OTRs		COTAs	
	1973	1986[b]	1973	1986[b]
Community mental health centers	4.2	1.7	0.0	4.3
Day-care center/program	1.4	1.0	1.2	4.4
HMO (including PPO/IPA)	0.3	0.3	0.7	0.1
Home health agency	0.9	4.5	0.2	0.9
Hospice		0.1		0.0
Outpatient clinic (freestanding)		2.4		0.6
Physician's Office		1.0		0.2
Private industry		0.7		0.7
Private practice	1.3	6.0	0.3	1.3
Public health agency	1.6	0.6	0.5	0.4
Residential care facility, including group home, independent living center		3.5		7.0
Retirement or senior center		0.3		1.0
School system (including private schools)	11.0	16.3	3.6	13.9
Sheltered workshop	0.7	0.3	1.4	0.9
Vocational or prevocational program		0.6		1.7
Voluntary agency (e.g., Easter Seal, UCP)		1.3		0.8

[a]Data from American Occupational Therapy Association, January 16, 1987.
[b]Preliminary data.

growing pressure for community health and therapeutic services. The trend toward deinstitutionalization increased the pressure; however, few funding mechanisms were available to pay for community care (3). The enactment of Title XVIII (Medicare) and Title XIX (Medicaid) were the beginnings of funding to support the delivery of community-based services. These acts were followed by the amendments to the Social Security Act in 1983 that established the prospective payment system for hospital care of Medicare recipients. Under Medicare provisions a client found to have continuing needs for therapy after a hospitalization can receive in-home services if a physician so orders and if the client is homebound and is considered to have potential for further improvement. Other pieces of legislation also spurred the development of community services. The Architectural Barriers Act of 1968 (section 504 of the Rehabilitation Act of 1973) mandated that community facilities be fully accessible to the disabled, and Title VII (another amendment to the Rehabilitation

act of 1973) created comprehensive independent living services to aid severely handicapped persons to live more independently in their homes and communities (4). All of these laws combined to encourage the development of services on the community level and provided funding to assist in this effort.

Although the growth of community-based occupational therapy services has been rapid, it has not been without problems. For many years, occupational therapy was not covered by Medicare if it was the only therapeutic service being given. Reimbursement for occupational therapy services was sometimes questioned by Medicare and by other third-party payers, and there was increasing demand for documentation of the effectiveness of occupational therapy intervention (5). These restrictions were eased in 1986 with the passage of amendments to the Medicare Act that permitted extended occupational therapy services to inpatients in skilled nursing facilities, provided Medicare coverage of occupational therapy services in rehabilitation agencies even if that were the only service being given, and enabled occupational therapists to become independent service providers for Medicare recipients. The latter provision opened the door to private practitioners to offer services to individual clients covered under Medicare and bill directly for their services. These changes (effective July 1, 1987) should increase the use of occupational therapy services for this client population (6).

This chapter describes several community-based occupational therapy services, introduces the student to concepts of community care, and illustrates the practice opportunities that are available. A case study is presented that shows the use of occupational therapy with a homebound client.

COMMUNITY PRACTICE SITES

HOME HEALTH AGENCIES

Most of the home care of clients receiving occupational therapy is coordinated by home health agencies. Medicare defines a home health agency as a public or private organization primarily engaged in providing skilled nursing care or other therapeutic services. To qualify under Medicare certification regulations, an agency must do the following:

- Provide at least one therapeutic service besides skilled nursing
- Have policies developed by at least one physician and one registered nurse
- Maintain records for all clients seen
- Employ professional personnel who meet established qualifications
- Provide for regular review of policies

Under Medicare guidelines any client services provided by a home health agency must be ordered by a physician. Clients must be homebound, and the services that are provided must not duplicate any other services. If a client is found to be in need of occupational therapy services the therapist will conduct an initial evaluation to determine the client's functional status and will then develop a written treatment plan to deal with the observed limitations. Documentation is required for each home visit. According to an AOTA position paper, occupational therapy home care is intended to assist the client to attain a maximum level of independent functioning in his or her own home and community. Home treatment may focus on 1) improving daily living skills, work or leisure skills, sensorimotor skills, cognitive skills, and psychosocial skills; 2) adapting the environment to allow for more effective functioning; or 3) preventing further limitations in function (3). Clients who are no longer making progress toward stated goals, who do not comply with the therapeutic program, or who have achieved maximum benefit must be discharged from active treatment.

Many OTRs and COTAs find home care particularly rewarding because a close relationship develops between therapist and client. Because clients are in their own environment, they have a greater sense of control over their lives and are often more ready to participate in therapy programs than when they were hospitalized. Home adaptations and equipment needs can be assessed more realistically in the home than anywhere else. Extra hours of therapy can be gained when home programs include a family member assisting the client in the practice of needed skills (7). Levine (8), who writes about the cultural aspects of home care, emphasizes that the occupational therapist who works in the client's home must plan a therapeutic program that takes into account the client's personal values and occupational roles. The therapist must refrain from judging the client's preferences and life-style and must establish goals and treatment methods that are meaningful to the client and the client's family. She suggests that the home care therapist try to enter the life of the client and caretaker as a participant/observer, taking her leads from them and adapting the therapeutic program to their specific needs.

Home health agencies can provide therapeutic services by hiring the appropriate professionals as part of their staff or by contracting with private practitioners who provide therapy on a fee-for-service basis. Because home health agency therapists must travel from one client's home to another, they need to be creative in their use of treatment equipment. These therapists will generally not have access to large pieces of equipment but may carry smaller portable items in their cars. Ordinary household items may be pressed into service for the therapy program. A can of vegetables can serve as a weight, and a rolling pin may be used to improve bilateral coordination and increase strength and range of motion. The medical model that is often the basis for hospital practice is less useful in home health care. Here function is the most important consideration, and a holistic approach that considers the social, personal, and environmental aspects of the client's life is more practical. Prevention is often an essential part of home care. The client must be aware of safety factors, must learn methods to perform tasks that will prevent reinjury, and must understand how to maintain health and well-being. Concepts of joint protection, energy conservation, stress management, and exercise are emphasized in preventive programs. These concepts must be carried over into the client's daily life for the maximum benefit (7).

Communication with other team members is more difficult when working in a home health agency, since each member may be visiting the client at a different time. Frequently telephone communications are used to keep team members in touch with one another, and written communications are even more important than usual. Time must be set aside for team meetings so that contributing disciplines can coordinate their care and effectively plan treatment (9).

A typical client visit lasts from 30 to 60 minutes; the number and frequency of visits will vary with the nature and severity of the client's condition. A typical Medicare-certified home health agency employs 27.9 staff members and contracts with another 7.7 health professionals for services (10). One agency conducted a chart review that showed that their clients averaged 7.25 occupational therapy visits at an average rate of two visits per week. Therapy was typically provided for a four- to eight-week period. In this agency, 79% of the clients treated by occupational therapists were able to remain at home, functioning either independently or with assistance (7).

The COTAs work in home health agencies as well as OTRs. The COTA must be supervised by an OTR and may not accept referrals for service independently. The COTAs may conduct routine assessments and frequently carry out the treatment plan that has been developed by the OTR. In home care, on-site supervision of COTAs is impractical, but they should receive periodic supervision during the implementation of the treatment program (11).

One disadvantage of working in home health care is that therapists tend to feel isolated from their peers. Therapists must be able to function independently, without frequent consultation from colleagues, but may feel the lack of the informal professional communication that is so easy and spontaneous in institutional settings. To combat the sense of isolation, the home care therapist must learn to "network" with other occupational therapists and professional colleagues. The home health therapist must be able to function with minimal supervision and few supplies and must be prepared to handle emergencies or conflicts that may occur in the client's home. It is necessary to be flexible so that work schedules and/or treatment procedures can be rearranged if necessary. The home health therapist must be a creative problem solver, since each client and environment will present different challenges. Above all, the home health therapist must have a background of broad clinical experience and be capable of dealing with problems in many areas of the client's life. Work in a home health agency is not easy but offers a challenging diversity to the skilled OTR or COTA (12).

INDEPENDENT LIVING CENTERS

Independent living centers are another type of community program in which occupational therapy can play an active role. In the 1960s and 1970s the concept of independent living for the disabled gained momentum, and in 1978 Congress amended the Rehabilitation Act of 1973 to include provisions for comprehensive services to encourage independent living. This action was the result of increased recognition that disabled people needed more than vocationally directed rehabilitation. The ability to enjoy a reasonable quality of life and to live independently or semi-independently in community settings was felt to be as important as employability for the handicapped. This legislation supported a variety of self-help programs intended to promote independent living for the disabled. One of the major provisions of the act was the establishment of independent living centers, defined as facilities offering a combination of services to encourage independence in family and community settings for the severely disabled population. State rehabilitation agencies (vocational rehabilitation) were

designated as the principle applicants for grant monies to establish and operate the centers. In 1982, 14 new grants were awarded to establish independent living centers and 97 established programs were continued. Some states had also developed local independent living programs funded through taxation, grants, fees for service, or third-party reimbursement sources.

Independent living programs vary considerably because they are intended to meet local needs. Some programs provide direct service, but a more common pattern is to utilize the services of agencies that already exist in communities. Independent living centers may follow three basic patterns:

1. The free-standing center: services are provided, adaptive housing assistance is given, and training in living skills may be offered
2. Transitional living programs: severely disabled clients are gradually enabled to live in less dependent or independent living arrangements
3. Residential programs: several disabled individuals live in a group housing unit and share attendant care and services

A key feature of all programs is a strong emphasis on consumer decision making. The disabled persons themselves plan and to some extent implement the program.

Occupational therapists have much to offer independent living programs because of their unique orientation toward adapting the environment to the needs of the handicapped person. The OTR and COTA may contribute to such programs by providing direct client service, consulting on programs, helping to initiate programs, and serving as advocates for the continuation of programs that enable handicapped persons to live in the community (4). Baum (13) notes, however, that occupational therapists have followed rather than led the independent living movement, even though their expertise gives them unique qualifications for leadership. She notes that occupational therapy was not mentioned as a primary service in these programs and urges that therapists direct their services toward integration of clients into community settings as well as toward vocational rehabilitation. Many severely disabled individuals may never be capable of competitive employment but can still live productive and fulfilling lives. Occupational therapists can be instrumental in helping them to do so and should take a more active role in promoting and contributing to independent living programs.

COMMUNITY SUPPORT SERVICES

A variety of services have developed to provide a smoother transition for clients as they move from hospital to community settings and to offer them support and assistance as they resume their customary roles in family and community life. Several programs are briefly described as examples of community support services in which occupational therapy plays a contributing role.

Some rehabilitation hospitals have developed programs to assess a patient's ability to function at home before he or she actually leaves the hospital. In one such program, the occupational therapist routinely accompanied the patient on a home visit prior to discharge for a preliminary assessment to identify architectural barriers, safety hazards, or other features that might be obstacles to the patient's ability to live comfortably at home. Because hospital patients are being discharged earlier than in the past, the hospital now bears greater responsibility to ensure a trouble-free transition from one environment to the other (14).

In another part of the country a Home Health Care Department was created in a large university medical center. The department provided home care to clients within a 40-mile radius of the medical center and referred those from outlying areas to agencies in their own communities. The occupational therapists involved found that clients were often more cooperative and better motivated to participate in home therapy programs than they had been in the hospital. Family members were asked to assist with the continuation of therapy programs, since clients were visited only two or three times a week. A loan closet of equipment was available so that clients could avoid purchasing expensive equipment that was only needed for a short period. The OTRs traveled with "therapy kits" containing essential pieces of equipment and made do with household items to serve some equipment needs. This hospital-based program provided good carryover for discharged patients and offered them needed support during their convalescence (15).

Project Open House represents still another type of community support service. Two occupational therapists helped develop a project for modifying the homes of disabled persons where architectural barriers existed. The therapists observed that the therapeutic gains made by many disabled people through rehabilitation programs were negated on their return home if architectural features confined them to the house or made it difficult for them to carry out necessary daily tasks. In this project the occupational therapist visited the home of a disabled client, assessed both the client's level of functioning and the home environment, and made plans to modify the home for increased convenience and accessibility. Even small modifications made a big difference in a client's level of independence. Typical modifications included the installation of ramps or mechanical lifting devices to avoid stairs; widening doorways; installing grab bars, tub seats, and hand-held showers in bathrooms; adapting kitchens for increased safety and convenience; lowering closet rods to within wheelchair reach; and installing bed rails or built-in platform beds. Project Open House found that an average one-time expenditure of $1,000 could make the difference between the disabled client being able to remain at home or becoming institutionalized. Because institutional costs are estimated at up to $128,000 per individual per year, this was a considerable saving (16).

Another private rehabilitation agency developed a program to restore the work capacity of injured workers. Representatives from major insurance carriers contracted with the agency to provide rehabilitative services for clients who had sustained industrial injuries. The insurance companies were seeking a rapid and effective way to return injured workers to their employment. The occupational therapists who were involved in this program found that in addition to knowing rehabilitation concepts, they also needed to learn about ergonomics, management theory, and labor relations in order to work effectively with industrial injuries. They performed work-tolerance tests, explored the worker's physical abilities, and looked at the demands of the job the worker had done before his or her injury. In some cases modifications could be suggested that would make it possible for the injured worker to resume the job. Clients were also taught the use of proper body mechanics, appropriate movement patterns, and pacing techniques so that reinjury could be avoided. The rehabilitation of injured workers is an expanding area of occupational therapy practice; in this agency occupational therapists were valuable contributors to the success of the program (17).

PRIVATE PRACTICE

More OTRs and COTAs are choosing to provide their services as private practitioners. Occupational therapy practices may be located in hospitals, medical centers, shopping centers, downtown office centers, or office buildings for health professionals. The private practitioner contracts to deliver services for a fee and establishes a small business to provide specific services. A therapist may contract with a facility to see patients of the facility, with agencies to see referred patients in their homes, or with individual clients whose physician has requested occupational therapy services. Various types of private practice exist. An individual practice consists of a single therapist providing contracted services. An associate practice has one therapist who serves as director and who employs other professional and technical staff members of the same professional group. In a group practice a variety of health professionals may be employed to offer more comprehensive services. A private practice may also be structured as a partnership between two or more therapists (18). Private practitioners must be business oriented, because they must make a profit to remain in business. They need to set financial goals for their business, just as they set treatment goals for their clients. The private practitioner establishes a set of specific services to be offered and then sets a fee schedule accordingly. Fees may be based on a set fee per visit, on units of time (15-minute or hourly intervals are common), or on the prevailing rates for the geographic area. According to Frazian (19), in 1986 an average 15-minute unit charge for individual occupational therapy assessment or treatment services ranged between $15 and $20. Private practitioners tend to make as much or more income as therapists employed in institutional settings. In addition they have direct control over their time, which institutional employees do not. Tulanian, Hammond, and Tulanian (20) have identified a number of differences between private practitioners (contractors) and institutional or agency employees (Table 15.2).

These authors note that while there is great independence of action in private practice, there is also great responsibility. Smith (21) confirms this in her discussion of private practice. She points out that the therapist has full control over the philosophy of the practice, the quality of care that is given, and the size of the practice. The financial rewards can be attractive, and one's time is more flexible than that of an employee. On the other hand, the professional and financial success of the private practice rests squarely on the shoulders of the therapist. It takes time and effort to build a reputation and a flourishing practice. The first few months or years may be difficult, and one must have sufficient cap-

ital to survive this establishment period. In private practice, if one is ill or takes a few days off, one does not earn income.

Most private practitioners agree that a therapist should have several years of clinical experience in traditional settings before entering into a private practice. One must have good clinical skills and be knowledgeable about current theory and procedures in the practice area. The needs of the community should be thoroughly explored before a private practice is established. One should be willing to take some financial risks and be prepared to work hard to establish the business on a sound footing. Knowledge of current business practices and procedures is as necessary to the private practitioner as is expertise in occupational therapy (21). The growth of private practice in occupational therapy is expected to continue, and the 1985 AOTA Manpower Report recommended that educational resources be developed for occupational therapists in topics such

Table 15.2.
Differences Between the Private Contractor and Employee[a]

Contractor	Employee
Paid by the service (pay includes paperwork, preparation, travel)	Paid by the hour
Paid lump sum per day travel fees	Paid by the mile
Therapist maintains time records, calculates amount due, submits bill for reimbursement	Facility keeps time records, computes salary, and pays on designated paydays
Provides own equipment or pays for use of equipment	Equipment provided by employer
Provides own liability and property damage insurance	Facility provides liability and property damage coverage
No taxes are withdrawn from paychecks; responsible for state and federal taxes, social security	Facility computes and deducts payroll taxes
Chooses own hours	Hours set by facility
No vacation or sick leave; no health insurance or workers compensation provided	Vacation and sick leave; health insurance and workers compensation provided by employer
Therapist chooses type of treatment to be given	Supervisor can specify type of treatment
Therapist provides own continuing education	Continuing education may be provided by employer
Therapist provides own space or pays for use of space	Facility provides space
Therapist bills third parties or pays for facility's billing service	Facility provides all billing services
Therapist has no mail slot or bulletin board space unless facility is reimbursed for these	Therapist provided with mail slot and bulletin board space for messages
Therapist provides for own secretarial services	Therapist uses facility's secretarial services
Therapist provides own name tag and personal business cards; may not use facility's business card	Therapist uses name tags and business cards of facility

From Tulanian M, Hammond S, Tulanian S: *The Business Management of Private Practice: Occupational Therapy, Physical Therapy*. Middletown, CA, Applied Educational Systems, 1985, pp. 11–12.

as marketing, systems behavior and networking, productivity, cost accounting, and application of computer technology (1). Such knowledge will benefit not only the private practitioner but also therapists who administer programs in institutional settings.

The COTAs as well as OTRs have been involved in private practice, although in smaller numbers. An enterprising COTA in St. Paul, Minnesota, founded a private agency, Supportive Care Service, in the early 1980s and provided services to help elderly clients remain in their own homes as long as possible. This service met a specific community need and now employs additional COTAs to staff the program (22).

TEAM MEMBERS

The OTRs and COTAs working in the community may work with public health nurses, visiting nurses, physical therapists, social workers, and home health aides. Significantly, nonprofessionals provide 70% of the services in home health care (10). The home health aide who assists with bathing and daily care may have the most frequent contact with homebound clients and may be a valuable ally for the OTR and COTA. Family members also contribute much to the therapeutic programs of clients and often are considered full members of the health care team.

TRENDS AND OPPORTUNITIES IN COMMUNITY PRACTICE

A report compiled by the General Accounting Office in 1983 made the following predictions regarding home health care:

- There is a massive unmet need for home health care in the 1980s.

- An estimated 5.5 million individuals require home health services, and Congress has been asked to consider adding a comprehensive home health benefit to the Medicare and Medicaid programs.
- Home health care is bearing the brunt of the effects of earlier patient discharges from hospitals due to the prospective payment system for Medicare recipients.
- There will be an increase in the purchase of home health equipment, a need for more training of home care staff in advanced medical techniques, and an increased demand for rehabilitation services.
- Rural home health services will increase, with hospitals contracting with home health staff.
- There is likely to be increased pediatric home health care, although at present a reimbursement mechanism is lacking.
- There may be increased incentives from insurance companies for clients to use home care, and broadened insurance coverage for homemaker and home health aide services.
- There will be one-stop shopping for home care products and services (10).

Community-based care will expand and take over many functions that were formerly carried out in the hospital. Occupational therapists and therapy assistants will need to learn new roles and ways of delivering their services in community environments. Occupational therapy personnel will need to aggressively market their services to homebound clients, the chronically ill, the elderly, and the severely handicapped. Hospital personnel face an increased responsibility for careful discharge planning and for referring clients for follow-up services if necessary. Referral networks between occupational therapists who work in hospitals and community programs will greatly improve the continuity of care for their clients and will help to ease the isolation of community-based therapists. Occupational therapists may create their own day programs, learning centers, work evaluation clinics, and neonatal treatment centers.

The OTRs and COTAs can also contribute to the development of community services in their area. Service on community boards, governmental committees, and the boards of local service agencies is one way occupational therapists can extend their skills to benefit the community at large. Such emerging areas of health care as rehabilitation of injured workers, hospice care, and case management of long-term care clients offer new opportunities for occupational therapy personnel. The community-based therapist of the future will be an individual who is able to accept new responsibilities, work with minimal supervision, and creatively apply occupational therapy theory and principles to new client groups and in new practice sites (23). The community will be where the action is in the health care of the future.

The case study that follows illustrates a typical case seen by a home health care staff.

CASE STUDY:
VENOUS ULCERS AND OBESITY

Midland Medical Center is a large hospital and medical center serving a heavily populated metropolitan area. Its occupational therapy department provides a variety of inpatient services and also participates in the hospital's home health care service. Occupational therapy services are provided through this unit to homebound clients whose ability to perform self-care, work, and/or leisure tasks has been impaired. A nurse makes the initial home visit to determine the client's needs and then makes appropriate referrals for service. A physician's referral must be obtained before occupational therapy services can be initiated. Both OTRs and COTAs work in the home care service through a contractual agreement between the occupational therapy department, the medical center, and the home health care service. A standard charge of $33 per visit is made for occupational therapy visits.

The initial occupational therapy visit is made by an OTR who evaluates the client's status and needs. If the client is found to have a need for occupational therapy services and shows potential for benefiting from the services, the OTR develops a treatment plan. If the services of an OTR are not required, a COTA is assigned to carry out the treatment plan. The OTR and COTA meet initially to review the treatment plan and at weekly intervals thereafter to review progress toward treatment goals and to modify the treatment plan if needed. Daily notes are required by the OTR or COTA who makes the home visits, with monthly reassessment of the client's status by the OTR. A discharge note is written by the OTR when maximum benefit has been achieved or when the client discontinues the program.

Mary is a 70-year-old woman who worked as a candy wrapper in a large candy company prior to her retirement. Mary had two years of high school education and came from a lower middle income family. She never married; however, Mary raised her sister's daughter when the sister died shortly after the child's birth. Mary has lived with her niece ever since a hospitalization in 1985, and the niece is now Mary's primary caretaker.

A nurse from the home health service opened Mary's case in May of 1985. Mary had chronic venous ulcers on both legs and was extremely obese. Her obesity caused valve incompetency and blood tended to pool in her legs, causing swelling and ulcerations. Mary was first referred for physical therapy treatment, but after four months of treatment little progress had been made. As a last resort she was referred to occupational therapy for evaluation of her functional status and her ability to perform self-care tasks.

The OTR performed an initial assessment that showed that Mary was independent in grooming, some hygiene tasks, and in dressing her upper body. She had difficulty with bed mobility and with all transfers. Her standing tolerance was limited, and she did not ambulate. Mary ate all her meals from a bedside table and performed her limited self-care activities in bed. She required a bedpan for toileting. Rolling to the left or right in bed required the use of bed rails. She was able to get from a seated position to standing only by having her bed raised to its highest level and having her niece stabilize a walker while Mary held onto it and pulled up to stand. Her standing tolerance was only 1 minute and 45 seconds. Mary was afraid of falling and did not initially trust the COTA who was assigned to her case.

Mary was self-conscious about her weight. She was aware that her obesity contributed to the development of her leg ulcers but was not on a diet and did not perform any exercise. The nurse had been unable to weigh her, as the scales did not register high enough for Mary's weight. Mary viewed herself as an invalid confined to her bed and seemed content to watch TV or look out of her large picture window. Mary showed adequate strength and range of motion in both arms and had no deficits in fine-motor function. No sensory limitations were present and she was cognitively intact.

The OTR developed a treatment plan for Mary that concentrated on promoting her ability to dress the lower part of her body independently, to use proper body mechanics so that she could rise to a standing position, to improve her ability to transfer, to increase her standing tolerance, to train the niece to assist in her program, and possibly to develop some ability to ambulate. Visits by the COTA were scheduled for twice a week, with the OTR to be kept informed of any

changes in Mary's status. The OTR visited Mary once a month to reevaluate her abilities and to assess progress. The OTR was also in communication with Mary's home care nurse regarding her program. The treatment plan was implemented in late September. A commode chair was obtained for Mary's room. The COTA taught Mary correct body mechanics for rising from sitting to standing, and each week her bed was lowered by a half inch until it reached a height of 20 inches (the height of the commode chair). Work on ambulation with a walker was begun so that Mary could eventually walk to the commode chair and back to her bed. Her ability to rise to a standing position improved, but she continued to have trouble lowering herself down to a sitting position.

By October of 1985 Mary could stand using the walker for up to 7 minutes at a time. She began to practice slight movement while standing, shifting her weight and stepping from side to side. Her niece helped her practice these skills and monitored her standing time. By November, Mary had begun to show an interest in dressing and began to put on her shoes and a dress rather than spending the day in a hospital gown. She was now able to walk four feet to the sofa and back with assistance. Gradually she began to walk to the commode chair, which was 18 feet from her bed. By December she was showing increased socialization and helped to wrap Christmas presents. The COTA now taught her to walk with a side step into the kitchen. Once there she was able to walk to the sink, operate the stove, remove items from the refrigerator, and make herself a cup of coffee. Her niece encouraged her by placing a sturdy bench near the kitchen door so that she could rest and by asking her to help with light chores. In late December, Mary was discharged from the home care service. She was now independent in getting to a standing position, could ambulate the length of her apartment with supervision, could use most kitchen appliances safely and independently, and could transfer onto the bed, the commode chair, and the kitchen bench without assistance. Her standing tolerance had reached 10 minutes. She was able to dress her lower body independently and no longer required her niece's help for most self-care tasks. Her mental attitude had improved, and she took a more active interest in neighborhood events. Mary's niece was grateful for her aunt's increased ability to care for her own needs and for her improved motivation to participate in daily homemaking activities.

DISCUSSION QUESTIONS

1. What kinds of community services are available in your area for the homebound, the severely disabled, or the chronically ill? How are these services supported?

2. In community practice, the OTR and COTA often work with clients in their homes. In what ways might the dynamics of a therapeutic relationship be different when working in the client's home rather than in a clinic?

3. Interview an elderly or homebound person in your community and find out what support services he or she might find most useful.

4. Collect newspaper clippings that describe new community health programs. How could occupational therapists and therapy assistants contribute to these programs?

5. Are any occupational therapists in your area engaged in private practice? If so, how did they get started? What is the scope of their practice? Why do they prefer private practice over traditional employment?

6. A therapist working in the community needs to be tuned in to local politics and issues in order to be sensitive to community needs. How could a therapist become acquainted with the political issues of a community that is new to her?

7. When working in home care it is often important to have the client practice skills in between the therapist's visits. How can the OTR or COTA ensure that the client correctly carries out the therapy activities?

REFERENCES

1. Ad Hoc Commission on Occupational Therapy Manpower: Occupational Therapy Manpower: A Plan for Progress. Rockville, MD, American Occupational Therapy Association, 1985, pp 55–59.
2. Research information division. Home health. Part I. Occup Ther News 39(10):7, 1985.
3. Practice division. Home Health. Rockville, MD, American Occupational Therapy Association, 1985, pp 25–40.
4. Practice division. Independent Living. Rockville, MD, American Occupational Therapy Association, 1984, pp 13–23.
5. Bracciano A: Medicare reimbursement of occupational therapy in home health care. Gerontology Special Interest Newsletter 8(4):3–6, 1985.
6. Provisions of Medicare amendment expand coverage for occupational therapy. Occup Ther News 40(12):4, 1986.
7. MaCrae A: Occupational therapy in a Medicare-approved home health agency. AJOT 38:721–725, 1984.
8. Levine R: The cultural aspects of home care delivery. AJOT 38:734–738, 1984.
9. Trossman P: Administrative and professional issues for the occupational therapist in home health care. AJOT 38:726–733, 1984.
10. Research information division, Home health. Part II. Occup Ther News 39(11):7, 1985.
11. I'm glad you asked. Occup Ther News 35(9): 1981.
12. Groves J: Home health. In Davis L, Kirkland M (eds): The Role of Occupational Therapy with the Elderly (ROTE). Rockville, MD, American Occupational Therapy Association, 1986, 153–170.
13. Baum C: Nationally speaking: independent living. A critical role for occupational therapy. AJOT 34:773–774, 1980.
14. Mason M: The home visit: a step from hospital to home. In: The Roles of Occupational Therapists in Continuity of Care. Binghamton, NY, Haworth, 1985, pp 39–49.

15. Borg N: Home care occupational therapy: a vital link to independence. In: *The Roles of Occupational Therapists in Continuity of Care.* Binghamton, NY, Haworth, 1985, pp 51–61.

16. Colvin M, Korn T: Eliminating barriers to the disabled. *AJOT* 38:748–753, 1984.

17. DeRenne-Stephan C: Industry and injuries: arena for occupational therapy. In: *The Roles of Occupational Therapists in Continuity of Care.* Binghamton, NY, Haworth, 1985, pp 127–134.

18. Frazian B: Establishing and administrating a private practice in a hospital setting. In: *Private Practice Information Packet.* Rockville, MD, American Occupational Therapy Association, 1986, pp 26–30.

19. Frazian B: Private practice update. In: *Private Practice Information Packet.* Rockville, MD, American Occupational Therapy Association, 1986, pp 31–33.

20. Tulanian M, Hammond S, Tulanian S: *The Business Management of Private Practice: Occupational Therapy, Physical Therapy.* Middletown, CA, Applied Educational Systems, 1985, pp 1–39.

21. Smith S: Private practices, home Care, and consultation for the occupational therapist. In: *Private Practice Information Packet.* Rockville, MD,

American Occupational Therapy Association, 1986, pp 55–58.

22. COTA Share. *Occup Ther News* 38(4):7, 38(11):7, 1984.

23. Taira E: After treatment what? New roles for occupational therapists in the community. In: *The Roles of Occupational Therapists in Continuity of Care,* Binghamton, NY, Haworth, 1985, pp 13–23.

SUGGESTED READINGS

Anderson H: *The Disabled Homemaker.* Springfield, IL, Charles C Thomas, 1981.

Crewe N, Zolak K: *Independent Living for Physically Disabled People.* San Francisco, Jossey-Bass, 1983.

Official position paper: occupational therapy's role in independent living or alternative living situations. *AJOT* 35:812–814, 1981.

Official position paper: the role of the occupational therapist in home health care. *AJOT* 35:809–810, 1981.

Special issue on home health care. *AJOT* 38:11, 1984.

Special issue on home health care. *Gerontology Special Interest Section Newsletter* 8:1–6, 1985.

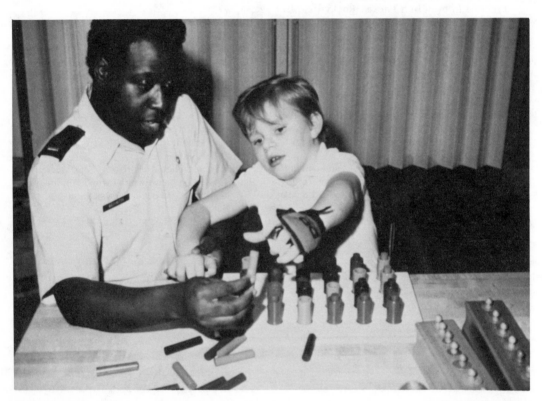

Courtesy AOTA

SIXTEEN

Indirect Service Careers in Occupational Therapy

The preceding chapters discussed careers in occupational therapy that involve providing direct service to clients. There are a number of occupational therapy careers, however, that do not involve direct client service. Professionals in these careers provide supportive or supplementary services that meet a variety of professional or client-related needs. These careers can be grouped under the general heading of indirect service careers. The beginning student in occupational therapy should be aware of these additional career options, even though they demand either advanced clinical expertise, advanced levels of education, or both.

Most OTRs and COTAs begin their careers as clinicians in a direct service role. As they gain experience and add to their knowledge and skills through continuing education programs or graduate study, they often move on to jobs that involve higher levels of responsibility. Figure 16.1 is an adaptation of Colman's schematic depiction of some of these patterns of career development (1).

This chapter explores some of the career options in indirect service roles and the trends that are expected to influence these careers in the future.

MANAGEMENT

The occupational therapy manager directs the activities of an occupational therapy service program. As administrator of the program, the manager is responsible for mobilizing the human and material resources of the program in order to meet the goals of the organization in which it is housed. The manager has a variety of roles to fulfill. As chief liaison between the staff members and the administration of the organization, the manager interprets the organization's policies to the staff and implements the service program in accordance with those policies. The manager represents the needs of the program to the organization's administration. Good communication and interpersonal skills are essential tools for the program manager. Because the manager is accountable for the overall operation of the occupational therapy program, he or she must lead the staff in developing long-range plans

177

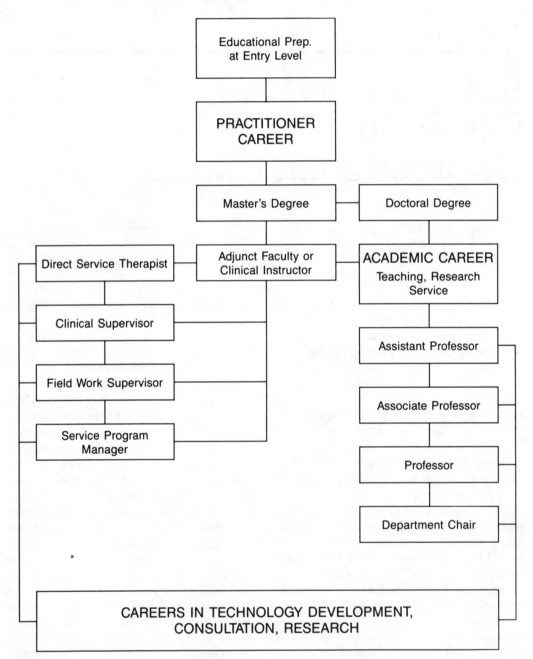

Figure 16.1. Adapted from Colman W: Organizational roles and relationships. In Bair J, Gray M (eds): *The Occupational Therapy Manager*. Rockville, MD, American Occupational Therapy Association, 1985, p. 205.

and must think far ahead of present needs. Together the program manager and staff develop program goals, policies, and procedures and establish standards of care. The manager is responsible for staffing the program, organizing the staffing patterns, and establishing lines of responsibility. The manager supervises the work of program staff and deals with any personnel problems that may arise. If the service program provides student education, the manager may also be responsible for developing and implementing a student program and supervising student performance. Supervision of related personnel (COTAs, aides, clerical staff, or volunteers) may also be part of the manager's responsibility.

Occupational therapy managers are accountable for the fiscal management of their programs and must provide the kind of documentation of service that is demanded by the administration for cost accounting and fiscal control. The manager participates in the development of the program budget and monitors expenditures. A knowledge of cost accounting and financial analysis is important for today's program managers (2). The manager also oversees the clinical service program and directs quality assurance studies to determine whether the service program is functioning effectively (3). The program manager may also serve a coordinating role, ensuring that the occupational therapy program does not duplicate services offered by other departments and works cooperatively with them.

Most occupational therapy managers rise to that position through years of experience working in their institution or organization. Beginning as staff therapists, they may later accept additional responsibilities as supervisors or take on limited administrative functions. As they gain experience in working within the organization, on-the-job training and continuing education may prepare them for higher level management responsibilities. Some

managers seek additional education in health care management to do their jobs more effectively.

In 1986 AOTA reported that 2390 of its members belonged to the Special Interest Section on Administration and Management. In the first issue of the special interest section's newsletter(4), occupational therapy managers commented that they found their service programs were being strongly affected by demographic, sociological, political, environmental, and technological changes. They believed that their jobs had changed significantly during the past few years as major changes occurred in health care delivery and reimbursement of services. Many expressed a need to acquire advanced skills in business administration and requested continuing education in marketing, reimbursement, quality control, budgeting, and program development.

Occupational therapy continues to be a human service field, but it is being forced to become more cost conscious and business oriented. In the future occupational therapy managers will probably need advanced education in business administration and management. The role of occupational therapy program manager is an advanced career option that requires both clinical experience and administrative skills. The 1985 AOTA Manpower Study(5) predicted an even greater emphasis on data-based management, documentation, and accountability in the future. Computers are increasingly being used to record and store clinical and financial data. As higher levels of productivity are demanded by health care organizations, more skilled and accountable management will be needed in occupational therapy service programs.

EDUCATION

There is a serious shortage of occupational therapy educators in the United

States today. According to 1985 data(5), there were only 566 occupational therapists serving as faculty members in OTR entry-level educational programs. Another 182 persons were teaching in technical level programs. Educational programs have continued to develop, with 61 colleges and universities offering entry-level OTR education in 1985 and 58 colleges or technical institutes offering COTA education (6). The number of available faculty has not increased accordingly. Part of the reason for this discrepancy is that in the 1980s many colleges and universities began to expect that potential faculty members would hold a PhD or equivalent doctoral degree to qualify for a faculty position. Only about 140 occupational therapists held doctoral degrees in 1984, so the supply lagged far behind the demand. In COTA education the master's degree was considered the major qualification for faculty, and about 4000 OTRs held master's degrees in 1984, making a larger pool of prospective faculty available for COTA programs. The AOTA actively encouraged graduate study for OTRs by offering graduate fellowships, but the pool of doctoral degree holders continues to be small within the field.

Most occupational therapy faculty members come from the ranks of clinicians. They have often entered graduate study to add to their professional knowledge and clinical skills, but some find that the academic setting is appealing and offers a satisfying and interesting career option. Mitchell (7) describes a pattern of career development from clinician to faculty member and discusses how the faculty role differs from the clinical role. The novice faculty member must learn to prepare courses, remain current with developments in the field, conduct research, and serve on department and college committees. The clinician's primary focus of attention is the client and the client's needs. In the academic setting, the focus

is on student needs; the new faculty member must help students develop the knowledge and skills that will allow them to function effectively in the clinical setting. In occupational therapy, education is a joint venture by academic faculty and fieldwork educators. Clinicians who provide fieldwork experiences for students play an important role in the educational process and contribute to the educational program through serving as role models and offering direct experience in subjects the student has studied in the classroom. Occupational therapy clinicians, both OTRs and COTAs, may serve as adjunct faculty or clinical instructors in academic programs and may provide guest lectures, teach courses, or supervise students in level I fieldwork.

The individual who accepts a faculty position in a college or university has three responsibilities: teaching, research, and service. Initially a good deal of time is spent developing courses, designing appropriate learning experiences for students, and assessing student progress. The faculty member must establish a research program and is expected to publish results that will add to the knowledge base of the field. Service on college and university committees, as well as professional and public service, is expected. The new faculty member must learn these new roles and master the art of teaching.

Career advancement takes place through promotion from assistant to associate professor, the rank at which tenure is awarded at most colleges and universities. Attainment of tenure depends on how well the faculty member fulfills his or her threefold responsibilities. Occupational therapy faculty have often found achieving tenured rank difficult for many reasons. As a service field, occupational therapy tends to encourage the development of clinical skills rather than research skills. The profession has not always valued research and scholarship as highly as have the more traditional academic disciplines; only recently have occupational therapists begun to earn doctoral degrees in larger numbers. In 1984 only 45% of occupational therapy faculty members were tenured at their institutions. Faculty turnover has occurred at a rate of approximately 10% per year. Some faculty return to clinical positions, while others accept positions in other academic programs. It will be critical to occupational therapy education for educators to earn tenure in greater numbers. Masagatani and Grant(8) offer some helpful suggestions for faculty members to develop the necessary skills and accomplishments to qualify for tenured rank.

Once tenure is achieved, the occupational therapy faculty member may eventually be promoted to the rank of full professor. This is the highest academic rank and usually reflects national and international recognition in the field. Full professors are regarded as authorities in their discipline and are the senior members of an educational program's faculty. The tenured faculty member may fulfill the additional position of department chair. The role of a chairman of an academic department is comparable with that of a service program manager, but the goals and priorities of clinical and academic organizations are quite different. Colleges and universities are communities of scholars whose primary mission is the development and dissemination of knowledge. The department chair must recruit and hire new faculty members, develop and maintain a curriculum that is current with developments in the field, promote faculty research and engage in research activities, manage the finances and resources of the academic program, and participate in college and university committees. If the shortage of occupational therapy faculty members is serious, the shortage of chairs of academic departments is even more severe (9).

Because of the current and projected shortfalls in occupational therapy personnel, the 1985 AOTA Manpower Report(5) made the following recommendations:

1. Encourage the expansion of the occupational therapy educational system through the development of new educational programs in under-served areas of the country; encourage non-traditional education programs; promote more entry-level master's degree programs.
2. Recruit more students into occupational therapy educational programs; and
3. Increase the numbers of qualified occupational therapy faculty.

Expansion of occupational therapy education is needed in order to meet the manpower needs of the next decade. There will be an increased demand for occupational therapy faculty at all levels—technical, entry-level professional, and graduate education.

RESEARCH

Research has been a high priority in occupational therapy for the past two decades. The need to relate practice to theory and to show scientific evidence of the effectiveness of occupational therapy services has given rise to an increased demand for occupational therapy research. The problem again has been one of manpower. Researchers are highly educated individuals who have mastered the tools of scholarly inquiry. They are skilled in identifying researchable questions of significance to their field and in developing methods for studying these questions. This specialized skill can only be gained through a research-oriented doctoral degree program, but only a very small number of occupational therapists have completed this level of education. There is a large gap between the number of researchers needed in occupational therapy and the number presently available. Students who have an interest in the scientific study of occupational therapy problems should be strongly encouraged to continue their education to the doctoral level.

Although much of the research published in occupational therapy (and in other fields) is the product of university faculty members, there is a strong need for clinicians to take part in research activities as well. The OTRs and COTAs practicing in clinical settings can contribute to research efforts by participating in collaborative studies with faculty members, by collecting data on specific types of client problems and occupational therapy interventions, and by utilizing information gained from research reports in professional journals. Dunn (10) emphasizes the fact that clinicians can and do develop into researchers. They often face constraints from their administration, however, over the time spent in research activity that the administrator may feel should more properly be devoted to client service. Establishing a partnership between clinicians and faculty researchers may be the best solution to this dilemma. Dunn further suggests that clinicians can contribute to research by contributing money to research foundations, responding to research surveys, and supporting the efforts of their professional organizations to provide funding and resources for research in occupational therapy.

There are also constraints on faculty members who engage in research. Teaching often makes heavy demands on their time, and they may be more concerned about maintaining their clinical skills than in developing the necessary research skills. Labovitz (11) suggests that faculty members may wish to begin their research career as a collaborator, either with colleagues or students. They can also teach their students to value research information and encourage them to develop some of the basic attitudes and interests of the researcher.

To be successful in a research career, an individual needs to have an inquiring mind and be able to look at problems critically and objectively. A good statistical background is necessary to analyze research data effectively, and computer skills are useful. Most importantly, the occupational therapy researcher must be familiar with the theories and basic principles of the field and able to identify research problems that will add to the knowledge of occupational therapy theory and practice. A career in research will bring professional recognition as well as personal satisfaction to the individual who is interested in solving problems that until now have remained unsolved.

CONSULTATION

Experienced occupational therapists who come from either a clinical or an academic background may be self-employed as consultants to organizations that request their services. An AOTA publication on private practice and consultation (12) defines consultation as giving advice, assistance, or an opinion based on professional knowledge, skill, or judgment. Consultation usually pertains to the application of occupational therapy treatment or to collaborative health programming. Thornton(13) emphasizes that consultants come from outside of organizations and that their purpose is to help the people within achieve the organizations' goals and purposes. The advice offered by consultants may be accepted or rejected by organizations. Consultants work, often on a contract basis, for the owners of organizations who hire them and share their expertise with the members of the organizations. The consultant's job is to listen and observe, identify the problems, and help the members of the organizations find ways to solve those problems. Consultants perform their role by working through other people. They consult about their discipline or area of expertise. Consultants are troubleshooters whose services may be sought for help with establishing, implementing, or evaluating occupational therapy services.

Occupational therapy consultants have pioneered in the development of new practice specialties in the field and have created jobs that were later filled by OTRs and COTAs. In some states consultants were used by school districts to help set up occupational therapy programs in public schools. Later these programs were operated by occupational therapy personnel employed by the school system. Some types of occupational therapy home health services were initiated in the same way. Occupational therapy consultants are often able to break new ground and develop new areas of practice (14). Consultants are agents of planned change and frequently function as educators or facilitators in order to make things happen. Consultants can only recommend change, however. It is up to the organization to decide whether to follow through on the suggestions.

Occupational therapy consultants may be found in private practice, in school systems, in industry, in occupational therapy departments of hospitals or rehabilitation centers, and in academic programs. Because of the varied environments in which consultation takes place, consultants must be creative and flexible. They must have broad clinical experience and a good knowledge of current trends and issues in health care. Maturity, a sense of humor, and good timing are also important characteristics for anyone who is considering a career as a consultant. Smith (15) discusses some of the things to consider before becoming a consultant. She suggests that one should assess the depth of one's professional expertise, consider

the ethical issues involved in consultation, and look for the reasons that underlie an organization's request for consultative services.

Consultation is considered an advanced career in occupational therapy because of the broad range of experience and depth of knowledge that it requires. Epstein (14) believes that the need for consultants and private practitioners working at the forefront of practice will increase dramatically in the next few years. Gilfoyle (16), in her 1984 Slagle lecture to members of the American Occupational Therapy Association, looked at the directions that occupational therapy practice might take and predicted that new service delivery patterns involving consultation, monitoring, and collaborative programming would be imperative in the future. For the experienced occupational therapy clinician or faculty member, consultation offers opportunities to develop and implement innovative programming ideas.

TECHNOLOGY DEVELOPMENT

The rapid development and proliferation of technology has affected occupational therapy practice, just as it has affected many other fields. Already technological advances are being put to work in occupational therapy clinics. There are now many clinics using the computer as a tool in retraining cognitive skills. Complex electronic control systems have been developed that enable severely handicapped individuals to control their immediate environment. Voice-activated input units allow handicapped workers to perform jobs that were previously closed to them. Computerized systems of motor control that may enable paralyzed individuals to walk and resume many of their daily activities are on the horizon. In the management of occupational therapy services the computer has also become a necessary tool. Most health care organizations now use computerized billing, record keeping, and data analysis, and academic institutions are looking at computerized learning applications. Computers and satellite communications may eventually allow us to consult, present professional papers, teach, and observe programs in other parts of the world.

Occupational therapy personnel who have advanced knowledge of computer applications could be in the forefront of this revolution. Because occupational therapists are skilled in activity analysis and adaptation, they are in a good position to work with biomedical engineers to develop new technological aids that can minimize many of the functional limitations imposed by handicapping conditions. Burke (17) suggests that such technology can effectively be applied to our knowledge of human occupation and to our work with individuals who have physical or psychosocial disorders.

Few occupational therapists have entered this field of technological development, but interest in it is increasing. In 1985, 40 occupational therapists attended the annual conference of the Rehabilitation Engineering Society of North America (RESNA) and heard papers presented on such topics as prosthetics and orthotics, sensory aids, computer applications, robotics, seating and positioning, powered mobility, augmentative communication, and technology transfer (18). In 1986, RESNA changed its name to the Association for the Advancement of Rehabilitation Technology to better reflect the interdisciplinary nature of its members. Occupational therapists are becoming actively involved in this and other organizations concerned with technology development. As a new advanced career for occupational therapists, it will no doubt demand advanced education to acquire computer and engineering skills, but for those persons who wish to combine an interest in occupational therapy with an interest in equipment design, the field of technology development may provide exciting opportunities and challenges.

SUMMARY

In all of the indirect service careers discussed in this chapter, additional education or experience beyond the entry level is needed. Occupational therapy personnel move through various stages in the course of their careers (Fig. 16.1). Although all begin as practitioners, many move on fairly quickly to positions that require higher levels of skill and greater responsibility. Some individuals may prefer to remain in clinical work, while others may move on to an academic career. Clinicians may enter a graduate program to gain more expertise in a specialized area of practice or to prepare themselves for a career in management, consultation, technology development, or research. Although it is often recommended that graduates of entry-level educational programs acquire some clinical experience before entering graduate study, it is also acceptable to enter a graduate program immediately after completing entry-level education. This choice must be made based on the individual's career goals and expectations. As knowledge and skills increase, the indirect service careers in occupational therapy open up new horizons to the practitioner. Students are advised to consider their long-range career goals even while they are enrolled in entry-level education and plan their career pattern in accordance with their interests and abilities.

DISCUSSION QUESTIONS

1. Invite one or more OTRs who are employed in indirect service careers to your class. Ask them to share their

experiences with you. How did they enter their advanced occupational therapy career? What sort of rewards or satisfactions has it brought them?

2. Do any of the indirect service careers interest you? If so, why? How could you prepare yourself for this career?

3. Many COTAs and OTRs are reluctant to give up their clinical role in favor of an indirect service career. Would it be possible to combine a direct service role with an indirect service career? Suggest some ways of doing this.

4. Can you think of other indirect service careers that exist now or may develop in occupational therapy? Give some examples.

REFERENCES

1. Colman W: Organizational roles and relationships. In Bair J, Gray M (eds): *The Occupational Therapy Manager.* Rockville, MD, American Occupational Therapy Association, 1985, pp 201–205.

2. Laase S: Financial management. In Bair J, Gray M (eds): *The Occupational Therapy Manager.* Rockville, MD, American Occupational Therapy Association, 1985, pp 83–122.

3. Joe B: Quality assurance. In Bair J, Gray M (eds): *The Occupational Therapy Manager.* Rockville, MD, American Occupational Therapy Association, 1985, pp 251–265.

4. Smith B, Scammahorn G: The occupational therapy manager: old title, new job, different needs. *Administration and Management Special Interest Section Newsletter* 1(1):1, 2, 4, 1985.

5. Ad Hoc Commission on Occupational Therapy Manpower. *Occupational Therapy Manpower: A Plan for Progress.* Rockville, MD, American Occupational Therapy Association, 1985, pp 26, 41–49, 57–59, 61–64.

6. Research Information and Evaluation Division. *1986 Education Data Survey.* Rockville, MD, American Occupational Therapy Association, 1986, pp 1, 9.

7. Mitchell M: Professional development: clinician to academician. *AJOT* 39:368–373, 1985.

8. Masagatani G, Grant H: Managing an academic career. *AJOT* 40:83–88, 1986.

9. Sieg K: Chairing the academic occupational therapy department: a job analysis. *AJOT* 40:89–95, 1986.

10. Dunn W: Occupational therapy's challenge: caregiving and research. *AJOT* 39:259–264, 1985.

11. Labovitz D: Faculty research. A pluralistic approach. *AJOT* 40:207–208, 1986.

12. The occupational therapist as a consultant. *Private Practice Information Packet.* Rockville, MD, American Occupational Therapy Association, 1986, pp 37.

13. Thornton P: An approach to consultation. *Private Practice Information Packet.* Rockville, MD, American Occupational Therapy Association, 1986, pp 40–49.

14. Epstein C: Consultation: Communicating and facilitating. In Bair J, Gray M (eds): *The Occupational Therapy Manager.* Rockville, MD, American Occupational Therapy Association, 1985, pp 299–321.

15. Smith, S: Private practice—home care—consultation for the occupational therapist. *Private Practice Information Packet.* Rockville, MD, American Occupational Therapy Association, 1986, pp 55–58.

16. Gilfoyle E: Eleanor Clarke Slagle Lecturship, 1984: Transformation of a Profession. *AJOT* 38:575–584, 1984.

17. Burke J: Occupational therapy: a focus for roles in practice. *AJOT* 38:24–28, 1984.

18. RESNA Conference features occupational therapists. *Occup Ther News* 40(9):5, 1986.

Current Trends and Future Outlook

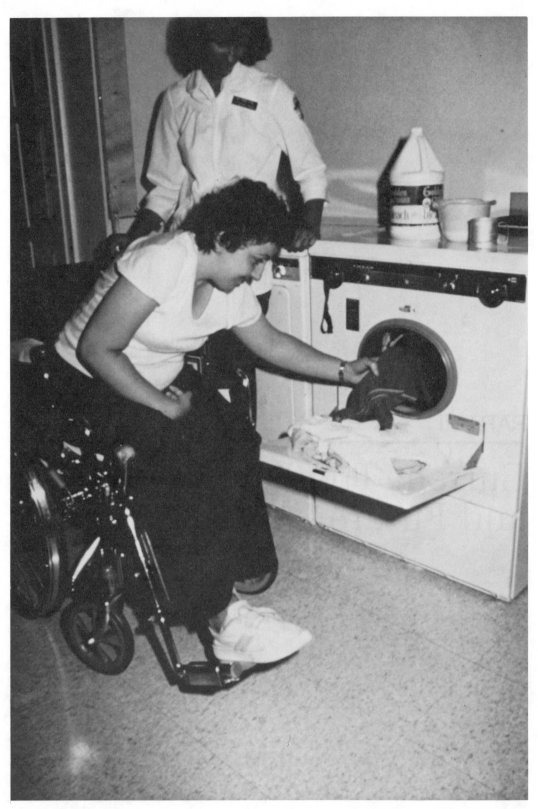

SEVENTEEN

Professional Organizations

In any profession practitioners inevitably feel the need to join forces with their colleagues in order to educate the public about the field, to achieve acceptance and recognition by outside groups, and to promote the advancement of the profession. Professional organizations help to achieve these goals and provide a variety of services that are helpful to their members. In occupational therapy, professional organizations have developed at the state, national, and international level. In this chapter we look at the professional organizations at each level to see what they contribute to the field and how they support the activities of their members.

THE AMERICAN OCCUPATIONAL THERAPY ASSOCIATION

In 1917 a small group of early pioneers in occupational therapy met to discuss forming a national organization that could unify the isolated occupational therapists then practicing and encourage the planned development of the new field. The founding members included George Barton, an architect who had suffered from tuberculosis and other health problems and who became convinced from personal experience that therapeutic activity could aid in recovery from physical and mental disorders. His secretary, Isabel Newton, also attended the planning meeting. Other founding members were Susan Johnson, a craftsperson and early occupational therapy educator; Eleanor Clarke Slagle, an early student of curative occupations who later developed occupational therapy programs in Maryland and Illinois; Susan Tracy, a nurse who recognized the value of occupation for hospitalized patients and who taught an early course on that topic; Thomas Kidner, a British architect who developed a system of vocational rehabilitation for disabled Canadian veterans of World War I; and Dr. William Rush Dunton, Jr., a psychiatrist who promoted the use of occupation as part of the treatment program for the mentally ill. This diverse group of people shared a common interest in the use of occupation as a therapeutic tool, and they agreed to establish the National Society for the Promotion of Occupational Therapy on March 15, 1917. Barton was elected the first president of the society, with Slagle serving as vice president. The new organization took on the tasks of defining the field, expanding the practice of occupational therapy from the mental hospitals where it had originated into other areas of rehabilitation, and promoting the use of occupation as therapy.

In 1921 the name of the society was changed to the American Occupational Therapy Association (AOTA), and that name has endured to the present. In the early 1920s physicians and hospital administrators were beginning to seek occupational therapists to work in hospitals and urged the association to maintain a registry of qualified practitioners. Before doing so, however, the association undertook to establish minimum educational standards for occupational therapists. This was achieved in 1923, with a minimum of 12 months of training, including 3 months of required hospital practice. The young association had also begun to publish a journal. The Archives of Occupational Therapy, first published in 1922, was owned and edited by Dr. Dunton. In 1925 its title was changed to Occupational Therapy and Rehabilitation, and subscription to the journal became a member benefit of the organization. In 1926 the organization's House of Delegates voted to establish a registry of qualified occupational therapists, and in 1932 the first registry was published with 318 names listed. In the same year the association moved from temporary quarters to rented office space in New York City and employed a secretary to help manage its affairs (1).

In 1931 the AOTA assumed another responsibility: accrediting occupational therapy educational programs. This function was shared with the American Medical Association. As a result of the initial visits to schools, new educational standards were developed; these were adopted in 1935. In 1945 the association reconsidered the question of professional qualifications and developed a written essay examination that all potential occupational therapists were required to take and pass in order to qualify. The examination

was revised in 1947 and was changed to a multiple-choice format. In the same year the association began to publish a new professional journal, the American Journal of Occupational Therapy, which eventually replaced Occupational Therapy and Rehabilitation as the official publication of the association.

By 1950 the association had begun to award honors and recognitions to those members who had made significant contributions to the field. In 1955 the association outgrew its office space and moved to a new location in New York City. During this period there was an increasing demand for occupational therapy personnel, and in an effort to meet his demand the AOTA developed educational standards for programs preparing occupational therapy assistants. In 1959 the association took on the additional function of reviewing and approving COTA educational programs. In the early 1960s the organization was restructured to improve its efficiency and ability to respond to member concerns. A major focus during this period was the encouragement of state licensure for OTRs and COTAs. The association aided state organizations in writing licensure acts and provided consultation as state groups moved their practice acts through the legislative process. The AOTA was also becoming more active in legislative matters on the federal level and represented the interests of occupational therapists when bills concerning health care funding and programming were being considered by Congress. In 1972 the national office of the association was moved to Washington, D.C., to facilitate participation in legislative matters; AOTA later purchased its own building for use as organizational headquarters (1).

GOALS AND FUNCTIONS OF AOTA

According to its bylaws, the purpose of the AOTA is "to act as an advocate for occupational therapy in order to enhance the health of the public in its medical, community, and educational environments through research, education, action, service, and the establishment and enforcement of standards"(2). In 1975 the organization's Delegate Assembly adopted a long range plan that was intended to guide the activities of the association in the years to come. The following are some of the goals identified in that document:

---

1. To provide opportunities for the expression of member concerns, to anticipate emerging issues, to facilitate decision making, and to expedite the translation of those decisions into action.
2. To support the development of research and knowledge bases for the practice of occupational therapy, and to promote the dissemination and sharing of such information.
3. To facilitate and support an educational system for occupational therapy which responds to current needs, anticipates, plans for, and accommodates to change.
4. To promote occupational therapy as a viable health profession.
5. To promote an understanding of occupational therapy which will have a strong and significant impact on health policy and health care.
6. To facilitate the formation of partnerships with consumers to promote optimal health conditions for the public. (3)

STRUCTURE AND MEMBERSHIP

From an initial membership of 40 persons in 1917, the AOTA had grown to a membership of 40,000 in 1985 (4). Its current activities are the result of a partnership between a paid national office staff and occupational therapy personnel who volunteer to serve on committees and commissions or who hold elected office within the organization. Figure 17.1 shows

the organization of the AOTA national office.

Eighty-five staff members are employed in the various divisions of the organization to carry out its day-to-day activities. An Executive Director is responsible for supervising the operations of the national office and for implementing the policies established by the AOTA Representative Assembly. The Executive Director represents the association at the national level and serves as spokesperson for the organization to outside groups.

The voluntary sector of the organization consists of the individual members (OTRs, COTAs, and students) of the association. Members are represented on the two major action bodies of the organization, the Representative Assembly and the Executive Board. Figure 17.2 shows the structure of the voluntary sector of AOTA. The Representative Assembly is the legislative and policy-making body of the association and is composed of representatives and alternates who are elected from state organizations through a system of proportional representation. Those states with less than 5% of the total association's voting membership are entitled to one elected representative and one alternate. States that have between 5% and 10% of the association's total membership may have two representatives and two alternates, and states with more than 10% may have three representatives and three alternates. Representatives and alternates serve for a three-year term or until successors have been elected. The Representative Assembly elects its own officers of speaker, vice speaker, and recorder. This body meets annually and formulates and approves policies for the association, approves its budget, fixes membership fees, and approves position statements on behalf of the association (2).

The Representative Assembly maintains three standing commissions and an intercommission council that promotes communication and interaction between

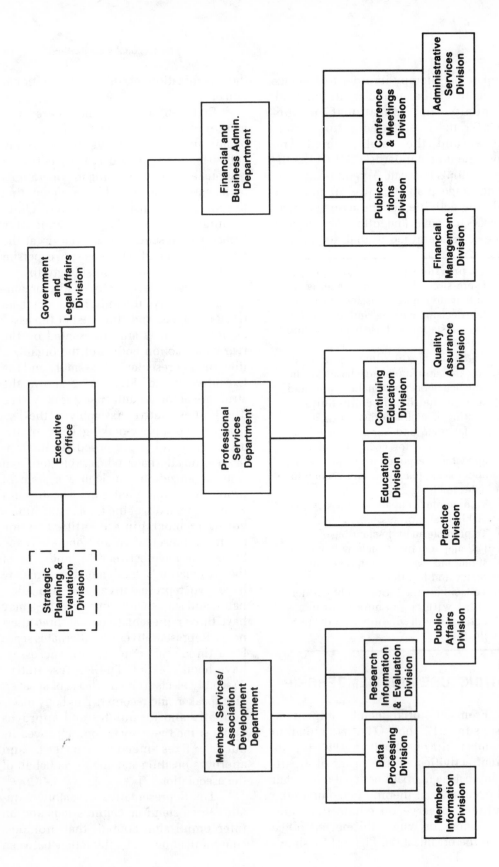

Figure 17.1 National office organization, the American Occupational Therapy Association, May 1982. [From AOTA *Member Handbook*. Rockville, MD, American Occupational Therapy Association, 1980, p A9 (revised 1982).]

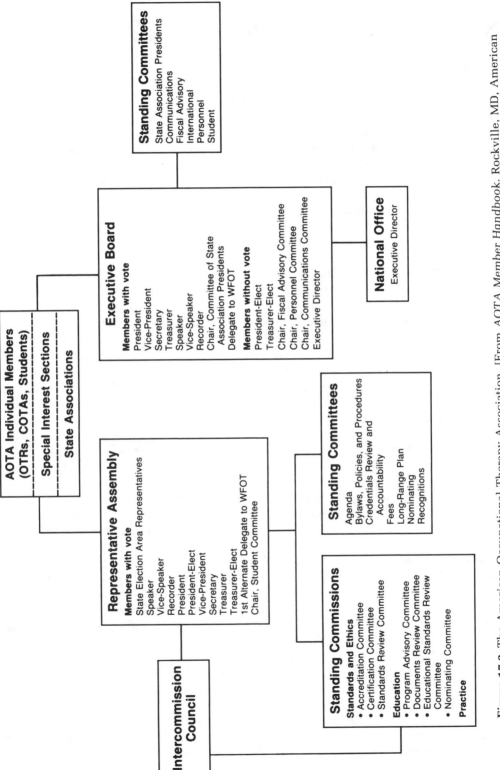

Figure 17.2 The American Occupational Therapy Association. [From *AOTA Member Handbook*. Rockville, MD, American Occupational Therapy Association, 1980 (revised 1982).]

the commissions. The three commissions have specific areas of function. The Commission on Standards and Ethics recommends the approval of necessary standards and ethics documents to the Representative Assembly. It reviews all standards and position papers for the association and enforces the standards and ethics of the organization. The Commission on Education promotes quality education and educational standards for programs preparing OTRs and COTAs relative to educator, student, and consumer needs. The Commission on Practice promotes quality occupational therapy practice and develops practice standards for OTRs and COTAs relative to practitioner and consumer needs. These commissions meet at set times during the year to conduct their business and report back to the Representative Assembly. In addition to these bodies, the Representative Assembly maintains a group of standing committees that are charged with specific tasks related to the affairs of the association. In 1986 certification of qualified OTRs and COTAs was removed from the functions of AOTA and was placed under the jurisdiction of the National Certification Board. This group is separate from AOTA and monitors and controls the certification process.

The second action body of the organization is the Executive Board. This group is charged with managing the affairs of the association and consists of its elected officers, the chairman of the Committee of State Association Presidents, and the association's delegate to the World Federation of Occupational Therapists. Five additional office holders and the AOTA Executive Director attend board meetings but have no vote. The Executive Board carries out the ongoing activities of the organization and implements the policies approved by the Representative Assembly. It monitors the finances of the association, prepares the budget, manages the national office, supervises grants and contracts, and

prepares and approves plans of action. The Executive Board also maintains a number of standing committees that carry out specific functions.

Seven special interest sections have been formed to promote communication between members working in specialized areas of practice. They include the areas of administration and management, developmental disabilities, gerontology, mental health, physical disabilities, sensory integration, and work programs.

MEMBERSHIP BENEFITS

Subscription to the *American Journal of Occupational Therapy* and other publications of the association, membership in a special interest section, voting privileges in the association, and the right to hold office and to participate on committees and commissions of the association have been traditional membership benefits of the AOTA. In 1986, AOTA announced an expanded list of benefits for its members (5). They include an information service network, computer access to the association's occupational therapy library, publication of an employment bulletin, an honors and recognitions program, an improved insurance program, and a financial benefits program that finances loans, scholarships, and research grants. The 1985 annual report of the association described the ways in which the organization was mobilizing to meet the projected manpower needs of the field, preparing its members to serve new markets, lobbying to improve consumer access to occupational therapy services, and informing the public about occupational therapy's roles in health care and rehabilitation. In addition to its efforts to influence health legislation through lobbying, the association's political action committee raised $30,000 in 1985 and supported 39 candidates for public office (4).

Members play an active role in the AOTA. They may raise issues for discussion, formulate resolutions to be considered by the Representative Assembly, instruct their state delegates in voting on specific issues, and utilize the resources of the association to obtain information about occupational therapy education and practice. The national office staff provides the support services needed to keep the association running smoothly and effectively. The office staff and the members of the association work together to fulfill the goals of the organization.

THE AMERICAN OCCUPATIONAL THERAPY FOUNDATION

A second national organization in occupational therapy is the American Occupational Therapy Foundation. Created in 1965, the foundation was established for charitable, scientific, literary, and educational purposes. As a philanthropic organization, the foundation accepts donations and bequests from AOTA members and friends of occupational therapy. With these funds it supports a program of scholarship awards for OTR and COTA students in entry-level programs and graduate fellowships for students in advanced degree programs. Another major activity is the publication of monographs, public information materials, and the *Occupational Therapy Journal of Research* in order to increase public understanding of occupational therapy and to disseminate the results of scientific research conducted within the field. Promotion of occupational therapy research is a goal of the foundation, and it awards research grants to investigators who submit well-documented research proposals for review. A further interest of the foundation is the maintenance of an occupational therapy library. Donations to the library are actively encouraged, and the collection now num-

bers approximately 2000 volumes. Library materials are available to researchers and soon will be accessible by computer.

The American Occupational Therapy Foundation is a charitable organization that receives monies through donations and utilizes these funds to benefit occupational therapy students, practitioners, and researchers. It is entirely separate from the AOTA and has its own elected officers who administer its programs (6).

STATE OCCUPATIONAL THERAPY ORGANIZATIONS

State occupational therapy associations are the grass roots level of the AOTA. The AOTA bylaws (2) provide for the recognition of state associations that have at least 10 voting members and that submit a set of bylaws for approval by the Committee of State Association Presidents of AOTA. State associations may elect delegates and alternates to the Representative Assembly and thus play a role in the development and implementation of policies at the national level. The purpose of state organizations is to collaborate with the AOTA and to carry out on the local level activities that advance the objectives of that organization. Once constituted, state associations may elect their own officers and carry out their own program of activities. Many state associations hold annual conferences, sponsor continuing education programs, provide information services to their members, and organize study groups and special interest groups. Today each of the 50 states has a state occupational therapy association, as do the District of Columbia and Puerto Rico. State associations may carry out AOTA projects on a local level and are active in communicating their concerns and needs to the national organization. A strong partnership has been established between state

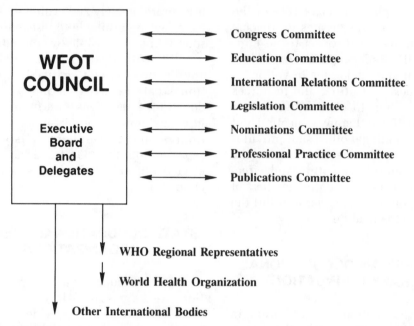

Figure 17.3 Organization of the World Federation of Occupational Therapists. (From *World Federation of Occupational Therapists*, WFOT, 1986.)

and national associations, with each level supporting the work of the other.

WORLD FEDERATION OF OCCUPATIONAL THERAPISTS

Discussions about the formation of an international occupational therapy organization began in 1951, and in 1952 delegates from nine countries met in Great Britain to hold a planning meeting. The organization that resulted from their efforts was named the World Federation of Occupational Therapists (WFOT); in 1986 it included 31 member countries or territories and 5 associate member countries. Full membership requires that a country have a professional occupational therapy association of at least 12 members who are citizens of that country, have a constitution,

and have an educational program in occupational therapy that meets WFOT standards. Associate membership requires a membership of four qualified occupational therapists who are citizens of the country. Figure 17.3 shows the structure of the WFOT.

The WFOT has identified its major objectives as follows:

1. To act as the official international organization for the promotion of occupational therapy; to hold international congresses.
2. To promote international cooperation among occupational therapy associations, occupational therapists, and between them and other allied professional groups.
3. To maintain the ethics of the profession and to advance the practice and standards of occupational therapy.

4. To promote internationally recognized standards for education of occupational therapists.
5. To facilitate the international exchange and placement of therapists and students.
6. To facilitate the exchange of information and publications, and to promote research. (7)

Individual membership in the WFOT is open to any qualified occupational therapist who is a member in good standing of a full or an associate member organization. The ongoing business of the federation is carried on by a council that meets every two years. A joint congress and council meeting are held every four years. In council meetings, each member country is represented by a delegate and has one vote. A number of standing committees carry on specific tasks assigned by the council and report on their work at the next council meeting. Much of the committee work is conducted by correspondence, since members live and work in different parts of the world. The congresses that are sponsored by the WFOT are international meetings at which papers are presented on topics relevant to occupational therapy. Professional and commercial exhibits are displayed, and film programs are shown. Social activities are included as well to promote friendship and communication between participants. Congresses are scheduled at different locations every four years and are planned and publicized well in advance.

Among the current activities of the WFOT are approving educational programs in occupational therapy that meet WFOT standards, creating opportunities for international experiences for occupational therapists and students, maintaining liaisons with international health organizations, encouraging the development of occupational therapy services in underserved areas of the world, and publishing monographs, bulletins, and congress proceedings. The WFOT makes valuable contributions to occupational therapy practice and education on an international scale and provides a connecting link between the national associations of member countries.

SUMMARY

The professional organizations that have been described provide critical support and development services to their members and promote occupational therapy practice, education, and research on local, national, and international levels. These organizations are the voice of occupational therapy to people and organizations outside the field and represent the interests of OTRs, COTAs, students, and consumers of occupational therapy services. It is largely because of the efforts of these organizations that occupational therapy has received positive recognition and acceptance by other health care professions, by legislators, and by the general public. Professional organizations have contributed substantially to the advancement of occupational therapy and will continue to do so. As new challenges arise, the professional organizations will be prepared to initiate policies and actions that will benefit occupational therapy personnel and the clients whom they serve.

DISCUSSION QUESTIONS

1. Invite an officer or member of the Occupational Therapy Association in your state to visit your class. What are the issues that this organization is currently discussing? What actions is the organization taking?

2. How does the state organization relate to the AOTA?

3. Do professional organizations contribute to their members' sense of professional identity? How?

4. Does your curriculum have a student professional organization? If so, what activities is it involved in?

5. Many OTRs and COTAs belong to other organizations in addition to occupational therapy organizations. Interview some OTRs or COTAs and find out what non-OT organizations they belong to and why.

6. Are you a student member of the AOTA? What are some of the membership benefits for students?

REFERENCES

1. Reed K, Sanderson S: Development of a professional organization. In: *Concepts of Occupational Therapy*, ed 2. Baltimore, MD, Williams & Wilkins, 1983, pp 182–193.
2. Bylaws. In: *AOTA Member Handbook*. Rockville, MD, American Occupational Therapy Association, 1980, pp E1–E9.
3. Long range plan. In: *AOTA Member Handbook*. Rockville, MD, American Occupational Therapy Association, 1980, p A3–A4.
4. *The Five Minute Annual Report*. Rockville, MD, American Occupational Therapy Association, 1985, pp 1–6.
5. AOTA member benefits expanded for 1987. *Occup Ther News* 40(9):4, 1986.
6. *1985 Annual Report*. Rockville, MD, American Occupational Therapy Foundation, 1985, pp 1–2.
7. *World Federation of Occupational Therapists*. WFOT, Graphic Services, University of Western Ontario, London, Ont., 1986.

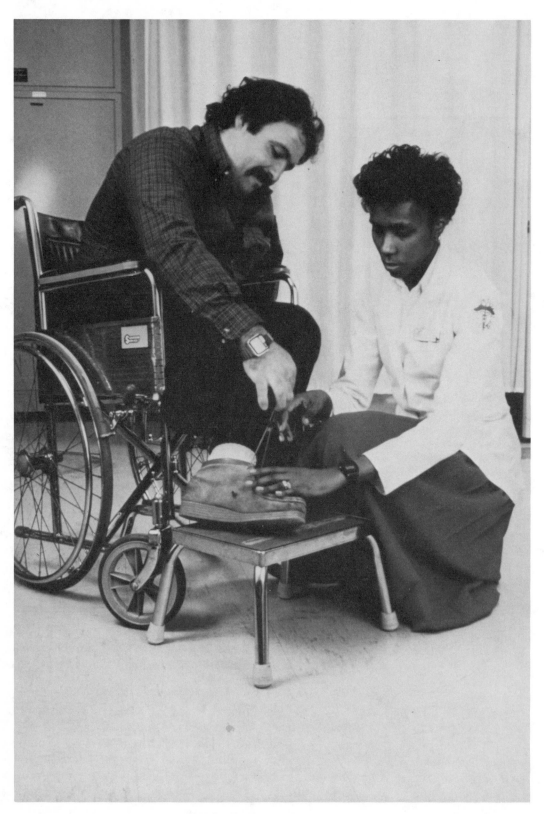

EIGHTEEN

International Occupational Therapy

Although the United States has the largest number of practicing occupational therapists, occupational therapy is truly an international field. In 1986, 31 countries or territories had occupational therapy associations and were full members of the World Federation of Occupational Therapists (WFOT). Five additional countries held associate memberships in the WFOT, and negotiations were underway with Malta, Pakistan, and Greece for future membership. Occupational therapists are practicing their profession in many parts of the world and have been able to adapt occupational therapy concepts and therapeutic approaches to different cultures and environments. This chapter introduces the student to occupational therapy on an international scale and presents some examples of practice in countries outside the United States.

Table 18.1 provides information about occupational therapy organizations around the world that are members or associate members of the WFOT (1). Many of these organizations publish a journal to keep their members informed of professional developments. A total of 217 schools were educating occupational therapists in 30 different countries in 1985 (2). Educa-

tional programs outside the United States must meet standards established by the WFOT in order to be approved by them. These educational standards are somewhat broader than those used in the United States and contain some content areas not required by the Educational Essentials of the American Occupational Therapy Association. In many foreign educational programs for the occupational therapist, the credentials awarded are different from those in the United States. Although some programs award a baccalaureate degree, others offer a diploma or certificate in occupational therapy or give a technician title. Many educational programs abroad are located in technical schools or in hospital-based training schools. These institutions do not grant degrees but provide technical education in specialized fields. Most foreign occupational therapy educational programs are three or four years in length and provide concentrated education in occupational therapy theory and practice. Some countries also offer postgraduate educational programs.

The largest number of occupational therapists practicing abroad seem to be employed in institutional settings. In a growing number of countries (Australia,

Table 18.1.
Incomplete List of WFOT Member Organizations and Their Current Activities[a]

Country or Territory	Name of Organization	Number of Qualified OTR Members	Total Membership	Number of Schools	Journal	Recent Developments
Argentina	Association Argentine de Terapestas Ocupacionales			2		
Australia	Australian Assoc. of Occupational Therapists	1,790	1,914	5	Australian Occupational Therapy Journal	Significant advancements in private practice and occupational health and safety.
Austria	Verband der Diplomiertan Beschaltigungs- and Arbietstherapeuten, Osterreichs	259	320	3	ERGO	
Belgium	Federation Nationale Belge Des Ergotherapeuten			8		
Canada	Canadian Assoc. of Occupational Therapists (CAOT)	3,549	3,520	11	Canadian Journal of Occupational Therapy	Field trial of CAOT certification exam; first exam held in 1986.
Chile	Colegio de Terapeutas Ocupacionales de Chile A.G.		1			
China, Republic of	Occupational Therapists Assoc. of Republic of China	32		2	Chinese Journal of Occupational Therapy	Admitted to full membership in WFOT in 1986.
Columbia	Association Columbiana de Terapia Occupational	151		2	Accion	
Denmark	Egopterapeutforeningen	1,961	2,718	6	Ergoterapeuten	
Federal Republic of Germany	Verband der Beschaftingungs-und Arbietstherapeuten	1,925	1,709	21	Beschaftigungstherapie und Rehabilitation	
Finland	Suomen Toimintaterapeutit Finlands Ergotherapeuter/Ry			3	Toiminaterapeutti	
France	Association Nationale de Ergotherapeutes			8	Journal d'Ergotherapie	
Hong Kong	Hong Kong Assoc. of Occupational Therapists	153	158	1	Journal of the Hong Kong Assoc. of Occupational Therapists	
Iceland	Icelandic Occupational Therapy Assoc.				Blad-Id	Admitted to full membership in WFOT in 1986.

Country	Association				Journal	Notes
India	All-India Occupational Therapists Assoc.	308	316	5	*Indian Journal of Occupational Therapy*	Celebrated 25 years as an organization in 1986.
Ireland	Assoc. of Occupational Therapists of Ireland			1	*O.T. Ireland*	A four-year honors degree program in OT opened in 1986 at Trinity College, Dublin University.
Israel	Israel Assoc. of Occupational Therapists	623	623	3		
Italy[b]	Associazione Italiana de Terapia Occupazionale				*Notizie AITO*	
Japan	Japanese Assoc. of Occupational Therapists	1,709	1,394	28	*Sagyo Ryoho* (Occupational Therapy)	Opening of a new school and opening of new assoc. office. Promotion of reimbursement through national health insurance and creation of administrative positions for OTs in the national hospitals.
Kenya	Kenya Occupational Therapy Assoc.			1		
Malaysia[b]	Malaysian Occupational Therapy Assoc.					
The Netherlands	Nederlandse Vereniging voor Ergotherapie	787	814	3	*Nederlandse Tijd-Schrift voor Ergo therapie*	
New Zealand	New Zealand Assoc. of Occupational Therapists			1	*Journal of the NZ Assoc. of Occupational Therapists*	
Norway	Norsk Ergoterapeut Forbund	900	828	2	*Ergoterapeuten*	
Philippines	Occupational Therapy Assoc. Philippines			1		
Portugal	Associacao Portuguesa de Terapia Ocupacional			1	*Boletin de Assoc. Portugal de Terapia Ocupational*	
Singapore[b]	Singapore Assoc. of Occupational Therapists	30				
South Africa	South African Assoc. of Occupational Therapists	547		7	*South African Journal of Occupational Therapy*	
Spain	Asoc. Espanola de Terapia Ocupacional			1	*Boletin Asoc. Espanola de Terapia Ocupation*	
Sweden	Forbundet Sveriges Arbetsterapeuten	3,569		8	*Arbetsterapeuten*	Has 24 local branches that meet regularly.
Switzerland	Verband Schweizerischer Ergo therapeuten			3	*Zeitschrift fur Ergotherapie*	

Table 18.1. (Continued)
Incomplete List of WFOT Member Organizations and Their Current Activities[a]

Country or Territory	Name of Organization	Number of Qualified OTR Members	Total Membership	Number of Schools	Journal	Recent Developments
United Kingdom	British Assoc. of Occupational Therapists	6,137	7,133	16	*British Journal of Occupational Therapy*	Second European Congress held in London in July, 1985, with delegates from 29 countries attending.
United States of America	American Occupational Therapy Assoc.	30,892	41,096	61	*American Journal of Occupational Therapy*	Held continuing education programs in vocational readiness, gerontology, and mental health. Accredited 4 new educational programs; continued activity in legislative and political areas and in marketing of OT services.
Venezuela	Asoc. Venezolana de Terapeutas Ocupacionales			2	*Boletin Informativo de la Associacion*	
Zimbabwe[b]	Zimbabwean Assoc. of Occupational Therapists					A new occupational therapy school will open in 1987–1988.

[a]Data supplied from annual reports (1985–1986) from member organizations, J. Barker, President, WFOT.
[b]Associate members of WFOT.

Canada, Belgium, Denmark, Israel, India, the United Kingdom, Norway, New Zealand, Sweden, Switzerland, and South Africa), however, there is a strong trend toward community-based practice while at the same time the traditional focus on hospital care is maintained. These countries are also experiencing an increased emphasis on geriatric care, are applying occupational therapy concepts to industrial settings, and are seeing more therapists engaged in private practice. The developing countries tend to have predominantly hospital-based practice and are more inclined to follow the medical model (J. Barker, WFOT president, personal communication).

Little information is available on the number of foreign therapists specializing in limited areas of practice. The WFOT conducted a survey of its member organizations in 1984 to determine the number of people who practiced as "single medium therapists." This term referred to individuals who had completed an advanced educational program in the therapeutic use of a specialized medium (art, music, drama, sport, recreation). The survey showed that 19 WFOT member organizations had such therapists working in their countries and 8 countries had training courses in the use of specialized media (3).

Private practice and consultation appear to be increasing in WFOT member countries. A 1984 WFOT survey revealed that 25 of the 29 member organizations had therapists who were self-employed as private practitioners or consultants. Only 14 countries reported problems with such practices. Nine countries noted that there were some regulations affecting private practice of occupational therapy in their countries. Some national organizations commented that occupational therapy practice in their countries was limited to institutional employment and that they were working to have this changed. Others noted the necessity for a medical prescrip-

tion for occupational therapy services in their country and felt that this requirement might slow the development of private practices. Countries that had nationalized health care systems pointed out that it was often difficult for private practitioners of occupational therapy to find a place in the health care system (4).

There seems to be no exact equivalent to the certified occupational therapy assistant outside the United States. Technicians exist, but training is variable and these technicians may function only in specialized areas of practice, such as gerontology. Only 11 of the WFOT member organizations reported having trained support staff available in 1980. Of those who did, the support staff ranged from aides with minimal on-the-job training to technical assistants with the over three years of training (5).

To understand what occupational therapists are doing in other countries, let's look at what some member organizations have reported in WFOT publications in the past three years.

JAPAN

Occupational therapy in Japan is 20 years old, with 2000 occupational therapists now practicing and 28 government-approved schools preparing occupational therapists. A 1984 survey conducted by the Japanese Association of Occupational Therapists showed that 66.3% of their members were female and 33.7% male. Most were employed by national or state hospitals or by rehabilitation facilities that were part of a national health and welfare system. Of those therapists surveyed, 32.5% were employed in general hospitals, 13.4% in mental hospitals, 13.1% in specialized rehabilitation hospitals, 10.9% in children's facilities, and 10% in occupational therapy schools. Occupational therapists in Japan are issued national licenses after passing a qualifying examination at the end of their academic work. With changes in Japan's national health insurance for the disabled, occupational therapists are now expanding their practice into geriatrics, community-based programming, and convalescent facilities (6).

ICELAND

Occupational therapy practice in Iceland dates from 1974, when several Icelandic graduates of European occupational therapy schools returned to augment the work of a single therapist who had been practicing before that time. A national occupational therapy organization was formed in 1976 and now has 50 members. Iceland has at this time no occupational therapy school, but developing one is a high priority of the professional organization. In 1976 the profession association conducted a survey to determine future personnel needs and found that approximately 100 therapists were likely to be needed in the foreseeable future. Icelandic therapists are increasingly participating in research activities and are investigating questions related to client problems that they frequently encounter in practice (7).

ZIMBABWE

This southeastern African country (former Rhodesia) now has 24 occupational therapists practicing in pediatrics, physical medicine, and psychiatry. Because there are few specialized treatment facilities, most practice as generalists with an emphasis on community-based rehabilitation. A rehabilitation school is planned at the University of Zimbabwe and will offer both occupational and physical therapy educational programs (8).

CHILE

In 1986 Chilean therapists studied the model of human occupation in a series of workshops taught by one of their colleagues who studied with Prof. Kielhofner at Boston University. The workshops were sponsored by the University of Chile and covered both theory and application of the model. Fifty therapists attended and later continued their discussions in monthly study groups. The model was believed to have broad application in existing clinical programs (9).

HONG KONG

Following a government study of population needs in Hong Kong in 1978, social welfare services were vastly expanded. Among the changes made were expansions and improvements of rehabilitation facilities and services. It was also recognized that more educational programs to prepare greater numbers of medical and health care workers were needed. As a result, the Hong Kong Polytechnic now offers educational programs in occupational therapy and a number of health-related fields. Education for all handicapped children was mandated by the government in the same year, and increased funding was made available for paramedical and social work services in schools for handicapped children. By 1981 these programs were under way, but the government recognized that there was still a shortfall in services available to the mentally handicapped and the formerly mentally ill. Occupational therapy services in these areas have expanded in recent years. In 1979 there were only 25 occupational therapists practicing in Hong Kong. By 1985 that number had risen to 200 qualified therapists, most of whom were educated locally. Another 206 students were enrolled in the professional diploma course in occupational therapy at the Hong Kong Polytechnic in 1985. Areas of emphasis in current practice include industrial accidents, treatment of burns, and the provision of community support services for the chronically mentally ill. In 1986, community facilities were a better market for occupational therapy services than were hospitals and other institutional settings (10).

DENMARK

The history of occupational therapy in Denmark goes back 50 years. In 1986 there were approximately 1800 therapists practicing. Of these, 550 were employed in medical institutions for the treatment of physical disorders, 300 worked in psychiatric facilities, and 650 were employed in the primary health service. Another 70 persons were working with industrial conditions, and 60 people were employed in occupational therapy educational programs. Education in occupational therapy consists of a three-year curriculum that emphasizes treatment, care, and preventive medicine. A six-week project of a scientific nature is required of each student prior to graduation. Since 1980 a one-year advanced educational program in administration and educational techniques has been available. Continuing education courses are organized each year by the professional association to help members update their knowledge and skills (11).

AUSTRALIA

Occupational therapy in Australia dates from 1942 and by 1986 had five schools preparing practitioners. All of the schools had graduate as well as undergraduate educational programs. Occupa-

tional therapists are employed mainly in hospitals or specialized treatment centers; however, therapists are also practicing in county or community health centers, nursing homes, in industry, and as consultants or private practitioners. Australian occupational therapists offer a wide variety of services and are increasingly participating in clinical research (12).

PORTUGAL

Carvalho and Simoes (13) described the establishment of the first private rehabilitation center in Portugal in a 1985 paper. The center was developed by two occupational therapists, two physical therapists, and a speech therapist. This group was discouraged after having worked for many years in an antiquated institution and decided to risk developing a private modern rehabilitation facility. They located in a large country house that could be remodeled to suit their needs and that had access to good public transportation. The house was purchased, and in their free time the team members and their families cleaned and reconstructed the building. Team members also contacted the necessary social and medical services, hospitals, physicians, lawyers, and government representatives whose help was needed to make the new center work. The center opened in 1984 with two administrators, one an occupational therapist and the other a physical therapist. Two full-time and three part-time employees helped to staff the center, which provides rehabilitation services for patients with rheumatic diseases, CVA (cerebrovascular accident), trauma, learning disabilities, and degenerative neurological diseases. Although the center is small, it is functioning well. The team members who developed the center were satisfied with the outcome and encouraged others to take the risks that are necessary to develop a new program or facility.

KENYA

Occupational therapy services have been available in Kenya since 1971. Most therapists are government employees, because the existing training program is located in a government college of health professions and admitted students are on government scholarships. Occupational therapy services have yet to develop in missionary and private hospitals within the country. From an initial emphasis on tropical medicine, health services are now expanding into other areas. Because occupational therapy has developed so recently in Kenya, its services are not yet well understood by medical practitioners; therapists find it necessary to educate the medical community and the general public about their contributions to health care. As health care facilities expand and occupational therapy becomes more common, this problem is expected to be eased (14).

INDONESIA

Like many developing countries, Indonesia faced the problem of how to bring rehabilitation services to its disabled citizens who lived in remote rural areas. By 1980, 26 government-administered rehabilitation centers had been developed within the country and these were supplemented by another 100 institutions that were operated by voluntary organizations. Most of these programs, however, were located in urban areas and had no outreach programs. After studying the problem the government decided to develop noninstitutional community-based rehabilitation services that would be accessible to people in the outlying rural areas. A pilot project was initiated that established four regional

base stations. These stations provided assessment and counseling services, training, and employment assistance. They also offered training in daily living skills and supplied technical aids to disabled persons when needed. The pilot program was so successful that 120 smaller base stations were later established throughout the country. By 1984 these stations were serving 20,000 disabled persons, and it was anticipated that this number would increase annually. In 1982 certain non-government institutions were designated to provide backup services to the community-based programs. A mobile rehabilitation unit was also developed. To meet the needs of the expanded program, training courses were established for managers, field staff, and technicians. By 1984 the programs had demonstrated their value and were cost-effective. The project was the result of successful collaboration between government, voluntary organizations, and United Nations technical agencies. Responsive communities also contributed much to the success of these decentralized rehabilitation programs (15).

WORK AND STUDY OPPORTUNITIES ABROAD

Many students and therapists in the United States are interested in the possibility of working abroad or studying occupational therapy abroad. The World Federation of Occupational Therapists offered some practical advice to therapists who wish to work in a foreign country in their 1984 publication *Information on Requirements for Employment of Occupational Therapists in Member Countries of WFOT* (16). This publication points out that although working abroad can be a uniquely enriching experience, one should ask the following basic questions of oneself before undertaking such a venture.

1. Do you have a speaking knowledge of the language of the host country? (This is essential for adequate communication with patients and staff in the workplace and also for daily living.)
2. Are you able to adapt to all kinds of conditions? (Although occupational therapy concepts are similar around the world, working conditions and equipment are not.)
3. How good is your emotional and physical health? (You must be able to adapt to changes in climate, nutrition, working hours, and attitudes.)
4. How good is your professional knowledge? (A therapist should have at least one year of clinical experience and preferably more before attempting to work aboard. You will be regarded as an expert and should be prepared to function as such.)
5. How well do you know your own country? (As a therapist working abroad you will unofficially represent your country. You should be prepared to answer questions on subjects such as your government, the educational system, cultural patterns, and political issues.)
6. How much do you know about sources of financial support for overseas assignments? (It is always best to seek financial support from resources within your own country. Are you familiar with the salary scale and the standard of living in the host country?)
7. Have you investigated the financial implications of taking money out of one country and into another? (Many countries have restrictions on the amount of money that can be brought in.)

The WFOT publication goes on to provide specific information on the immigration requirements and educational requirements to practice in each of its member countries.

For students or therapists wishing to visit occupational therapy programs abroad or to work for a limited period of time, a variety of resources are available. Some occupational therapy schools have established their own exchange programs with counterpart schools in another country. Several countries sponsor friendship tours for foreign therapists. New Zealand, the Federal Republic of Germany, Denmark, and the United States offer such arrangements, but visitors are expected to pay their own transportation costs. A number of voluntary organizations that have an interest in rehabilitation offer opportunities for exchange programs between rehabilitation professionals. Partners of the Americas, the American Refugee Committee, and Rehabilitation International are examples of such organizations. The United States Department of Defense employs some occupational therapists to provide services to handicapped children who are military dependents and are stationed abroad. Some church groups offer missionary opportunities for those who wish to contribute their professional skills to church-sponsored hospitals and clinics abroad. Government agencies such as the Peace Corps recruit occupational therapists to serve two-year terms of duty in countries that request assistance in developing rehabilitation services. Finally, private foundations offer some support for study or work abroad in professional fields. The student or therapist interested in such possibilities should thoroughly research potential funding sources before making a commitment to foreign study or employment. The American Occupational Therapy Association can provide a detailed listing of such sources on request (17).

INTERNATIONAL CONFERENCES

The international congresses sponsored by the WFOT every four years offer occupational therapists and therapy assistants an opportunity to meet and talk with their colleagues from WFOT member countries. The next congress is scheduled for 1990. Regional international meetings are also beginning to develop. The Second European Congress of Occupational Therapists was held in London in July 1985. It focused on clinical developments in the field, occupational therapy in the community, the organization of occupational therapy services, and developments in occupational therapy education. The congress was attended by delegates from 29 countries. An Inter-Nordic Occupational Therapy Seminar was held in Sweden in 1984, with 150 delegates attending from five Nordic countries. A similar regional conference was held in Brazil in 1985 for occupational therapists from Latin American countries. In the future more regional conferences may be held to discuss specific topics of concern to occupational therapists in certain parts of the world.

SUMMARY

Occupational therapy is growing and developing throughout the world, and therapists here and abroad are eager for communication and interchange with their colleagues in other countries. A variety of opportunities exist for travel, study, or employment in countries outside the United States. Therapists are advised to plan such experiences carefully so that maximum benefit will be obtained both by the individual and by the host country. The World Federation of Occupational Therapists provides a connecting link between occupational therapy organizations in its member countries and offers communication and exchange opportunities through its publications and international congresses. As the number of occupational therapists increases around

the world, opportunities for exchange programs between schools and between occupational therapy organizations should expand.

DISCUSSION QUESTIONS

1. Have you ever considered work or study outside the United States? If so, what countries interest you?

2. If you have the opportunity, invite a foreign-educated occupational therapist to attend your class. How was their education different from yours? What is practice like in their country?

3. Do you think that the development of rehabilitation services is a high priority of governments in developing countries? Why or why not?

4. Do you think that work, self-care, or leisure activities might vary with the culture and the country? Why? How might they be different?

5. How might client attitudes toward rehabilitation and achievement of independent functioning vary from culture to culture?

6. Have any of your faculty members attended a WFOT International Conference? If so, ask them to share their experiences with you.

7. Could your student occupational therapy association contact and exchange information with students of a foreign occupational therapy school?

8. Could your curriculum host a foreign occupational therapy educator or clinician who wishes to visit the United States?

REFERENCES

1. *Annual Reports of Member Organizations*. World Federation of Occupational Therapists, 1985.
2. *List of WFOT-Approved Schools*. World Federation of Occupational Therapists, 1985.
3. Professional Practice Committee: *Survey on Single Medium Therapists*. World Federation of Occupational Therapists, 1984.
4. *Survey on Private Practice and Consultation*. World Federation of Occupational Therapists, 1984.
5. *Survey on Recognized Training of Support Staff*. World Federation of Occupational Therapists, 1980.
6. Sato T: The past and present situation of occupational therapists in Japan. *WFOT Bull* 13:2–4, 1986.
7. Knutsson H: An overview of research activities by Icelandic occupational therapists. *WFOT Bull* 13:5–6, 1986.
8. News from national associations: Zimbabwe. *WFOT Bull* 13:31, 1986.
9. De la Heras C: The model of human occupation being taught in South America. *Occup Ther News* 41(1):8, 1987.
10. Sinclair K: Development of occupational therapy in Hong Kong. *WFOT Bull* 13:13–14, 1985.
11. Research activities in Denmark. *WFOT Bull* 13:13,1986.
12. Western Australian Association of Occupational Therapists: *Occupational Therapy in Western Australia*. Dalglish, Western Australia, 1986, pp 1–3.
13. Carvalho C, Simoes R: Establishment of a rehabilitation center in Portugal. *WFOT Bull* 11:33–35, 1985.
14. Shimali I: Problems in the delivery of occupational therapy services. *WFOT Bull* 14:24–25, 1986.
15. *A community-based approach in vocational rehabilitation—Indonesia's Experience*. *WFOT Bull* 9:35–38, 1984.
16. Publications Committee: *Information on Requirements for the Employment of Occupational Therapists in the Member Countries of WFOT*. World Federation of Occupational Therapists, 1984, pp 1–39.
17. *Opportunities for International Experiences*. Rockville, MD, American Occupational Therapy Association, 1985, pp 1–8.

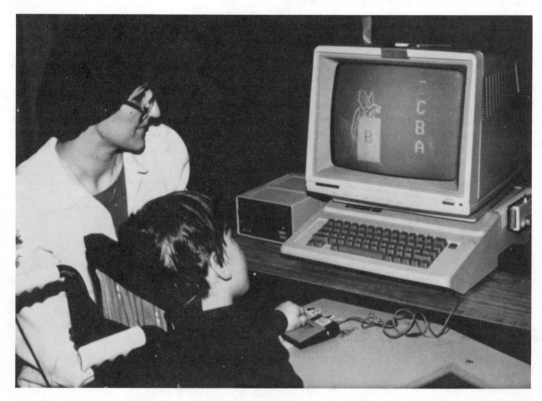

Courtesy AOTA

NINETEEN

Current Trends in the Field

Occupational therapy has grown and developed a great deal since its beginnings in the early years of the twentieth century. Each succeeding generation of occupational therapists has faced new challenges and has adapted the traditions of the field to meet new needs and conditions. In the 1980s, occupational therapy continues to face challenges, some of which may influence profound changes in the profession. This chapter examines the current status of occupational therapy in the United States and reviews some of the issues of concern to OTRs and COTAs in the 1980s. Let us begin by looking at some of the societal changes that are affecting health care in the United States.

SOCIETAL CHANGES

A comprehensive study of occupational therapy personnel was conducted by the American Occupational Therapy Association in 1984 and reviewed some of the societal changes that will influence health care and occupational therapy services in the future (1). The report noted that significant demographic changes have taken place in American society that are changing the clientele seen by occupational therapists and therapy assistants. A dramatic increase in the older population is occurring, and at the same time there is a reduction in the proportion of young people in American society. Government figures project that the over 65 population will increase by 24.5% by 1990. This increase is over twice the rate of increase projected for the population as a whole. The number of persons aged 75 years and older is expected to increase by 37.9%. The "frail elderly" (over age 85) are also expected to show a rapid increase in numbers. Americans are living longer and are enjoying good health longer than ever before. As the baby-boom generation (born in the decade after World War II) reaches maturity, the proportion of children in the population will markedly increase. By 1990 the population of children under five years of age is expected to increase by 16.7%. The teenage and young adult population, however, is declining but is expected to rise slowly during the 1990s. The clients served by occupational therapists in future years will reflect these changes within the population.

In addition to demographic changes there have also been changes in the health status of some groups within American society. The "wellness movement" of the 1970s and 1980s caused many Americans to become more conscious of their personal responsibilities in health maintenance and prevention. Increased attention to good nutrition, exercise, and avoidance of substances that can cause negative health effects improved the general health of many people. This movement, however, was largely limited to the middle class. Death rates for cardiovascular disease are declining among the adult population in the United States. Deaths from cancer and automobile accidents are continuing to rise. As the population ages, chronic diseases and disability are expected to be seen with greater frequency. Government statistics show that between 18% and 43% of the noninstitutionalized elderly have physical limitations.

THE CHANGING HEALTH CARE SCENE

At this writing, more than 100 allied health occupations exist, and the number of people practicing in these fields doubled between 1966 and 1978. Even so, there continue to be personnel shortages in some allied health fields. It is unlikely that the supply will catch up with the demand until the year 2000. The number of active physicians, however, is increasing, and a surplus is expected by 1990. This oversupply of physicians may help to redistribute health care services to underserved areas of the country. It may also tend to create increased competition between some allied health practitioners and physicians.

Mental health services are utilized by only 15% of the population in a single year. The number of outpatient clinics and mental health agencies is increasing; these programs are dealing with clients who are experiencing stress, employment problems, marital problems, or who are having

difficulty coping with daily life. A major shift has occurred from long-term custodial care for psychiatric disorders to outpatient and community care. Long-term health care facilities are rapidly expanding to meet the needs of the older, chronically ill segment of the population. This trend is expected to continue. The American Health Care Association predicts that 3% more nursing home beds will be needed annually to maintain current levels of service (1).

The prospective payment system adopted by Congress in 1983 as an attempt to curtail costs of the Medicare program is likely to be extended to outpatient services, home health services, physician payments, mental health services, skilled nursing care, and those children's hospitals and rehabilitation facilities that were initially excluded. Although all the effects of this change are not predictable, it may mean reductions in staff and financial cutbacks by many health care institutions. The number of health maintenance organizations (HMOs) is growing rapidly, and this movement toward prepayment of health care represents another effort at cost-containment and better fiscal control of health care services.

Because hospital services will be increasingly limited to acute care, alternative delivery systems are developing to fill the gap. New outpatient programs, urgent care clinics, fitness programs, women's health centers, home health programs, and specialized clinics for the treatment of specific disorders are being rapidly organized. Such programs are expected to continue to develop during the 1990s (1).

OCCUPATIONAL THERAPY PERSONNEL AND EMPLOYMENT PATTERNS

According to the 1985 AOTA manpower report, the occupational therapy work force grew 230% between 1966 and 1978. Growth has slowed since that time, however, and there is a significant shortage of occupational therapy personnel for present and future needs. The United States Bureau of Labor Statistics projects that a 60% increase in occupational therapy personnel is needed to meet the needs of the population within the next decade. There is also a maldistribution of occupational therapy personnel within the United States that is more pronounced for COTAs than for OTRs. Areas of greatest shortage are the Southeast (for both OTRs and COTAs) and the West (for COTAs). The fact that 95% of occupational therapy practitioners are female appears to influence the employment patterns within the field. There is a constant turnover of personnel as therapists leave the work force (presumably to raise a family) and then return later. Male therapists, however, tend to remain in the work force all through their working lives.

The proportion of minority therapists continues to be very low—about 7% to 8% of all occupational therapists—and has remained at that level since 1973. Currently over 14% of OTRs hold advanced degrees, with the remainder holding baccalaureate degrees. Seventy-five percent of all COTAs hold associate degrees. The number of OTRs with advanced degrees has increased fivefold since 1970, and this increase is expected to continue. Therapists who enter the field with a master's degree are more likely to remain in the work force full time, whereas baccalaureate degree OTRs show a higher frequency of part-time employment.

Employment frequency among OTRs and COTAs has increased steadily since 1970. There are greater numbers of OTRs working full time. The proportion of full-time COTAs has remained constant in the last few years. Future personnel needs are expected to be particularly high in school systems, in the new alternative health care programs, and in home health services. The demand for OTRs by hospitals has continued to increase, but the demand for COTAs in such facilities appears to be leveling off. The number of foreign-educated OTRs who become certified in the United States is increasing, but this group continues to be a very small proportion of the occupational therapy population. The increase in foreign-educated therapists has had no noticeable effect on the personnel supply or on employment.

Hospitals continue to be the most common work setting for both OTRs and COTAs, but this may change as hospitals limit their services to acute care. The 1985 AOTA manpower report showed a 4-fold increase in the number of occupational therapists working in home health care and a 2½-fold increase in private practitioners. Public and private schools were the second largest employment site for OTRs and the third largest for COTAs in 1985. (Skilled nursing homes and intermediate care facilities were the second largest employment site for COTAs.) As the health care delivery system changes, we can expect to see more OTRs and COTAs employed in community-based programs with fewer employed in inpatient facilities (1). In the future, HMOs may become large-scale employers of OTRs. Final Medicare regulations for HMOs were published in 1985 and included coverage of comprehensive rehabilitation facility services, including occupational therapy. This may open the door to OTRs to provide their services to HMOs on a contract basis (2).

SALARY LEVELS

What kind of a salary can an OTR or COTA expect? In 1986 the United States Bureau of Labor Statistics published the results of a wage survey of hospital health care professionals in 23 metropolitan areas. This study showed an average hourly wage for hospital-based OTRs that ranged from

$9.77 to $14.31. No hourly wage figures were reported for COTAs (3).

In 1984, *Occupational Therapy News* published figures on the annual income levels for OTRs and COTAs who were employed on a full-time basis. According to this report, the average salary for OTRs in 1982 was $20,351, with reported incomes ranging from $8,000 to over $40,000 per year. The average income for COTAs was $12,864, with an income range from $8,000 to $40,000 (4). (Only one person was at the $40,000 level.) In a later issue, salaries were reported by employment setting. In this breakdown, colleges and universities, HMOs, private practice, public health, and research facilities led the list with the highest salary levels for OTRs. They were followed by community agencies, general and specialized hospitals, and residential care facilities. The lowest salary levels were reported for school systems, sheltered workshops, skilled nursing homes, and voluntary agencies. The highest salaries for COTAs were found in colleges, HMOs, hospitals, private industry, private practice, rehabilitation hospitals, and residential care facilities. Lower salaries were being paid by day-care centers, independent living centers, school systems, sheltered workshops, skilled nursing homes, and voluntary agencies. When salary levels were analyzed in terms of geographic location, the highest salaries for both OTRs and COTAs were found in Alaska, California, Nebraska, and Nevada. States on the low end of the salary scale included Idaho, Massachusetts, New Hampshire, New Mexico, Rhode Island, South Dakota, Utah, Vermont, Virginia, and Puerto Rico (5).

PRACTICE TRENDS IN OCCUPATIONAL THERAPY

Bell (6) discussed the changing nature of occupational therapy practice in 1985 and noted that the strenuous efforts to contain health care costs were resulting in the development of alternative delivery systems of health care. At the same time there was an increased demand for accountability by health care providers. This meant that occupational therapists, along with other providers, were expected to set measurable treatment objectives for their clients and to document progress toward the achievement of these objectives in a timely and cost-effective manner. Occupational therapy departments were faced with increasing demands for productivity. Health care reimbursers were beginning to use the independent functioning of the client as a criteria for judging the effectiveness of services, and occupational therapy was in a strong position to document its contribution toward this goal. Preventive services were more cost-effective than treatment services. As a result of these changes, OTRs and COTAs learned new documentation and management skills. Therapists found it more necessary than ever to consult and communicate with one another to improve the quality of client care and to facilitate the movement of clients from one level of health care to another. Bell predicts that the occupational therapy practice skills of the 1980s and 90s need to include strong management skills; effective communication abilities; the ability to collaborate with other health professionals and agencies; consultative, supervisory, and leadership skills; and a sound knowledge of business and management techniques.

An area of occupational therapy practice that had been neglected in recent decades was that of prevocational evaluation and training. In the mid-1980s interest in this practice area was revived and work programs began to develop in occupational therapy clinics. In 1985 a Work Programs Special Interest Section was formed. Many occupational therapists were seeing work adjustment and vocational evaluation as an important professional role and were moving quickly to reestablish themselves in this practice area (7).

An increasing degree of specialization was being seen in occupational therapy practice in the 1980s. Special Interest Sections, which had been created by AOTA to improve communication between OTRs and COTAs practicing in specialized areas, were attracting large groups of members. In 1986 AOTA reported the following membership figures for the Special Interest Sections (8).

Administration and management	2,390
Developmental disabilities	6,812
Gerontology	3,648
Mental health	4,838
Physical Disabilities	11,024
Work Programs	Not reported

An increased emphasis on research was also being seen in occupational therapy practice and education. As more funding became available for research, more investigations were begun. Occupational therapy educational programs were beginning to offer courses in research methodology, and more graduate degree programs were requiring research projects of their students.

Another trend was the growing emphasis on data-based management, documentation, and accountability. This trend grew out of the new federal requirements for documentation under the Medicare program and from private reimbursers who were demanding the same accountability. Client and management records were now being computerized, and therapists were learning how to use new data-management systems. All of these changes required new skills of practitioners, and educational programs were adding content areas to their curricula so that students would be prepared for the clinical environments of the 1980s (1).

EFFECTS OF CHANGING REIMBURSEMENT PATTERNS

In 1985 Baum (9) discussed the ways in which changing reimbursement mechanisms were influencing occupational therapy practice. She noted that as hospitals moved to the prospective payment system, health care decisions were more frequently being made on the basis of cost factors rather than on the quality of patient care. Under the new system, hospitals were being rewarded for providing fewer services for patients and for earlier discharges. They were being forced to actively compete with one another for patients and were expected to show higher productivity levels for staff members. In an effort to compete, many hospitals developed vertical referral systems that could provide a continuum of care for clients. Baum argues that for occupational therapy to survive under the prospective payment system it is necessary for therapists to expand their services within a hospital's vertical referral system and broaden their community involvement. She suggests a number of strategies for occupational therapists to expand their services, including the redesign of programs so that they provide specific skill training for clients or specialized treatment for clients with particular disabilities. Creation of new markets for occupational therapy services is another strategy urged by Baum. Table 19.1 shows some potential occupational therapy services that she suggests could be developed by hospital-based programs.

Baum further recommends that occupational therapists explore new sources of reimbursement for their services. She suggests that potential sources might include self-payment by those able to pay for their own care, workers compensation funds, liability insurance funds, corporate funds, HMOs, public health funds, and social security funds. Baum states that occupational therapists must determine the

Table 19.1.
Potential Occupational Therapy Services[a]

Occupational Therapy	Hospital	Physician Practice	Industry	Public System	Public
Inpatient triage	X				
Home health	X	X		X	
Skilled nursing	X	X			X
Hospice	X	X			X
Wellness programs	X	X	X	X	X
Designated beds	X				
Rehabilitation facilities	X	X		X	X
Life skills evaluation/training	X	X		X	X
Work evaluation/training	X	X	X	X	X
Industrial consultation	X	X	X	X	X
Driving evaluation/training	X	X		X	X
Technology services	X	X	X	X	X
Community services			X	X	X
Public school services				X	

[a]From Baum C: Growth, renewal, and challenge: an important era for occupational therapy. *AJOT* 39:780, 1985.

efficacy of their services and must be able to show reimbursers and others the effect that occupation has on performance (9).

TRENDS IN OCCUPATIONAL THERAPY EDUCATION

Just as with occupational therapy practice, societal changes were influencing changes in occupational therapy education in the 1980s. Higher educational institutions were experiencing budget shortfalls, and public funds to support higher education were growing scarcer. As the number of young adults in the population declined there were fewer college-age students. Enrollments declined in most colleges and universities as a result. These general trends were reflected in occupational therapy educational progams as well. While manpower experts were bemoaning the shortage of occupational therapy personnel and were urging educational programs to accept more students, the pool of prospective students was growing smaller. Occupational therapy schools were having difficulty recruiting students and financing their educational programs. The funding of the fieldwork phase of education

was a particular problem, because hospitals were more and more reluctant to bear the costs of clinical education for students in health care occupations. In addition there was increasing pressure to reassess the types and levels of education needed for allied health practitioners (10).

The 1985 AOTA manpower report looked at the status of occupational therapy education and found that the number of graduates from professional and technical programs had not increased since 1977. Enrollments appeared to be declining in certificate programs but were increasing in entry-level master's degree programs. The pool of applicants for technical educational programs was even smaller than that for professional programs. There was also a serious faculty shortage, particularly in programs preparing the OTR. Outside financial support for occupational therapy educational programs had declined 64% for the professional programs and 95% for the technical programs since 1977.

Because of increasing fiscal constraints, some occupational therapy educators were suggesting that AOTA assume the responsibility for the fieldwork phase of educational programs. Some felt that the assigning and scheduling of level II field-work could be better done on a national scale than by each program individually. Others saw level II fieldwork as an inter-related part of the educational program of each school and believed that responsi-bility for it should continue to lie with the educational programs. This controversy has not been resolved, and discussion over the merits of each plan continues (11).

OCCUPATIONAL THERAPY ISSUES OF THE 1980s

Many issues arose for occupational therapists in the 1980s that reflected the changes taking place in American society, in health care, and within the field. These issues help to set the stage for predictions of future trends in occupational therapy.

ENTRY LEVEL FOR OTRs

A group of leaders in occupational therapy has proposed that the entry point into the profession for OTRs be raised from the baccalaureate level to the master's degree level. The rationale behind this proposal has been outlined by Royeen (12), who made the following points:

- The increasing specialization of occupational therapy practice requires that practitioners have more specialized skills and a more advanced education.
- Clinical research and documenta-tion that is needed to give credi-bility to the claims of improved function as a result of occupational therapy treatment can only be car-ried out by practitioners with a graduate education.
- By moving to the master's degree entry level, the profession may attract a new breed of student who has completed a liberal arts degree,

thus alleviating the shortage of OTRs.
- Most of the health care profession-als with whom occupational ther-apists work are prepared at the master's degree level.
- As the health care system grows more complex and as additional demands are made for advanced skills, it makes sense to allow time for a more extended education and a move to the master's degree level.

Those who disagree believe that rais-ing the entry level will only increase health care costs, because higher salaries will be demanded by master's degree graduates. They fear that occupational therapists will price themselves out of the market and will have difficulty finding employment. The issue of a higher entry level for OTRs has arisen periodically, but the discussion appears to have reached a new level of intensity in the 1980s.

OCCUPATIONAL THERAPY AS AN ACADEMIC DISCIPLINE

In a 1985 paper, Tanguay (13) pointed out that although occupational therapy is a profession, it has not developed as an academic discipline. The result is that many educational programs in colleges or universities have been unable to meet the standards of university departments. Only a minority of occupational therapy faculty members hold a doctoral degree, and rel-atively few are involved in the generation of knowledge through organized research programs. For these and other reasons, occupational therapy faculty members fre-quently fail to achieve tenure in their col-lege or university. This poses serious problems for educational programs and for the field as a whole. For occupational ther-apy to achieve respectibility within the academic community, it must produce doctoral faculty members and professional leaders, subject its traditional beliefs and practices to scientific scrutiny through research, and nurture the development of scholars who can contribute to the knowledge base of the field (13). This point of view was reinforced by Austin (14) in a presentation to occupational therapy educators in 1986. Austin pointed out that any discipline must have a constantly expanding body of knowledge to remain a viable profession and an academic discipline, and he urged occupational therapy educators to live up to the expectations of their academic institutions.

This issue is closely related to the preceding one. If OTRs were prepared at the master's degree level, more of them would be likely to continue their education in doctoral programs and would expand the number of faculty members and researchers available. Occupational therapy is unlikely to survive in colleges and universities as funds grow more limited, unless it can show that it is a genuine academic field of study. Its faculty members must be equivalent in educational preparation and skills to those in other university departments. If this is not achieved, occupational therapy educational programs may be dropped from the fields of study available at institutions of higher education.

RESEARCH NEEDS IN OCCUPATIONAL THERAPY

The critical need for research in occupational therapy was identified repeatedly in the 1970s and 1980s by leaders in the field. In a presentation to occupational therapy educators in 1986, Ottenbacher (15) asked those assembled whether occupational therapy wished to develop as an applied technology or as an applied science. He pointed out that if the latter course is chosen, occupational therapists will need to place less emphasis on technology and more on the "why" ques-

tions of the field. Health professions, including occupational therapy, have often tended to discourage those members who have the interest and potential for conducting research and encourage those interested in providing direct client services. According to Ottenbacher, that practice must change if occupational therapy is to survive and meet the challenges of the years ahead. We must not only engage in research, we must also teach students to value scientific inquiry (15). Most leaders of the field agree that research into the basic questions of the field is an absolute necessity. Most of the problems occupational therapists are facing today can only be solved through systematic study and analysis.

THE OCCUPATIONAL THERAPY IDENTITY CRISIS

In her 1984 Slagle Lecture to members of the American Occupational Therapy Association, Gilfoyle (16) admitted that for the past few decades occupational therapy has been in an identity crisis. Occupational therapy values, the scope of its practice, and its educational requirements have been questioned. There have been serious differences of opinion about the legitimate "territory" of the profession, its philosophical base, and the ability of the field to survive the changes taking place in health care. Gilfoyle held that occupational therapy in the 1980s is in a period of paradigm shift—a change in the ways of thinking about old concepts. She examined some of the traditional occupational therapy beliefs and concluded that the traditional values of the field concerning the importance of occupation and the value of the occupational process are as valid today as they ever were. She suggested, however, that occupational therapy may have outgrown the medical model that was so much a part of its early development. The model of human occupation, Gilfoyle proposed, might prove more useful to occupational therapy in communicating its basic philosophy and beliefs as therapists adapt their practices to changing health care environments.

West (17), in another 1984 conference presentation, agreed. She suggested use of the term "occupation" as the common core of occupational therapy and urged that therapists describe themselves as serving "the occupational needs of man." She further suggested that occupational therapy focus on "occupational performance dysfunction" rather than disabilities. This change, she asserted, would help to unite occupational therapists working in the different specialty areas of practice, since all are working to reduce performance dysfunction. Finally, West noted, occupational therapists should not lose sight of the basic concept of "mind-body-environment interrelationships activated through occupation." By organizing these concepts into a science of occupation, she proposed, the profession would be able to unify its practice and clearly identify its role in health and health care.

DEVELOPMENT OF A UNIFIED THEORETICAL BASE

Throughout the 1970s and 1980s occupational therapists were seeking a theoretical framework that would provide unity and cohesion for occupational therapy. One school of thought held that a single unifying theory should be developed, an all-encompassing set of beliefs that would be equally relevant to therapists working in all of the specialty areas of practice. Another school of thought subscribed to the idea that multiple theories were needed to adequately explain the varied aspects of the field. Arguing for the latter approach, Mosey (18) pointed out that occupational therapy is a diverse profession and deals with people of different ages and with different limitations.

A single comprehensive theory, she warned, might be so vague that it would offer little guidance for practice. The use of multiple theories would recognize the importance of all elements of the profession and better suit a field with as much variability as occupational therapy. Mosey proposed a taxonomy (a classification system) that would include multiple theories that could be used to explain aspects of occupational therapy within a loosely organized theoretical framework. According to Mosey, occupational therapy is too broad a field to expect that a single theory could explain all aspects of its practice.

Others disagreed. Katz (19) proposed that the core of occupational therapy be considered to be human occupation, as described by Kielhofner, Burke, Barris, and others. Human occupation, said Katz, is the key concept of occupational therapy and includes all of the relevant elements with which the field is concerned. According to proponents of this point of view, the primary concern of the occupational therapist is an individual's occupational role performance. Adoption of this single theoretical model would provide the field with a comprehensive framework for guiding clinical practice and for further theoretical development.

The debate over an appropriate theoretical model for occupational therapy practice continues. As the field develops and as occupational therapy methods are subjected to critical assessment we may evolve a model of practice that will clearly describe the parameters of the field in terms that can be accepted by most of its clinicians, educators, and researchers.

OCCUPATIONAL THERAPY IN A HIGH-TECH SOCIETY

Many occupational therapy leaders have commented on the rapid advent of technology in health care and the impact that this is likely to have on the field.

Already occupational therapy clinics have incorporated the use of electronic biofeedback devices for relief of chronic pain, as a training device for correcting movement disorders, and as an aid to muscle relaxation. The most promising of all technical devices, the computer, has quickly been adopted as a necessary tool in client treatment and in the management of occupational therapy programs. We need to remind ourselves, however, that these new technologies are only additional tools to enable us to help clients achieve needed occupational behaviors. Burke (20) suggests that occupational therapists are likely to become part of bioengineering teams developing new technological aids, because of their expertise in activity analysis and adaptation. When entering the world of high-tech, however, occupational therapists need to remember Ottenbacher's question (15): "Does occupational therapy wish to become an applied technology or an applied science?" Development of technology alone will not promote development of the field, but when accompanied by scientific research and theory development, it may yield great benefits. All of these components are needed to evolve a science of occupational therapy. At the present time the development of technology appears to be outdistancing the development of theory, which should guide its use.

Many issues confront occupational therapy personnel in the 1980s. It is critical for professional leaders and the occupational therapy community to continue a dialogue in order to develop effective policies to guide the future directions of the field.

DISCUSSION QUESTIONS

1. What are some of the ways that the profession can influence students to enter the specialty areas that will be most needed in the 1990s?

2. Will there be more competition between allied health professionals in the 1990s? How might this be seen?

3. If the pool of college-age students is growing smaller, from where are the future OTRs going to come?

4. Discuss the possibilities that Baum suggests as potential new service areas for occupational therapy. How might some of these areas be developed?

5. Would raising the entry-level education of the OTR to the master's degree level increase or decrease the number of graduates? What effects might this change have on the practice of occupational therapy?

6. Can occupational therapy be explained by a single comprehensive theory? Why or why not?

REFERENCES

1. Ad Hoc Commission on Occupational Therapy Manpower: *Occupational Therapy Manpower: A Plan for Progress.* Rockville, MD, American Occupational Therapy Association, 1985, pp 11–39.
2. New medicare regulations for HMOs open door for occupational therapy services. *Occup Ther News* 39(4):1, 1985.
3. Bureau of Labor Statistics reports on hospital wage survey. *Occup Ther News* 40(10):5, 1986.
4. Annual professional income. Part I. *Occup Ther News* 38(8):5, 1984.
5. Annual professional income. Part II. *Occup Ther News* 38(9):5, 1984.
6. Bell E: The changing faces of practice. *AJOT* 39:637–639, 1985.
7. Work programs SIS a success. *Occup Ther News* 40(9):3, 1986.
8. Annual Report of the American Occupational Therapy Association, Inc. *Occup Ther News* 40(8):12–13, 1986.
9. Baum C: Growth, renewal, and challenge: an important era for occupational therapy. *AJOT* 39:778–790, 1985.
10. Del Polito C: Future trends and opportunities—An assessment of environmental factors affecting health professions' education. In: *Proceedings. Target 2000: Occupational Therapy Education.*

Rockville, MD, American Occupational Therapy Association, 1986, pp 45–51.

11. Anderson R, Cuthbert M, Prendergast N, Levine R: Debate: Resolved, Level II fieldwork should become the responsibility of the professional organization. In: *Proceedings. Target 2000: Occupational Therapy Education.* Rockville, MD, American Occupational Therapy Association, 1986, pp 98–105.

12. Royeen C: The issue is: Entry level education in occupational therapy. *AJOT* 40:425–427, 1986.

13. Tanguay P: The issue is: Does occupational therapy belong in the university? *AJOT* 39:466–468, 1985.

14. Austin P: The university environment as it affects faculty today. In: *Proceedings. Target 2000: Occupational Therapy Education.* Rockville, MD,

American Occupational Therapy Assocation, 1986, pp 52–56.

15. Ottenbacher K: The importance of research to the viability of a profession. In: *Proceedings. Target 2000: Occupational Therapy Education.* Rockville, MD, American Occupational Therapy Association, 1986, pp 185–190.

16. Gilfoyle E: 1984: Transformation of a profession. *AJOT* 38:575–584. 1984.

17. West W: A reaffirmed philosophy and practice of occupational therapy. *AJOT* 38:15–23, 1984.

18. Mosey A: A monistic or a pluralistic approach to professional identity? *AJOT* 39:504–509, 1985.

19. Katz N: Occupational therapy's domain of concern: reconsidered. *AJOT* 39:518–524, 1985.

20. Burke J: Occupational therapy: a focus on roles in practice. *AJOT* 38:24–28, 1984.

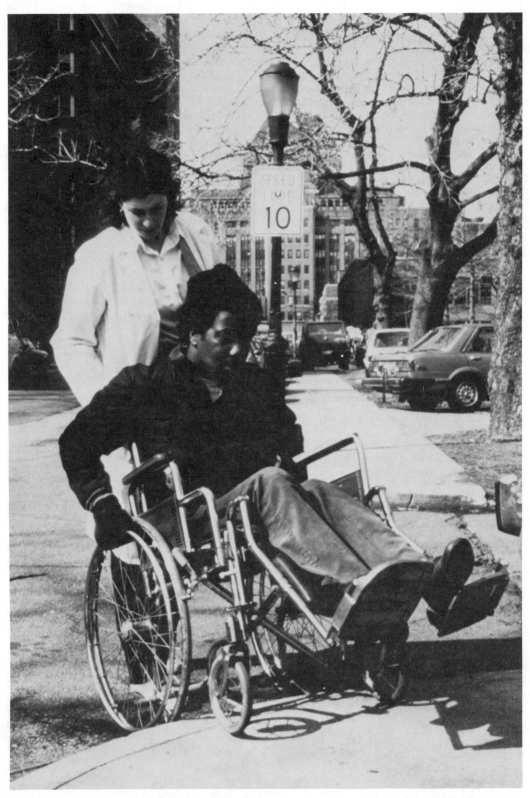

Courtesy AOTA

TWENTY

Future Outlook for Occupational Therapy

In this final chapter we look at some of the predictions that have been made for future developments in health care and in occupational therapy. Forecasting the future is hazardous. All projections should be considered only possibilities based on present conditions. These possibilities may be influenced by societal changes, revised professional attitudes and policies, and changing patterns of health care. Like all health care fields, occupational therapy is in a period of transition as health care delivery and reimbursement mechanisms take new forms. It is only possible to speculate on the long-term results of such changes.

CHANGING PATTERNS OF HEALTH CARE DELIVERY

The health care industry in the United States accounted for 12% of the gross national product in 1986 and is expected to rise to over 20% by the next century. We are seeing a shift from a nonprofit social welfare model of health care to a for-profit business model. Health care organizations are integrating and expanding their services both vertically and horizontally. The physician's role is changing. A technology explosion is changing the methods of diagnosing and treating disease and disability. Finally, the government is disengaging itself from direct involvement in health care. All of these changes that were in progress in 1986 are expected to continue well into the next decade.

Roth (1) predicts that the following changes will take place by the year 2010 (1).

- Health care will move from the illness end of the continuum to the wellness end.
- Health care services will largely be in the hands of large medical conglomerates that will provide multiple levels of service.
- There is likely to be a three-tiered system of health care: one for those who can pay their own costs; one for those who have insurance; and one for those with no personal resources who depend on government aid. The latter group will lack adequate health services and emergency care.
- Community hospitals will be a thing of the past.
- Health care conglomerates may develop their own medical schools

and training programs, just as General Motors trains its own skilled workers.

- Physicians will function largely as skilled technicians and will lose status and prestige as their income drops and their professional power declines.
- The diseases of the elderly will receive greater attention. The aging population will have political power and will demand attention to its problems.
- Because of rapid advances in technology, many routine medical tests will be carried out at home and will be transmitted by computer to the health care organization for analysis.
- The frequency of surgery will be dramatically reduced as chemotherapy, radiation, and nuclear magnetic resonance techniques are perfected. These methods will offer noninvasive diagnostic and treatment procedures for many diseases.
- The government will limit its expenditures for health care and will refuse to involve itself in making health care policies.

EFFECTS ON OCCUPATIONAL THERAPY PRACTICE

If these changes do come about, how is occupational therapy going to fit into the health care spectrum of the future? In 1985, Jaffe (2) outlined some strategies for occupational therapists who wish to prepare for the anticipated changes. Among the suggestions made were the following:

- Development of cost-effective programs, with services being provided in collaboration with other professions and health agencies.

- Participation in studies to assess quality of care. Occupational therapy will need to prove that the health services it provides are effective in restoring or maintaining health.
- Participation in the making of health policy decisions for the future. Taking part in policy making and planning will ensure that the views and priorities of occupational therapists will be considered when health care issues are acted upon.
- Aggressive marketing of occupational therapy services and a more businesslike approach to the way services are packaged and delivered.
- Development of innovative and nontraditional roles in occupational therapy, and reaching out to underserved segments of the population who could benefit from occupational therapy intervention.
- Promotion of the occupational therapy role in wellness and health equally with the role of restoring function in the ill and disabled.

In 1984, Gilfoyle (3) looked at possible future directions of the field and saw the possibility of occupational therapy focusing its services in two major environments—medical and educational. Gilfoyle believes that the expansion of occupational therapy services will take place primarily in educational environments. As a result of changes occurring in health care delivery, Gilfoyle predicts that occupational therapy services will be affected in the following ways:

- Occupational therapy will continue to be practiced in organizational structures, with increased pressures to make these organizations cost-effective.

- New and more effective communication networks must be developed to insure continuity of care among the various health professionals.
- Demands for interagency collaboration will be imperative.
- Power and political issues operating within health and educational organizations will increase rather than decrease.
- New service delivery patterns, involving consultation and monitoring, as well as collaborative programming, will be imperative. (3)

The 1985 AOTA Manpower Report also provided some projections of how occupational therapy practice is likely to change in the future (4). This task force saw trends that are likely to increase the need for occupational therapy:

- More emphasis on health promotion and disease prevention.
- More occupational therapy involvement with cancer patients, as more survive the disease but have limited function.
- An increase in school-based occupational therapy as the number of handicapped children increases.
- Increased use of technology in medical treatment, requiring that occupational therapists help patients adapt to restricted environments.
- An increase in health maintenance programs, particularly for the elderly, with a corresponding increase in occupational therapy involvement with alternative residential arrangements for the elderly.
- The emergence of social health maintenance organizations, in which occupational therapists could function as case managers

and integrators of social/health care factors.
- Advances in technology that provide opportunities for more independent living by the elderly and a higher survival rate for impaired infants.
- Greater emphasis on the rehabilitation of head trauma cases.

Another set of trends was identified that could decrease the need for occupational therapy services. Among these trends were the following items:

- A declining incidence of cerebrovascular accidents, a diagnostic category that is the number one health problem seen by occupational therapists.
- Increased competition among health care providers for the shrinking health care dollars available from consumers and reimbursers.
- More requirements for prior approval by reimbursers before extensive rehabilitation programs can be initiated.
- A decline in the incidence of complications following cardiac emergencies because of improvements in coronary care.
- Increased personal expenditures for health care as insurance coverage becomes more limited.
- The movement of mental health services from institutional to community settings could decrease the number of occupational therapists employed in mental health programs or increase the demand if new jobs are created in community agencies and outpatient services.
- Extension of the Medicare prospective payment system to such areas as long-term care, home health programs, and rehabilitation services

may reduce the use of occupational therapy in these programs. However, occupational therapy could continue to provide services to these programs in new and different ways. The effect on occupational therapy personnel is unknown at this time.

EFFECTS ON OCCUPATIONAL THERAPY EDUCATION

Just as changes in health care are likely to affect occupational therapy practice, they will also influence patterns of occupational therapy education. Del Polito (5) identified some of the changes that occupational therapy educational programs may need to accommodate to in future years. Curricula will need to be flexible and adaptable, in order to reflect rapid changes in practice. Educational programs will need to be redesigned to accommodate the older, part-time student as well as the traditional college-age student. Multiple skills will be needed for occupational therapists to remain employable, so curricula must provide students with a broad knowledge base. Development of qualified faculty who can meet the accepted standards of colleges and universities for hiring and promotion will be a high priority, and faculty will need to stay in touch with the rapidly changing trends in health care. Interdisciplinary training is expected to become even more important to the education of all health professionals as team functions and interrelationships become more crucial in health care delivery.

After studying the current patterns of occupational therapy education, the task force that prepared the *AOTA 1985 Manpower Report* made a number of recommendations related to occupational therapy education (4). They stressed that the following actions are needed if occupational therapy is to meet future personnel needs.

- Expansion of the occupational therapy educational system in order to meet projected personnel needs.
- Development of new educational programs in underserved areas of the country (West and South).
- Encouragement of nontraditional programs to serve the needs of students who want part-time, weekend, or concentrated programs.
- Expansion of recruitment activities to encourage more students to enter occupational therapy educational programs.
- An increase in the number of qualified occupational therapy faculty.
- Expansion of continuing education programs in order to help practitioners meet changing population needs and changing service delivery patterns.
- Adoption of curricula that will ensure that occupational therapy education produces graduates who are prepared to practice in new service environments and assume new professional roles.
- Modification of the credentialing policies in occupational therapy to enable additional personnel to join the occupational therapy work force.

If some or all of these recommendations are carried out, occupational therapy will be in a better position to respond to the need for personnel and for changes in practice as we move into the 1990s and beyond.

MAINTAINING TRADITIONAL VALUES IN A CHANGING SOCIETY

Englehardt (6) notes that advances in technology invariably give rise to questions of ethics and values. Health care fields, in particular, need to consider their traditional values in deciding how to apply technological advances. Will occupational therapy values and principles continue to be relevant? The answer given by occupational therapy leaders is a resounding "yes!" In 1986 Bing (7) reviewed some of the major concepts of the field as they were stated by its founders and pioneers and concluded that these ideas continue to express the basic philosophy of occupational therapy. "We will find comfort, safety, and stability . . . in those decades-old fundamentals and principles developed by our founders and practiced by our pioneers and each succeeding generation of therapists," said Bing, a former president of AOTA. "The belief system that has emerged . . . will continue to develop as time moves on" (7).

Another former president of AOTA agreed. Johnson (8) elaborated further on the impact of societal and health care changes on traditional occupational therapy values. She outlined six occupational therapy values that express basic beliefs about the field.

1. The value of the individual as a total person;
2. The value of purposeful activity and occupation in producing change and recovery;
3. The value of goal-oriented activity designed for a given individual's skills and abilities;
4. The value of permitting patients to choose meaningful activities . . . which parallel those they might normally engage in;
5. The value of seeing the individual interacting within the framework of the environment; and
6. The value we place on ourselves, our feelings, and our interactions with patients/clients as vital, integral, and caring components of the therapeutic process.

These values, which appear and reappear throughout the occupational therapy literature, continue to be meaningful to occupational therapists. Johnson notes that occupational therapists have been highly successful in adapting their tools, techniques, and values to new categories of clients. The repertoire of occupational therapists has expanded to include splinting and orthotics, use of self, prevocational exploration, and neuro-developmental and kinesiological theories and techniques. Perhaps occupational therapists have overadapted, Johnson suggests. As a result there is an increased demand for their services, but some of the new directions taken seem to be the result of external forces rather than the application of our traditional values. Overadaptation to the changing health care scene has had some negative consequences, Johnson believes. Inadequate preparation for today's stressful clinical environments can lead to new therapists feeling overwhelmed by the demands being placed on them. Occupational therapy has not provided adequate nurturing or recognition for those of its members who work as administrators, clinical specialists, researchers, or curriculum directors. Practitioners have been so busy selling their clinical skills that they have neglected to do the work necessary to substantiate the effectiveness of those skills. Finally, the field has become so concerned with personnel shortages that it has neglected its conceptual issues. The goal for the future, says Johnson, should be to "understand the cause of dysfunction; diagnose dysfunction as it affects performance and occupation; to identify and establish the appropriate program and process for specific individuals that will result in adaptation and . . . reintegration; and to bring about change in society and technology so that both share the responsibility for adapting to the needs of humans . . ." (8) Johnson sees occupational therapy as facing a conflict between a desire to retain traditional values and a recognition of the importance of science and research.

Therapists, however, are worried about where an emphasis on science and research will take the field. Will occupational therapy continue to hold its humanistic values in a world where every fact must be proven and every method put to the test? Johnson concludes that the two points of view can be reconciled and that by doing so the profession will acquire new competence. "The process of adaptation will bring about change, but integration can provide us with a unity and a wholeness which we have not yet achieved" (8).

As occupational therapy faces its second century, it is preparing to meet new challenges and expectations. Occupational therapists and therapy assistants will be able to successfully adapt to the changing health care scene. When questioning their contributions to the health care of the future, Dunn (9) suggests that occupational therapists ask themselves, "What business are we really in?" The answer is that occupational therapy is still in the business it has always been in—that of facilitating life-long independence in individuals. Its methods have changed and will continue to change; its work sites may be different from those of the past, but the concerns of occupational therapists remain the same. Occupational therapy is in the business of helping people adapt to physical, psychosocial, and environmental changes in their lives, and it moves into the twenty-first century prepared to take its place as an active contributor to health and health care.

DISCUSSION QUESTIONS

1. What will happen if community hospitals close? Where will people in small towns and rural areas receive hospital care? What effects might this have on individuals and families?

2. If there is no insurance coverage for the health care of low-income groups, how will they receive care?

3. Will the recommended changes in occupational therapy educational patterns result in more graduates? Why or why not?

4. What is likely to happen if occupational therapists are not available in large enough numbers to meet projected personnel needs?

5. How will the projected needs for occupational therapy personnel affect your future as an occupational therapist or therapy assistant?

6. Where may OTRs and COTAs be working in the next century? Discuss possible work sites and health care needs that they could fulfill.

REFERENCES

1. Roth B: Health care 2010: the shape of things to come. *SCAN* 5–7, 1986.
2. Jaffe E: Nationally speaking: transition in health care—critical planning for the 1990s. *AJOT* 39: 499–503, 1985.
3. Gilfoyle E: 1984: transformation of a profession. *AJOT* 38:575–584, 1984.
4. Ad Hoc Commission on Occupational Therapy Manpower: *Occupational Therapy Manpower: A Plan for Progress.* Rockville, MD, American Occupational Therapy Association, 1985, pp. 58–59, 61–64.
5. Del Polito C: Future trends and opportunities—an assessment of environmental factors affecting health professions' education. In: *Proceedings. Target 2000: occupational Therapy Education.* Rockville, MD, American Occupational Therapy Association, 1986, pp. 45–51.
6. Englehardt T: The importance of values in shaping professional directions and behaviors. In: *Proceedings. Target 2000: Occupational Therapy Education.* Rockville, MD, American Occupational Therapy Association, 1986, pp. 39–44.
7. Bing R: Nationally speaking: the Subject is health: not of facts, but of values. *AJOT* 40:667–671, 1986.
8. Johnson J: Old values—new directions: competence, adaptation, integration. *AJOT* 35:589–598, 1981.
9. Dunn W: Keynote address: challenging our energies—a focus on the future. Annual Conference of the Wisconsin Occupational Therapy Association, September 19–20, 1986.

Glossary

Activities of daily living (ADL) performance of self-care, work, and leisure activities

Acute of short duration. Used to describe the first phase of an illness or diseases that run a rapid course

Adductor pads pads at the sides of a wheelchair to hold the hips and legs toward the midline of the body

Affect emotional feeling, tone, or mood

AIDS acquired immune deficiency syndrome

Alzheimer's disease degeneration of the medium and smaller blood vessels of the brain

Ambulate to walk about

Ambulatory care medical care for patients who are able to get about

Amputation the surgical removal of a body part

Anxiety a state of worry or distress; apprehension

Aphasia impaired spoken communication or poor comprehension of speech due to dysfunction of the language centers in the brain

Arteriosclerosis a hardening or thickening of the walls of arteries resulting in decreased blood flow to the heart, the brain, or the extremities

Arthritis inflamation of the joints; may be seen in acute or chronic forms

Athetoid relating to athetosis, a condition characterized by fluctuating muscle tone and slow, involuntary movements

Augmentative communication communication through the use of mechanical devices that expand the individual's ability to communicate

Avocational relating to activities outside of one's work; leisure pursuits

Baseline information data on the patient's level of function when he or she is first seen by a health care worker

Behaviorist theory a branch of psychology that attempts to explain human behavior in terms of learning principles and conditioning

Bilateral on both sides of the body

Biofeedback training the use of electronic devices to help an individual learn to gain voluntary control over autonomic body functions

Biomechanics the science of the action of forces, internal or external, on the living body

Body mechanics application of physics principles to avoid undue stress on joints or body parts

Bone grafting transplanting bone tissue from one part of the body to another

Cardex information a card file at the nurses station on a hospital unit that contains summarized information about the status of patients on the unit

Cerebral pertaining to the two hemispheres of the brain

Cerebral arteriosclerosis narrowing of the blood vessels within the brain, which may result in headache, dizziness, insomnia, memory changes, or personality changes

Cerebral palsy a group of nonprogressive disorders characterized by disturbances in muscle tone and motor control

Cerebral vasular disease those diseases that

result from changes in the blood vessels supplying the brain

Certification a voluntary process whereby a nongovernmental agency documents that a person has qualified to practice a given profession

Cervical pertaining to the neck

Chart review the process of reading the patient's medical chart in order to better understand his or her condition

Chart rounds meetings at which the health care team reviews the status of its' patients and makes any necessary adjustments in the treatment program

Chronic of long duration. Used to describe conditions that are long-standing

Chronic brain syndrome permanent and generalized loss of cerebral function that may include disorientation, memory loss, confusion, and stereotyped behavior

Closed-head injury a head injury in which there is little or no damage to the skull

Cognitive functions the mental processes that are necessary to perform daily activities

Cognitive retraining a systematic method of helping a person to improve his or her understanding of concepts, ability to concentrate, memory, and orientation

Collaboration working cooperatively with others to achieve a mutual goal

Coma, comatose a state of profound unconsciousness from which the patient cannot be aroused

Commode a chair enclosing a chamber pot

Congenital anomalies structural abnormalities that are the result of birth defects or genetic disorders

Contracture a permanent muscular contraction that results in loss of function

Coordination the ability to use several groups of muscles in a combined way to smoothly execute complex movements

CPR cardiopulmonary resuscitation; an emergency technique to restore breathing and heart rate following an injury

Craniectomy the cutting out of a portion of the skull

Craniotomy making a surgical opening in the skull

Cuing strategies methods of offering a patient cues in order to help him or her perform a given task

Custodial institution one that provides the basic necessities of life but does not provide active treatment or training

CVA cerbrovascular accident; commonly known as a stroke. Bleeding, blockage of a vessel, or a blood clot in a vessel within the brain that results in paralysis, sensory loss, speech impairments, and other neurologic symptoms

Debridement the cutting out of dead tissue and foreign matter from a wound

Deinstitutionalization the movement to shift treatment services from large governmental institutions to local community-based programs

Depression a clinical condition in which the patient feels dejected and hopeless and may withdraw from social contacts

Developmental delay a condition in which a child is found to be functioning at a level below age or maturational expectations

Diabetes a metabolic disorder characterized by a deficient supply of insulin and an inability to metabolize carbohydrates

Diffuse brain damage widespread, generalized deficits in the brain

Dilation enlargement or opening of a hollow structure

DRGs diagnostic-related groups, which are now the basis for reimbursement for hospitalized Medicare recipients

Dysfunction disordered or impaired function

Egalitarian equal; the idea that all members of a group have equal rights in the group

Embolism an obstruction in a blood vessel, often by a blood clot

Energy conservation the application of energy-saving procedures to minimize energy output by the patient

Equilibrium balance

Existential pertaining to existence and individual experience

Extensor muscles those muscles that extend or straighten a limb or a body part

Eye tracking the ability to follow an object through the visual field using both eyes simultaneously

Flailing movements thrashing about wildly

Focal brain damage localized injury to a specific part of the brain

Fracture a broken bone or piece of cartilege

Freud's psychoanalytic theory a method of

therapy developed by Freud that emphasized bringing unconscious material to consciousness

Gastric pertaining to the stomach

Gastrointestinal referring to the stomach and the intestines; the digestive tract

Gastrostomy the surgical creation of an artificial opening into the stomach

Generic relating to or descriptive of an entire group or class

Geriatrics the branch of medicine that deals with the medical problems of the elderly

Gerontology the study of old age

Gestation the total length of a pregnancy

Hemiplegia paralysis of one side of the body

Holistic looking at a thing as a unified whole

Homonymous hemianopsia blindness for objects in one-half of the visual field, resulting from injury to one optic tract

Hospice programs programs providing care for terminally ill patients and emotional support for them and their families

Hyaline membrane disease respiratory distress syndrome of the newborn

Hydrocephalus a condition in which excessive fluid accumulates in the ventricles of the brain, thinning the brain tissue and causing the skull to enlarge

Hyperventilate to overbreathe, taking rapid shallow breaths that can sometimes cause fainting

Intensive care unit the hospital unit that provides extensive life support services for seriously ill and injured patients

Intracerebral contusion a bruising of the brain without rupture of the membranes surrounding it

Intrinsic pertaining to the essential nature of a thing; inherent

Intrinsic motivation motivation that comes from within the individual; self-motivation

Joint fusion a surgical procedure that fixes a joint in one position, rendering it immovable

Licensure official or legal permission from a governmental body to engage in a given occupation or to do or own a specified thing

Manual muscle test a method of evaluating the strength of individual muscles or groups of muscles

Motor planning the ability to plan and execute purposeful movements

Multiple sclerosis a chronic, progressive neurologic disease characterized by fluctuating periods of wellness and periods of serious impairment

Muscle tone the amount of mild, continuous contraction that is present in normal living muscles

Nasogastric tube a tube inserted through the nose for feeding a patient who is unable to take food by mouth

Neurodevelopmental referring to the gradual, progressive development of the nervous system

Neuromuscular pertaining to the nerves and the muscles

Neuromuscular facilitation and inhibition increasing or decreasing the activity of muscles through the specific application of sensory stimuli

Neuromuscular functions performance of motor behaviors

Neurophysiology the study of the functioning of the nervous system

Neurosis a psychological or behavioral disorder characterized by anxiety

Noninvasive techniques methods that do not require entering the body of the patient

Obesity a condition in which there is an abnormal amount of fat in body tissues

Organic mental disorders those conditions that are believed to be the result of physiological or structural change or damage

Orthopedics the branch of medicine concerned with restoring the function of the limbs and spine through medical, surgical, and physical methods

Orthotics splints, braces, or slings used to relieve pain, maintain the alignment of joints, protect joints, improve function, or decrease deformity

Palliative treatment treatment that reduces the symptoms but does not cure the disease

Paradigm an example or model

Parkinson's disease a degenerative disease of the central nervous system characterized by increasing rigidity, tremors, and slowness of movement

Pathology the anatomic or functional manifestations of disease

Perception   the brain's interpretation of information received through the senses

Performance components   the subskills necessary to perform daily life activities

Personality disorders   a group of mental disorders characterized by long-standing patterns of maladaptive behavior

Philanthropy   charitable activities intended to increase the well-being of humankind

Physiatrist   a physician who specializes in physical medicine and rehabilitation

Pneumonia   inflammation of the lungs

Polio   poliomyelitis, an acute viral disease that may result in paralysis and atrophy of muscle groups

Prevention   minimizing the possibility of disease, dysfunction, or disability

Prevocational evaluation   assessment of work-related abilities and the potential for employment

Primitive reflexes   a group of automatic movement patterns seen in newborn infants that are controlled at the spinal and brain stem levels

Progressive resistive exercise   exercise against an opposing force, in which the resistance is systematically increased in order to strengthen muscles

Prosthetics   artificial substitutes for missing body parts, such as artificial limbs

Psychodynamics   the theory of human behavior that emphasizes the unconscious motivation and the functional significance of emotion

Psychometric tests   tests that measure psychological variables such as intelligence, aptitude, or emotional disturbance

Pulmonary   pertaining to the lungs

Quality assurance program   a method of studying the outcomes of therapy in order to assess the effectiveness of services being provided and to recommend changes in service delivery if necessary

Range of motion   a person's maximum span of joint movement

Regression   a return to more primitive patterns of behavior

Rehabilitation   restoration, after a disease or injury, of the ability to function in a normal or near-normal manner

Reimbursement   to pay back or compensate someone

Remedial   intended to correct something

Resection   the surgical removal of a section or a part

Respiratory   pertaining to the lungs and the process of breathing

Rheumatoid arthritis   a chronic inflammatory condition affecting the joints that results in pain and swelling of joints with increasing stiffness and disability

Robotics   the science of mechnical devices that work automatically or by remote control

Sacrum   the last lumbar vertebra or tailbone

Schizophrenic disorders   a group of mental disorders characterized by flat or inappropriate affect, social isolation, and delusions or hallucinations

Seizure disorder   a condition in which there are periodic alterations in brain function, usually accompanied by motor, sensory, autonomic, or psychic symptoms

Sensory   referring to the senses

Sensory aids   devices to increase the efficiency of receiving sensory stimuli, such as hearing aids or eyeglasses

Sensory deprivation   lowering the amount of sensory signals from the environment, which may result in emotional, perceptual, and behavioral abnormalities in human beings

Sensory integration   the organization of sensory input for practical use; the ability to respond to sensory stimuli in a purposeful way

Spastic quadriplegia   a nonprogressive condition in which the muscles are excessively tight and all four limbs are affected

Spinal cord injury   damage to the spinal cord that may result in permanent paralysis and loss of sensation below the level of the injury

Spinal meningitis   inflammation of the membranes of the spinal cord

Standing tolerance   the ability to stand for a given period of time

Subdural hematoma   a blood clot underneath the outer membrane that covers the brain and causes pressure on the brain, resulting in neurological symptoms

Subtotal   incomplete

Tactile   pertaining to the sense of touch

Technology   the application of science to meet industrial or business objectives

Technology transfer   the transfer of technology from one field to another or from one application to another

Total hip arthroplasty   a surgical procedure in which an artificial hip joint is created

Tracheostomy   surgical creation of an opening into the windpipe

Traction   pulling against resistance

Trauma   an injury caused by harsh contact with an object

Tuberculosis   a bacterial disease most commonly affecting the lungs that results in fever and weight loss

Ulcer   a lesion on the surface of the skin or a mucous surface, usually with inflammation

Upper extremities   the hands, arms, and shoulders

Venous   pertaining to the veins

Ventricular hemorrhage   bleeding within the ventricles of the brain

Visual field cuts   a patient's inability to see a part of the environment when looking straight ahead

Visual perceptual disorder   impairment in the ability to analyze and interpret visual information

Vocational   pertaining to one's work

Vocational rehabilitation   a specialized field that is concerned with enabling disabled persons to resume productive employment

BIBLIOGRAPHY

Ayres A J: Sensory Integration and the Child. Los Angeles, Western Psychological Services, 1979.

Bair J, Gray M (eds): The Occupational Therapy Manager. Rockville, MD, American Occupational Therapy Association, 1985.

Boyd W, Sheldon H: Introduction to the Study of Disease, ed 8. Philadelphia, Lea & Febiger, 1980.

Chusid J G: Correlative Neuroanatomy and Functional Neurology, ed 19. Los Altos, CA, Lange Medical Publications, 1985.

Clark PN, Allen AS: Occupational Therapy for Children. St. Louis, CV Mosby, 1985.

Clark RG: Manter & Gatz's Essentials of Clinical Neuroanatomy and Neurophysiology ed 5. Philadelphia, FA Davis, 1975.

Hensyl WR (ed): Stedman's Medical Dictionary, ed 24. Baltimore, Williams & Wilkins, 1982.

Morris W (ed): American Heritage Dictionary of the English Language, New College Edition. Boston, Houghton Mifflin, 1981.

Occupational therapy definitions. In Reference Manual of the Official Documents of the American Occupational Therapy Association, Inc. Rockville, MD, American Occupational Therapy Association, 1985, pp. VII11–VII15.

Reed KL, Sanderson SR: Concepts of Occupational Therapy, ed 2. Baltimore, Williams & Wilkins, 1983.

Trombly C: Occupational Therapy for Physical Dysfunction, ed 2. Baltimore, Williams & Wilkins, 1983.

Appendix A

For further information about occupational therapy, contact the American Occupational Therapy Association, Inc., 1383 Piccard Drive, P.O. Box 1725, Rockville, MD, 20850-4375, telephone # (301) 948-9626.

The abbreviated directory below shows which office to contact for certain kinds of information

American Occupational Therapy Association Inc.

For information about:	Contact:
Student scholarships	American Occupational Therapy Foundation
General information	Public Affairs Division
AOTA publications	AOTA Products
Membership benefits	Membership Information
Career information	Public Affairs Division
Certification examination	American Occupational Therapy Certification Board
Student loan program	Membership Information
Current list of accredited educational programs	Education Division, Accreditation
Employment service program	Member Services
Fellowships	American Occupational Therapy Foundation
Films	AOTA Products
Foreign graduate certification	American Occupational Therapy Certification Board
Graduate education	Education Division

For information about:	Contact:
Information packets occupational therapy practice	AOTA Products
International issues	Executive Office
Job bulletin	Member services
Job descriptions	Practice Division
Legislation	Government and Legal Affairs Division
Library	Library
Licensure	Government and Legal Affairs Division
Manpower	Research Information and Evaluation
Position papers	Practice Division
Public information materials	Public Affairs Division
Recruitment materials	Public Affairs Division
Reimbursement issues	Government and Legal Affairs Division
Research grants	American Occupational Therapy Foundation
Roles and functions of occupational therapy personnel	Practice Division
Salaries of occupational therapy personnel	Research Information and Evaluation
Speakers network	Continuing Education, Practice Division
Standards of practice	Practice Division
State associations	Practice Division
Statistics	Research Information and Evaluation
Student newsletter	Education Division
World Federation of Occupational Therapists	Executive Office

APPENDIX B

The American Occupational Therapy Association, Inc.

Listing of Educational Programs in Occupational Therapy

November 1986

The Council on Postsecondary Accreditation and the U.S. Department of Education require that the list of accredited educational programs for the occupational therapist be published annually. In addition, the American Occupational Therapy Association publishes the list of approved educational programs for the occupational therapy assistant. These lists follow.

Professional Programs 1986–1987

The following *entry level* programs are accredited by the Committee on Allied Health Education and Accreditation of the American Medical Association in collaboration with the American Occupational Therapy Association. On-site evaluations for program accreditation are conducted at 5-year intervals for initial accreditation and 7-year intervals for reaccreditation. The dates on this list indicate the academic year the next evaluation is anticipated. for specific information, contact the program directly.

Key:
1   Baccalaureate program
2   Postbaccalaureate certificate program
2A   Certificate awarded to students in
      partial fulfillment of master's degree
3   Professional master's degree program
4   Combined BS/MS degree program
a   Public nonprofit
b   Private nonprofit

ALABAMA

1, a   **90/91**
**University of Alabama in
  Birmingham**
Regional Technical Institute,
  Room 114
University Station
Birmingham, AL 35294
Carroline Amari, MA, OTR,
  Director
Division of Occupational
  Therapy

1, b   **90/91**
Tuskegee University
Division of Allied Health
School of Nursing and Allied
  Health
Tuskegee, AL 36088
Marie L. Moore, MS, OTR,
  FAOTA, Director
Department of Occupational
  Therapy

ARKANSAS

1, a   **89/90**
University of Central Arkansas
PO Box U1761
Conway, AR 72032
Marian Q. Ross, MA, OTR/L,
  FAOTA, Chair
Department of Occupational
  Therapy

CALIFORNIA

1, b   **89/90**
Loma Linda University
School of Allied Health
  Professions
Loma Linda, CA 92350
Edwinna Marshall, MA, OTR,
  FAOTA, Chair
Department of Occupational
  Therapy

1, 2A, a   **90/91**
San Jose State University
School of Applied Arts and
  Sciences
One Washington Square
San Jose, CA 95192-0001
Lela A. Llorens, PhD, OTR,
  FAOTA, Chair
Department of Occupational
  Therapy (Priority given to Cal-
  ifornia residents)

1, 2A, 3, b   **88/89**
**University of Southern
  California**
12933 Erickson Avenue, Building
  30
Downey, CA 90242
Elizabeth J. Yerxa, EdD, OTR,
  FAOTA, Chair
Department of Occupational
  Therapy

COLORADO

1, 3, a   **86/87**
Colorado State University
100 Humanities Building
Fort Collins, CO 80523
Elnora M. Gilfoyle, DSc, OTR,
  FAOTA, Head
Department of Occupational
  Therapy

CONNECTICUT

1, 2*, b   **90/91**
Quinnipiac College
School of Allied Health and Nat-
  ural Sciences
Hamden, CT 06518
Muriel S. Schwartz, MS, OTR/L,
  Chairperson
Department of Occupational
  Therapy
*Program level pending
  accreditation

DISTRICT OF COLUMBIA

1, b   **86/87**
Howard University
College of Allied Health Sciences
6th & Bryant Streets, NW
Washington, DC 20059
Joyce B. Lane, MEd, OTR,
  FAOTA, Chair
Department of Occupational
  Therapy

FLORIDA

1, a   **86/87**
Florida International University
Miami, FL 33199
Susan H. Kaplan, MHS, OTR,
  Acting Chairperson
Department of Occupational
  Therapy

1, 3*, a   **86/87**
University of Florida
Box J164, JHMHC
Gainesville, FL 32610
Kay W. Sieg, MEd, OTR, Chair
Department of Occupational
  Therapy
*Program level pending
  accreditation

GEORGIA

1, a   **91/92**
Medical College of Georgia
School of Allied Health Services
Augusta, GA 30912
Nancy Prendergast, EdD, OTR/L,
  FAOTA, Chair
Department of Occupational
  Therapy

ILLINOIS

1, a   **90/91**
Chicago State University
College of Allied Health
95th Street at King Drive
Chicago, IL 60628
Artice W. Harmon, MPH, OTR,
  Director
Occupational Therapy Program

1, a   **91/92**
University of Illinois at Chicago
College of Associated Health
  Professions
Health Sciences Center
1919 West Taylor Street
Chicago, IL 60612
Gary Kielhofner, DPH, OTR,
  Head
Department of Occupational
  Therapy

3, b   **90/91**
**Rush University, Rush-
  Presbyterian-St. Luke's Medi-
  cal Center**
1753 West Congress Parkway
Chicago, IL 60612
Cynthia J. Hughes, MEd, OTR,
  Director
Department of Occupational
  Therapy

INDIANA

1, a   **88/89**
**Indiana University School of
  Medicine**
Division of Allied Health
  Sciences
1140 West Michigan Street
Indianapolis, IN 46223
Celestine Hamant, MS, OTR,
  FAOTA
Associate Professor and Director
Occupational Therapy

KANSAS

1, a   88/89
University of Kansas
School of Allied Health
4017 Hinch Hall
39th and Rainbow Boulevard
Kansas City, KS 66103
Winnie Dunn, PhD, OTR,
    FAOTA, Chair
Department of Occupational
    Therapy

KENTUCKY

1, a   87/88
Eastern Kentucky University
Wallace Building, Room 109
Richmond, KY 40475
Joy Anderson, MA, OTR,
    FAOTA, Chair
Department of Occupational
    Therapy

LOUISIANA

1, a   87/88
**Louisiana State University Medi-
    cal Center**
School of Allied Health
    Professions
1900 Gravier Street
New Orleans, LA 70112
M. Suzanne Poulton, MHS, L/
    OTR, Head
Department of Occupational
    Therapy
Offered: New Orleans,
    Shreveport*
*Pending accreditation

1, a   87/88
Northeast Louisiana University
School of Allied Health Sciences
Monroe, LA 71209
Lee Sens, MA, OTR, Director
Occupational Therapy Program

MAINE

1, b   90/91
University of New England
College of Arts and Sciences
Biddeford, ME 04005
Judith G. Kimball, PhD, OTR,
    FAOTA, Director
Division of Occupational
    Therapy

MARYLAND

1, a   87/88
Towson State University
Towson, MD 21204
Marie-Louise Blount, AM, OTR,
    Chair
Occupational Therapy
    Department

MASSACHUSETTS

1, 3, b   86/87
**Boston University, Sargent Col-
    lege of Allied Health
    Professions**
University Road
Boston, MA 02215
Anne Henderson, PhD, OTR,
    FAOTA, Chair
Department of Occupational
    Therapy

1, 3, b   89/90
**Tufts University-Boston School
    of Occupational Therapy**
Medford, MA 02155
Sharan L. Schwartzberg, EdD,
    OTR, FAOTA, Chairperson
Department of Occupational
    Therapy

MICHIGAN

1, a   90/91
Eastern Michigan University
Department of Associated Health
    Professions
328 King Hall
Ypsilanti, MI 48197
Ruth Ann Hansen, PhD, OTR,
    FAOTA, Program Director
Occupational Therapy Program

1, 2, a   86/87
Wayne State University
College of Pharmacy and Allied
    Health Professions
Detroit, MI 48202
Miriam C. Freeling, MA, OTR,
    FAOTA, Chair
Department of Occupational
    Therapy

1, 3, a   91/92
Western Michigan University
Kalamazoo, MI 49008
Claire Callan, EdS, OTR, Chair
Department of Occupational
    Therapy

MINNESOTA

1, a   86/87
University of Minnesota
Health Sciences Center
Box 388, Mayo Building
Minneapolis, MN 55455
Rondell S. Berkeland, MPH,
    OTR, Program Director
Program in Occupational
    Therapy

1, 2, b   86/87
College of St. Catherine
2004 Randolph Avenue
St. Paul, MN 55105
Sr. Miriam Joseph Cummings,
    MA, OTR, FAOTA, Director
Department of Occupational
    Therapy

MISSOURI

1*, 3, a**   88/89
University of Missouri-Columbia
Health Related Professions
124 Lewis Hall
Columbia, MO 65211
Diana J. Baldwin, MA, OTR,
    Director
Occupational Therapy
    Curriculum
*Preference given to Missouri
    residents
**Admission to this level is
    closed

1, b   89/90
Washington University
School of Medicine
4567 Scott Avenue
St. Louis, MO 63110
Mary Ann Boyle, PhD, OTR
Elias Michael Director
Program in Occupational
    Therapy

NEW HAMPSHIRE

1, a   89/90
University of New Hampshire
School of Health Studies
Hewitt Hall
Durham, NH 03824
Barbara Sussenberger, MS, OTR,
    Chair
Occupational Therapy
    Department

NEW JERSEY

1, 2, a   88/89
Kean College of New Jersey
Willis 311, Morris Avenue
Union, NJ 07083
Paula Kramer, MA, OTR,
    FAOTA, Chairperson
Occupational Therapy
    Department

NEW YORK

1, a   91/92
University of Buffalo, State University of New York
515 Stockton Kimball Tower
3435 Main Street
Buffalo, NY 14214
Karen E. Schanzenbacher, MS, OTR
Acting Chair and Assistant Professor
Department of Occupational Therapy

3, b   86/87
Columbia University
College of Physicians and Surgeons
630 West 168th Street
New York, NY 10032
Barbara Neuhaus, EdD, OTR, FAOTA, Director
Programs in Occupational Therapy

1, b   90/91
Dominican College of Blauvelt
10 Western Highway
Orangeburg, NY 10962
Kenneth Skrivanek, MA, OTR, Coordinator
Occupational Therapy Program

1, 3, b   88/89
New York University
Division of Health
34 Stuyvesant Street, Room 101
New York, NY 10003
Deborah R. Labovitz, PhD, OTR, FAOTA, Chair
Department of Occupational Therapy

1, a   87/88
State University of New York Health Science Center at Brooklyn
450 Clarkson Avenue, Box 81
Brooklyn, NY 11203
Patricia Trossman, MA, OTR, Chairman
Occupational Therapy Program

1, b   86/87
Utica College of Syracuse University
Division of Allied Health
Burrstone Road
Utica, NY 13502
Richard C. Wright, MS, OTR, Director
Curriculum in Occupational Therapy

1, a   86/87
York College of the City University of New York
Jamaica, NY 11451
Wimberly Edwards, MS, OTR, FAOTA, Coordinator
Occupational Therapy Program

NORTH CAROLINA

1, a   89/90
East Carolina University
School of Allied Health and Social Work
Greenville, NC 27834
Margaret Wittman, MS, OTR/L, Chair
Department of Occupational Therapy

3, a   92/93
University of North Carolina at Chapel Hill
Medical School, Wing E 222H
Chapel Hill, NC 27514
Cathy Nielson, MPH, OTR/L, Acting Director
Occupational Therapy Division

NORTH DAKOTA

1, a   89/90
University of North Dakota
Box 8036, University Station
Grand Forks, ND 58202
Sue McIntyre, MS, OTR, Chairperson
Department of Occupational Therapy

OHIO

1, 2, a   86/87
Cleveland State University
Health Sciences Department
College of Arts and Sciences
1983 East 24th Street
Cleveland, OH 44115
Julia Miller, MEd, OTR/L, Director
Occupational Therapy Program

1, 2, a   90/91
Ohio State University
School of Allied Medical Professions
1583 Perry Street
Columbus, OH 43210
H. Kay Grant, PhD, OTR/L, FAOTA, Director
Occupational Therapy Division

OKLAHOMA

1, a   92/93
University of Oklahoma Health Sciences Center
College of Allied Health
PO Box 26901
Oklahoma City, OK 73190
Sharon Sanderson Nelson, MPH, OTR, Chair
Department of Occupational Therapy

OREGON

1, b   90/91
Pacific University
2043 College Way
Forest Grove, OR 97116
Molly McEwen, MHS, OTR, Director
Occupational Therapy Department

PENNSYLVANIA

1, b   88/89
Elizabethtown College
Elizabethtown, PA 17022-0521
Robert K. Bing, EdD, OTR, FAOTA
Professor and Chairman
Department of Occupational Therapy

1, b   91/92
College Misericordia
Division of Allied Health Professions
Dallas, PA 18612
Jack Kasar, MS, OTR/L, Program Director
Occupational Therapy Program

1, b   89/90
University of Pittsburgh
School of Health Related Professions
204 Mineral Industries Building
Pittsburgh, PA 15260
Caroline R. Brayley, MEd, OTR/L, FAOTA, Director
Program in Occupational Therapy

1, 2A, 3, a, b   86/87
Temple University
College of Allied Health Professions
Health Sciences Campus
3307 North Broad Street
Philadelphia, PA 19140
Elizabeth G. Tiffany, MEd, OTR/L, FAOTA, Interim Chair
Department of Occupational Therapy

1, 2, b   90/91
Thomas Jefferson University
College of Allied Health Sciences
Edison Building, Room 820
130 South 9th Street
Philadelphia, PA 19107
Ruth Ellen Levine, EdD, OTR,
  FAOTA
Department of Occupational
  Therapy

PUERTO RICO

1*, a   92/93
University of Puerto Rico
Medical Sciences Campus
College of Health Related
  Professions
Physical and Occupational Ther-
  apy Department
GPO Box 5067
San Juan, PR 00936
Elsie Rodriguez de Vergara,
  ScD(c), OTR, Director
Occupational Therapy Program
*Does not accept nonresident
  students

SOUTH CAROLINA

1, a   88/89
**Medical University of South
  Carolina**
College of Health Related
  Professions
171 Ashley Avenue—Room 224
Charleston, SC 29425
Maralynne D. Mitcham, PhD,
  OTR/L
Associate Professor and
  Chairman
Occupational Therapy Educa-
  tional Department

TEXAS

1, a   92/93
**University of Texas Health Sci-
  ence Center at San Antonio**
7703 Floyd Curl Drive
San Antonio, TX 78284
Charles H. Christiansen, EdD,
  OTR, FAOTA
Professor and Director
Occupational Therapy Program

1, a   90/91
**University of Texas School of
  Allied Health Sciences at
  Galveston**
**University of Texas Medical
  Branch at Galveston**
Galveston, TX 77550
Donald A. Davidson, MA, OTR
Associate Professor and
  Chairman
Department of Occupational
  Therapy

1, a   89/90
**Texas Tech University Health
  Sciences Center**
School of Allied Health
Lubbock, TX 79430
Laurence N. Peake, PhD, OTR,
  FAOTA, Chair
Department of Occupational
  Therapy

1, 2, 3, a   92/93
Texas Woman's University
Box 23718, TWU Station
Denton, TX 76204
Grace E. Gilkeson, EdD, OTR,
  FAOTA, Dean
School of Occupational Therapy
Offered: Denton, Dallas, Houston

VIRGINIA

1, 3, a   92/93
**Virginia Commonwealth
  University**
Box 8, MCV Station
Richmond, VA 23298
M. Jeanne Madigan, EdD, OTR,
  FAOTA, Chair
Department of Occupational
  Therapy

WASHINGTON

1, 2, 3, b   86/87
University of Puget Sound
1500 North Warner
Tacoma, WA 98416
Margo B. Holm, PhD, OTR,
  Director
School of Occupational Therapy

1, a   87/88
University of Washington
School of Medicine, Department
  of Rehabilitation Medicine,
  RJ-30
Seattle, WA 98195
Elizabeth M. Kanny, MA, OTR,
  Head
Division of Occupational
  Therapy

WISCONSIN

1, b   87/88
Mount Mary College
2900 North Menomonee River
  Parkway
Milwaukee, WI 53222
Diana Bartels, MS, OTR, Acting
  Chairperson
Occupational Therapy
  Department

1, a   92/93
University of Wisconsin-Madison
1300 University Avenue
Madison, WI 53706
Rita Holstein, MS, OTR,
  Coordinator
Occupational Therapy Program

1, a   88/89
**University of Wisconsin-
  Milwaukee**
School of Allied Health
  Professions
PO Box 413
Milwaukee, WI 53201
Franklin Stein, PhD, OTR,
  Director
Occupational Therapy Program

Developing Professional Programs 1986–1987

The following *entry level* programs are in the developing stage and are not yet accredited by the Committee on Allied Health Education and Accreditation of the American Medical Association in collaboration with the American Occupational Therapy Association. The dates of the academic year for the initial on-site evaluation of the program appear in the listing. For specific information, contact the program directly.

INDIANA

3, b   86/87
University of Indianapolis
1400 East Hanna Avenue
Indianapolis, IN 46227
Zona R. Weeks, PhD, OTR,
   FAOTA, Chairperson
Occupational Therapy Program

MASSACHUSETTS

1, a   87/88
Worcester State College
486 Chandler Street
Worcester, MA 01602-2597
Donna M. Joss, EdD, OTR/L,
   Director
Occupational Therapy Program

NEBRASKA

1, b   86/87
Creighton University
School of Pharmacy and Allied
   Health Professions
Omaha, NE 68178
Patricia A. Gromak, MA, OTR/L,
   Acting Chairperson
Department of Occupational
   Therapy

NEW YORK

4*, b   90/91
D'Youville College
One D'Youville Square
320 Porter Avenue
Buffalo, NY 14201-1084
Linda DiJoseph, MS, OTR,
   FAOTA, Program Director
Occupational Therapy Program
*5-year program

1, b   88/89
Keuka College
Keuka Park, NY 14478-0098
Shirley Zurchauer, MSW, OTR,
   FAOTA
Chair, Division of Special
   Programs
Program in Occupational
   Therapy

Technical Programs 1986–1987

The following *entry level* programs are approved by the American Occupational Therapy Association. On-site evaluations for program approval are conducted at 5-year intervals for initial approval and 7-year intervals for reapproval. The dates on this list indicate the academic year the next evaluation is anticipated. For specific information, contact the program directly.

Key: **1**   Associate degree program   **a**   Public nonprofit
          2   Certificate program   **b**   Private nonprofit

ALABAMA

1, a   90/91
**University of Alabama in
   Birmingham**
Regional Technical Institute,
   Room 114
University Station
Birmingham, AL 35294
Carroline Amari, MA, OTR, ·
   Director
Division of Occupational
   Therapy

COLORADO

1, a   90/91
Pueblo Community College
900 West Orman Avenue
Pueblo, CO 81004
Terry R. Hawkins, MPH, OTR,
   Director
Occupational Therapy Assistant
   Program

CONNECTICUT

1, a   91/92
Manchester Community College
PO Box 1046, MS #19
Manchester, CT 06040
Brenda Smaga, MS, OTR/L,
   Coordinator
Occupational Therapy Assistant
   Program

FLORIDA

1, a   86/87
Palm Beach Junior College
4200 South Congress Avenue
Lake Worth, FL 33461
Sylvia Meeker, MS, OTR,
   Director
Occupational Therapy Assistant
   Program

HAWAII

1, a   92/93
Kapiolani Community College
Allied Health Department
4303 Diamond Head Road
Honolulu, HI 96816
Ann Kadoguchi, OTR, Director
Occupational Therapy Assistant
   Program

ILLINOIS

1, a   92/93
**Chicago City-Wide College/Cook
    County Hospital**
Health Services Institute at Cook
    County Hospital
1900 West Polk Street
Chicago, IL 60612
Susan Kennedy, MS, OTR/L, Pro-
    gram Director
Occupational Therapy Assistant
    Program

1*, a   86/87
Illinois Central College
East Peoria, IL 61635
Javan E. Walker, Jr., MA, OTR/L,
    Director
Occupational Therapy Assistant
    Program
*Does not accept out-of-state
    students

1, a   90/91
Thornton Community College
15800 South State Street
South Holland, IL 60473
Carolyn A. Yoss, OTR,
    Coordinator
Occupational Therapy Assistant
    Program

INDIANA

1, a   88/89
**Indiana University School of
    Medicine**
Division of Allied Health
    Sciences
Coleman Hall—311
1140 West Michigan Street
Indianapolis, IN 46223
Celestine Hamant, MS, OTR,
    FAOTA
Associate Professor and Director
Occupational Therapy

IOWA

1, a   89/90
Kirkwood Community College
PO Box 2068
6301 Kirkwood Boulevard
Cedar Rapids, IA 52406
Mary Ellen Dunford, OTR/L,
    Director
Occupational Therapy Assistant
    Program

KANSAS

1, 2, a   91/92
**Barton County Community
    College**
Great Bends, KS 67530
Judy White, OTR, Director
Occupational Therapy Assistant
    Program

LOUISIANA

1, a   87/88
Northeast Louisiana University
School of Allied Health Services
College of Pharmacy and Health
    Sciences
Monroe, LA 71209
Lee Sens, MA, OTR, Director
Occupational Therapy Assistant
    Program

MASSACHUSETTS

1, b   89/90
Becker Junior College
61 Sever Street
Worcester, MA 01609
Edith C. Fenton, MS, OTR/L,
    Coordinator
Occupational Therapy Assistant
    Program

1, a   87/88
North Shore Community College
3 Essex Street
Beverly, MA 01915
Sophia K. Fowler, L/OTR,
    Director
Occupational Therapy Assistant
    Program

1, 2, a   91/92
**Quinsigamond Community
    College**
670 West Boylston Street
Worcester, MA 01606
Elaine Fallon, MS, OTR,
    Coordinator
Occupational Therapy Assistant
    Program

MICHIGAN

1, a   92/93
Grand Rapids Junior College
143 Bostwick NE
Grand Rapids, MI 49503
Alice A. Donahue, MA, OTR,
    Director
Occupational Therapy Assisting
    Program

1, a   91/92
Schoolcraft College
1751 Radcliffe Street
Garden City, MI 48135-1197
Masline Horton, MS, EdSp, OTR
Professor/Coordinator
Occupational Therapy Assistant
    Program

1, a   87/88
**Wayne County Community
    College**
1001 West Fort Street
Detroit, MI 48226
Doris Y. Witherspoon, MA, OTR,
    Director
Occupational Therapy Assistant
    Program

MINNESOTA

1, a   89/90
**Anoka Vocational Technical
    Institute**
1355 West Main Street
Anoka, MN 55303
Julie Jepsen Thomas, MHE, OTR,
    Director
Occupational Therapy Assistant
    Program

2, a   92/93
**Duluth Area Vocational Techni-
    cal Institute**
2101 Trinity Road
Duluth, MN 55811
Julie A. Halom, OTR, Director
Occupational Therapy Assistant
    Program

1, b   92/93
**St. Mary's Campus of the College
    of St. Catherine**
2500 South Sixth Street
Minneapolis, MN 55454
Louise C. Fawcett, MHS, OTR,
    Director
Occupational Therapy Assistant
    Program

MISSOURI

1, a   90/91
Penn Valley Community College
3201 Southeast Trafficway
Kansas City, MO 64111
Kathryn Duvenci, MA, OTR,
    Director
Occupational Therapy Assistant
    Program

1, a   **89/90**
**St. Louis Community College at
   Meramec**
11333 Big Bend Boulevard
St. Louis, MO 63122
Carol Niman-Reed, MS, OTR,
   Director
Occupational Therapy Assistant
   Program

NEW HAMPSHIRE

1, a   **88/89**
**New Hampshire Vocational-
   Technical College**
Hanover Street Extension
Claremont, NH 03743
Deborah Lord, OTR, Director
Occupational Therapy Assistant
   Program

NEW JERSEY

1, a   **88/89**
Atlantic Community College
Allied Health Division
Mays Landing, NJ 08330
Angela J. Busillo, MEd, OTR,
   Director
Occupational Therapy Assistant
   Program

1, a   **86/87**
Union County College
1700 Raritan Road
Scotch Plains, NJ 07076
Carol Keating, MA, OTR, Pro-
   gram Director
Occupational Therapy Assistant
   Program

NEW YORK

1, a   **88/89**
Erie Community College
Main Street and Youngs Road
Buffalo, NY 14221
Sally Jo Harris, MS, OTR/L,
   Director
Occupational Therapy Assistant
   Program

1, a   **86/87**
**Herkimer County Community
   College**
Herkimer, NY 13350
Brice Kistler, OTR/L, Program
   Director
Occupational Therapy Assistant
   Program

1, a   **90/91**
LaGuardia Community College
31-10 Thomson Avenue
Long Island City, NY 11101
Naomi S. Greenberg, MPH, PhD,
   OTR, FAOTA, Director
Occupational Therapy Assistant
   Program

1, b   **92/93**
Maria College
700 New Scotland Avenue
Albany, NY 12208
Bearldean B. Burke, MA, OTR,
   FAOTA, Coordinator
Occupational Therapy Assistant
   Program

1, b   **87/88**
Maria Regina College
Applied Science Division
1024 Court Street
Syracuse, NY 13208
Sr. Thomas Marie Corcoran, MS,
   OTR, Director
Occupational Therapy Assistant
   Program

1, a   **88/89**
**Orange County Community
   College**
115 South Street
Middletown, NY 10940
Mary Sands, MSEd, OTR, Chair
Occupational Therapy Assistant
   Program

1, a   **92/93**
Rockland Community College
145 College Road
Suffern, NY 10901
Ellen Spergel, MS, OTR, Director
Occupational Therapy Assistant
   Program

NORTH CAROLINA
1, a   **88/89**

**Caldwell Community College
   and Technical Institute**
1000 Hickory Boulevard
Hudson, NC 28638
Lyndon Lackey, OTR/L,
   Coordinator
Occupational Therapy Assistant
   Program

1, a   **87/88**
Stanly Technical College
Route 4, Box 55
Albemarle, NC 28001
Noel S. Levan, MA, OTR, Pro-
   gram Director
Occupational Therapy Assistant
   Program

NORTH DAKOTA

1, a   **86/87**
**North Dakota State School of
   Science**
Wahpeton, ND 58075
Sr. Carolita Mauer, MA, OTR/L,
   Chair
Occupational Therapy Assistant
   Program

OHIO

1, a   **87/88**
Cuyahoga Community College
2900 Community College Avenue
Cleveland, OH 44115
Phyllis Zucker, OTR/L, Program
   Manager
Occupational Therapy Assistant
   Program

1, b   **90/91**
Lourdes College
6832 Convent Boulevard
Sylvania, OH 43560
Jean Thomas, MEd, OTR/L,
   Director
Occupational Therapy Assistant
   Program

1, a   **90/91**
Shawnee State University
940 Second Street
Portsmouth, OH 45662
Valerie J. Kramer, OTR, Program
   Director
Occupational Therapy Assistant
   Program

1, a   **89/90**
Stark Technical College
6200 Frank Avenue, NW
Canton, OH 44720
Johannes Kicken, MS, OTR,
   Director
Occupational Therapy Assistant
   Program

OKLAHOMA

1, a   **87/88**
**Oklahoma City Community
   College**
7777 South May Avenue
Oklahoma City, OK 73159
Margaret F. Roseboom, OTR,
   Coordinator
Occupational Therapy-
   Therapeutic Recreation Tech-
   nician Program

OREGON

1, a   **88/89**
Mount Hood Community College
26000 SE Stark Street
Gresham, OR 97030
Chris Hencinski, OTR,
    Coordinator
Occupational Therapy Assistant
    Program

PENNSYLVANIA

1, a   **89/90**
Community College of Allegheny
    County
Boyce Campus
595 Beatty Road
Monroeville, PA 15146
Richard L. Allison, MS, OTR/L,
    Director
Occupational Therapy Assistant
    Program

1, b   **91/92**
Harcum Junior College
Bryn Mawr, PA 19010
Jerald P. Stowell, MPH, OTR,
    Director
Occupational Therapy Assistant
    Program

1, a   **87/88**
Lehigh County Community
    College
2370 Main Street
Schnecksville, PA 18078
Haru Hirama, EdD, OTR,
    Coordinator
Occupational Therapy Assistant
    Program

1, b   **91/92**
Mount Aloysius Junior College
Cresson, PA 16630
Patricia Marvin, MA, OTR/L,
    Chair
Occupational Therapy Assistant
    Program

PUERTO RICO

1, a   **89/90**
Humacao University College
CUH Postal Station
Humacao, PR 00661
Milagros Marrero-Diaz, MPH,
    OTR, Program Director
Occupational Therapy Program

1, a   **91/92**
Ponce Technological University
    College
University of Puerto Rico
PO Box 7186
Ponce, PR 00732
Ana V. Ferran, PhD, OTR,
    Coordinator
Occupational Therapy Assistant
    Program

TENNESSEE

1, a   **92/93**
Nashville State Technical
    Institute
120 White Bridge Road
Nashville, TN 37209
Anne Drury, MS, OTR, Program
    Director
Occupational Therapy Assistant
    Program

TEXAS

2, a   **87/88**
Academy of Health Sciences,
    U.S. Army
Medicine & Surgery Division
Fort Sam Houston, TX 78234-
    6100
LTC Leah Palm, MA, OTR, Chief
Occupational Therapy Branch
(Limited to enlisted personnel in
    army and air force)

1, a   **89/90**
Austin Community College
Riverside Campus
5712 E. Riverside Drive
Austin, TX 78741
Martha Sue Carrell, OTR, Depart-
    ment Head
Occupational Therapy Assistant
    Program

2, a   **86/87**
Houston Community College
3100 Shenandoah
Houston, TX 77021
Linda Williams, MA, OTR,
    Coordinator
Occupational Therapy Assistant
    Program

1, a   **92/93**
St. Philip's College
2111 Nevada Street
San Antonio, TX 78203
Jana Cragg, OTR, Program
    Coordinator
Occupational Therapy Assistant
    Program

WASHINGTON

1, a   **89/90**
Green River Community College
12401 SE 320th Street
Auburn, WA 98002
Susan Noel Hepler, OTR/L
Acting Program Coordinator
Occupational Therapy Assistant
    Program

WISCONSIN

1, a   **86/87**
Fox Valley Technical Institute
1825 North Bluemound Drive
PO Box 2277
Appleton, WI 54913
Thomas H. Kraft, MEd, OTR,
    Coordinator
Occupational Therapy Assistant
    Program

1, a   **88/89**
Madison Area Technical Col-
    lege—TRUAX
Downtown Campus
3550 Anderson Street
Madison, WI 53704-2599
Toni Walski, MS, OTR, Director
Occupational Therapy Assistant
    Program

1, a   **87/88**
Milwaukee Area Technical
    College
1015 North 6th Street
Milwaukee, WI 53203
Suzanne L. Brown, MS, OTR,
    Coordinator
Occupational Therapy Assistant
    Program

Developing Technical Programs 1986–1987

The following *entry level* programs are in the developing stage and are not yet approved by the American Occupational Therapy Association. The dates of the academic year for the initial on-site evaluation of the program appear in the listing. For specific information, contact the program directly.

CALIFORNIA

2, a   88/89
North Santa Clara County
    Regional Occupational
    Program
1188 Wunderlich Drive
San Jose, CA 95129
Peg Bledsoe, MA, OTR, Acting
    Director
Occupational Therapy Assistant
    Program

GEORGIA

1, a   86/87
►**Medical College of Georgia**
School of Allied Health Sciences
Augusta, GA 30912
Nancy Prendergast, EdD, OTR/L,
    FAOTA, Chair
Department of Occupational
    Therapy

ILLINOIS

1, a   86/87
Parkland College
2400 West Bradley Avenue
Champaign, IL 61821-1899
Carol Ruch, OTR/L, Coordinator
Occupational Therapy Assistant
    Program

MARYLAND

1, a   86/87
Catonsville Community College
800 South Rolling Road
Baltimore, MD 21228
Judith Davis, MS, OTR,
    Coordinator
Occupational Therapy Assistant
    Program

MASSACHUSETTS

1, b   86/87
Mount Ida College
Junior College Division
777 Dedham Street
Newton Centre, MA 02159
Heather Moulton, OTR/L,
    Director
Occupational Therapy Assistant
    Program

MINNESOTA

1, a   87/88
Austin Community College
1600 8th Avenue, N.W.
Austin, MN 55912
Thomas H. Dillon, MA, OTR/L,
    Program Director
Occupational Therapy Assistant
    Program

OHIO

1, a   87/88
Cincinnati Technical College
3520 Central Parkway
Cincinnati, OH 45223
Joanne Phillips-Estes, OTR,
    Program Director
Occupational Therapy Assistant
    Program

PENNSYLVANIA

1, a   87/88
Williamsport Area Community
    College
1005 West Third Street
Williamsport, PA 17701-5799
Barbara N. Sims, OTR/L, Program
    Coordinator
Occupational Therapy Assistant
    Program

WASHINGTON

1, a   88/89
Yakima Valley Community
    College
Sixteenth Avenue and Nob Hill
    Boulevard
PO Box 1647
Yakima, WA 98907
Margaret Bryant, OTR, Acting
    Program Director
Occupational Therapy Assistant
    Program

Principles of Occupational Therapy Ethics

PREAMBLE

The American Occupational Therapy Association (AOTA) and its component members are committed to furthering man's ability to function fully within his total environment. To this end the occupational therapist renders service to clients in all stages of health and illness, to institutions, other professionals, colleagues, students and to the general public.

In furthering this commitment the American Occupational Therapy Association has established the Principles of Occupational Therapy Ethics. The Principles are intended for use by all occupational therapy personnel, including practitioners in all settings, administrators, educators, and students. Licensure laws and regulations should reflect and support these Principles which are intended to be action oriented, guiding and preventive rather than negative or merely disciplinary. The Principles, likewise, should influence the consulting, planning, and teaching of occupational therapists.

It should be noted that these Principles are intended only for internal use by the American Occupational Therapy Association as a guide to appropriate conduct of its members. The Principles are not intended to define a standard of care for patients or clients of a particular community.

Professional maturity will be demonstrated in applying these basic Principles while exercising the large measure of freedom which they provide and which is essential to responsible and creative occupational therapy service.

For the purpose of continuity the following definitions will support information in this document: Occupational therapist includes registered occupational therapists, certified occupational therapy assistants, occupational therapy students; clients include patients, students, and those to whom occupational therapy services are delivered.

I RELATED TO THE RECIPIENT OF SERVICE

The occupational therapist demonstrates a beneficent concern for the recipient of services and maintains a goal-directed relationship with the recipient which furthers the objectives for which it is established. Services are evaluated against objectives and accountability is maintained therefore. Respect shall be shown for the recipients' rights and the occupational therapist will preserve the confidence of the client relationship.

Guidelines: Recipients of occupational therapy services refer to clients, patients, students and the employers of occupational therapists, i.e., agencies, facilities, institutions, etc.

It is the professional responsibility of occupational therapists to provide services for clients without regard to race, creed, national origin, sex, handicap or religious affiliation. Occupational therapists recognize each client's individuality and worth as a unique person.

Services provided should be planned in concert with clients' involvement in goal-directed activities, in accordance with the overall habilitation or rehabilitation plan. Treatment objectives and the therapeutic process must be measurable to insure professional accountability.

Clients' and students' rights are to be protected as stipulated in the Federal Privacy Act of 1974, in addition to any specified rules, regulations or procedures as may be required by the employer.

The financial gain of occupational therapists should never be paramount to the delivery of services. Those occupational therapists who are compensated by virtue of being a direct service provider or vendor have the right to assess reasonable fees for profit.

Occupational therapists are obligated to provide the highest quality of service to the recipient. If further services would be beneficial to the client, the referring practitioner should be informed. It is also incumbent upon occupational therapists to recommend termination of services when established goals have been met, or when further services would not produce improved recipient performance.

Occupational therapy educators are obligated to provide the highest quality educational services supporting the AOTA "Essentials" and the current theory that supports service delivery.

II. RELATED TO COMPETENCE

The occupational therapist shall actively maintain and improve one's professional competence, represent it accurately, and function within its parameters.

Guidelines: Occupational therapists recognize the need for continuing education and where relevant, they obtain training, experience, self-study or counsel to assure competent occupational therapy services.

Occupational therapists accurately represent their competence, education, training, and experience. Occupational therapists must accurately represent their skills and should not provide services or instructions, either for pay or in a voluntary capacity, that are not within their demonstrated competencies.

Occupational therapists must recognize the skills necessary to manage a client or a position. If client needs exist that the therapist cannot effectively manage, the therapist should seek consultation or refer the client to an occupational therapist or another professional who can provide the required service.

III. RELATED TO RECORDS, REPORTS, GRADES AND RECOMMENDATIONS

The occupational therapist shall conform to local, state and federal laws and regulations, and regulations applicable to records and reports. The occupational therapist abides by the employing institution's rules. Objective data shall govern subjective data in evaluations, grades, recommendations, records and reports.

Guidelines: Occupational therapists realize that reports are a required function of any position. Occupational therapists accurately record information and report information as required by AOTA standards, facility standards and state and national laws.

Occupational therapists fulfilling a teaching role utilize objective data in determining student grades.

All data recorded in permanent files or records should be supported by the occupational therapist's observations or by objective measures of data collection.

Students' records can only be divulged as authorized by law or the students' consent for release of information.

IV. RELATED TO INTRA-PROFESSIONAL COLLEAGUES

The occupational therapist shall function with discretion and integrity in relations with other members of the profession and shall be concerned with the quality of their services. Upon becoming aware of objective evidence of a breach of ethics or substandard service, the occupational therapist shall take action according to established procedure.

Guidelines: Information gained or data gathered on a client shall only be divulged as expedient to other professional colleagues, students, referring practitioner, and employer. This includes data used in the course of in-service programs, professional meetings, prepared papers for presentation or publication, and educational materials. Undue invasion of privacy should be of utmost concern. Any reference to quality or service rendered by, or the integrity of a professional colleague will be expressed with due care to protect the reputation of that person.

It is the obligation of occupational therapists with first-hand knowledge of a breach of the ethical principles of this Association, by a colleague or student, to attempt to rectify the situation. If informal attempts fail, such activities or incidents against the ethical principles of this Association, should immediately be brought to the attention of the appropriate local, regional or national Association committee/commission on ethical standards.

Designated procedures should be followed and at all times the confidentiality of the information must be respected to protect the alleged party.

Practices by an employer which are in conflict with the ethical principles of this Association, should also be brought to the immediate attention of the appropriate body(ies).

Information gained in peer review procedures should be held within the realm of confidentiality and be dealt with according to established procedures.

Publication credit for material developed by colleagues must be given. Also, credit for materials used in the classroom, manuals, in-service training, and oral or written reports, for example, should acknowledge the name of the individual or group who developed the material.

V. RELATED TO OTHER PERSONNEL

The occupational therapist shall function with discretion and integrity in relations with personnel and cooperate with them as may be appropriate. Similarly, the occupational therapist expects others to demonstrate a high level of competence. Upon becoming aware of objective evidence of a breach of ethics or substandard service, the occupational therapist shall take action according to established procedure.

Guidelines: Occupational therapists understand the scope of education and practice of related professions, and make full use of all the professional, technical and administrative resources that best serve the interests of consumers.

Occupational therapists do not delegate to other personnel those client related services where the clinical skills and expertise of an occupational therapist is required. Other personnel or students may support treatment or educational goals, but must have demonstrated competency in each aspect of service to the occupational therapist before the responsibility can be delegated.

Occupational therapists who employ or supervise other professionals or technicians, or professionals or technicians in training, accept the obligation to facilitate their further development by providing suitable working conditions, consultation and experience opportunities.

Occupational therapists protect the privacy of all persons with whom professional collaboration occurs. If, however, an occupational therapist has first-hand knowledge of a colleague's performance which is in conflict with ethical standards, the therapist shall attempt to rectify the situation. Failing an informal solution, the occupational therapist shall utilize procedures established within the facility or agency, or to call the behavior to the attention of management, or utilize procedures established by the profession to handle such situations. Under no circumstances should the occupational therapist remain silent when a client, student or facility's status is in jeopardy.

VI. RELATED TO EMPLOYERS AND PAYERS

The occupational therapist shall render service with discretion and integrity and shall protect the property and property rights of the employers and payers.

Guidelines: Occupational therapists function within the parameter of the job description or the goals established mutually between the employer or agency, and the occupational therapist. Occupational therapists use the utmost integrity in all dealings with the facility, university/college or contracting agency. Established procedures are followed regarding purchasing and bids.

Occupational therapists recommend appropriate fees for services and gain necessary acceptance for fees from the facility, agency and payers. Fees must be based upon cost analysis or a factor that can be justified upon request.

Occupational therapists shall not use the property, such as supplies and equipment, of the employer for their own personal use and aggrandizement.

VII. Related to Education

The occupational therapist implements a commitment to the education of society and the consumer of health services as well as to the education of health personnel on matters of health which are within the purview of occupational therapy.

Guidelines: Occupational therapists do not only provide direct service to alleviate specific problems with clients, programs or a community, but in addition, include education of all phases of services which can be provided to the public. This should include education of situations and conditions for which the competency of occupational therapists is recognized to assist in alleviating barriers limiting a person's ability to function socially, emotionally, cognitively or physically.

The public includes not only individuals concerned with the well-being of a member of their family, but also federal, state and local governmental agencies, educational systems and social agencies dealing with the health and well-being of the public.

VIII. RELATED TO EVALUATION AND RESEARCH

Occupational therapists shall accept responsibility for evaluating, developing and refining service and the body of knowledge and skills which underlie the education and practice of occupational therapy and at all times protects the rights of subjects, clients, institutions and collaborators. The work of others shall be acknowledged.

Guidelines: Clients' families have the right to have, and occupational therapists have the responsibility to provide explanations of the nature, the purposes, and results of the occupational therapy services unless, as in some employment or treatment settings, there is an explicit exception to this right agreed upon in advance.

In reporting test results, occupational therapists indicate any reservations regarding validity or reliability resulting from testing circumstances or inappropriateness of the test norms for the person tested.

In performing research and reporting research results, occupational therapists must use accepted scientific methodology.

IX. RELATED TO THE PROFESSION

The occupational therapist shall be responsible for gaining information and understanding of the principles, policies and standards of the profession. The occupational therapist functions as a representative of the profession.

Guidelines: Occupational therapists should provide accurate information to the public about the profession and the services that can be provided. Occupational therapists should remain informed about changes in the profession and represent the profession accurately to the consumer.

Occupational therapists should conduct themselves in a manner befitting professionals. The profession is judged in part by the conduct of its members as they carry out their functions.

Occupational therapists should show support and loyalty to the Association by cooperating with the Representatives in collecting information regarding proposed Association policy, replying to official requests for information and supporting

the policies of the Association. It is the member's duty if he disagrees with an Association policy to work through existing channels to effect change.

Occupational therapists who engage in work or volunteer activities in addition to professional occupational therapy responsibilities, shall not violate the ethical principles of the Association in such activities.

X. RELATED TO ADVERTISING

Advertising by therapists under their professional title shall be in accordance with propriety and precedent in health professions.

Guidelines: Occupational therapists may provide information to the public about available services through procedures established by the employing facility or contracting agency. If an occupational therapist provides an independent service, it is appropriate to advertise those services.

The occupational therapist shall not use, or participate in the use of, any form of communication containing a false, fraudulent, misleading, deceptive, self-laudatory or unfair statement or claim. Testimonials or statements which promise a favorable result shall be avoided.

XI. RELATED TO LAW AND REGULATIONS

The occupational therapist shall seek to acquire information about applicable local, state, federal and institutional rules and shall function accordingly thereto.

Guidelines: Occupational therapists are obligated to function professionally as a practitioner within the limits of all laws related to the delivery of health services, and applicable to the practice of occupational therapy. Occupational therapists will not engage in any cruel, inhumane or degrading practices in the treatment of clients or in the education of students, or in supervision of others or in peer relationships with other individuals.

It is the responsibility of occupational therapists to make known to their employers, employees and colleagues, those laws applicable to the practice of occupational therapy and education of occupational therapists.

XII. RELATED TO MISCONDUCT

The occupational therapist shall not appear to act with impropriety nor engage in illegal conduct involving moral turpitude and will not circumvent the principles of occupational therapy ethics through actions of another.

Guidelines: As employees, occupational therapists refuse to participate in practices inconsistent with legal, moral and ethical standards regarding the treatment of employees or the public. For example, occupational therapists will not condone practices that are inhumane, or that result in illegal or otherwise unjustifiable discrimination on the basis of race, age, sex, religion, handicap or national origin in hiring, promotion or training.

In providing occupational therapy services, occupational therapists avoid any action that will violate or diminish the legal and civil rights of clients or of others who may be affected.

As practitioners and educators, occu-

pational therapists keep abreast of relevant federal, state, local and agency regulations and American Occupational Therapy Association Standards of Practice and education essentials concerning the conduct of their practice. They are concerned with developing such legal and quasi-legal regulations that support the interests of the public, students and the profession.

XIII. RELATED TO BIOETHICAL ISSUES AND PROBLEMS OF SOCIETY

The occupational therapist seeks information about the major health problems and issues to learn their implications for occupational therapy and for one's own services.

Guidelines: The principle is a philosophical statement that encourages occupational therapists to be global in their views of health in relationship to society.

Enforcement Procedures are available from the Division of Practice, 1383 Piccard Drive, Rockville, MD 20850. Complaints should be addressed to the Standards and Ethics Chair, 1383 Piccard Drive, Rockville, MD 20850.

Approved, April 1977

Approved, revised, April 1979

Reference: AOTA: Principles of Occupational Therapy Ethics. *Am J Occup Ther* 38(12):799–802, 1984

Appendix D

Standards of Practice for Occupational Therapy

PREFACE

These standards will assist the AOTA members in the management of occupational therapy services and will serve as a minimum standard for occupational therapy practice that is applicable to all client populations and the programs in which clients are served.

These standards are for qualified occupational therapists (OTRs) that are currently certified or licensed where required by the state.

STANDARD I: SCREENING

1. Occupational therapists have the responsibility to identify clients who may present problems in occupational performance (work, self-care, and play/leisure) that would require an evaluation.

2. Occupational therapists screen independently or as members of a team.

3. Screening methods shall be appropriate to the client's age, education, cultural background, medical status, and functional ability.

4. Screening methods may include interview, observation, testing and record review.

5. Occupational therapists shall communicate the screening results and recommendations to all appropriate individuals.

STANDARD II: REFERRAL

1. A client is appropriately referred to occupational therapy for remediation, maintenance, or prevention when the client has, or appears to have, a dysfunction or potential for dysfunction in occupational performance (work, self-care, play/leisure) or the performance components (sensorimotor, cognitive, psychosocial).

2. Clients shall be referred to occupational therapy for evaluation, design construction of, or training in therapeutic adaptations that include, but are not limited to, the physical environment, orthotics, prosthetics, and assistive and adaptive equipment.

3. Occupational therapists respond to a request for service and enter a case at their own professional discretion and on their own recognizance, and then assume full responsibility for the determination of the appropriate type, nature, and mode of service.

4. When physician referral is necessary to meet regulations (facility, state, federal, Joint Commission for Accreditation of Hospitals, licensure) or is required for third-party payment, the registered

occupational therapist enters a case at the request of a physician; assumes full responsibility for the occupational therapy assessment; and, in consultation with the physician, establishes the appropriate type, nature, and mode of service.

5. Registered occupational therapists shall refer clients to other appropriate resources when, in the judgment of the occupational therapist, the knowledge and expertise of another professional is required.

6. Occupational therapists have the responsibility to teach appropriate persons how to make occupational therapy referrals.

STANDARD III: EVALUATION

1. Occupational therapists shall evaluate the client's performance according to the Uniform Occupational Therapy Checklist (AOTA-Adopted, 1981).

2. Initial occupational therapy evaluations shall consider the client's medical, vocational, educational, activity, social history, and personal/family goals.

3. The occupational therapy evaluation shall include assessment of the functional abilities and deficits as related to the client's needs in the following areas:

   a. Occupational Performance: work, self-care, and play/leisure.

   b. Performance Components: sensorimotor, cognitive, psychosocial.

   c. Therapeutic adaptations and prevention.

4. Initial occupational therapy evaluations shall be completed and results documented within the time frames established by facilities, government agencies, and accreditation programs.

5. All evaluation methods shall be appropriate to the client's age, education, cultural and ethnic background, medical status, and functional ability.

6. The evaluation methods may include observation, interview, record review, and the use of evaluation techniques or tools.

7. When standardized evaluation tools are used, the tests should have normative data for the client characteristics. If normative data are not available, the results should be expressed in a descriptive report.

8. Collected evaluation data shall be analyzed and summarized to indicate the client's current status.

9. Occupational therapists shall document evaluation results in the client's record and indicate the specific evaluation tools and methods used.

10. Occupational therapists shall communicate evaluation results to the appropriate persons in the facility and community.

11. If the results of the evaluation indicate areas that require intervention by other professionals, the occupational therapist should refer the client to the appropriate service or request consultation.

STANDARD IV: INDIVIDUAL PROGRAM PLANNING

1. Occupational therapists shall use the results of the evaluation to develop an individual occupational therapy program that is:

   a. Stated in measurable and reasonable terms appropriate to the client's needs and goals and expected prognosis.

   b. Consistent with current principles and concepts of occupational therapy theory and practice.

2. The planning process shall include:

   a. Identifying short- and long-term goals.

   b. Collaborating with client, family, other professionals, and community resources.

   c. Selecting the media, methods, environment, and personnel needed to accomplish goals.

d. Determining the frequency and duration of occupational therapy services.

3. The initial program plan shall be prepared and documented within the time frames established by facilities, government agencies, and accreditation programs.

STANDARD V: INDIVIDUAL PROGRAM IMPLEMENTATION

1. Occupational therapists shall implement the program according to the program plan.

2. Occupational therapists shall formulate and implement program modifications consistent with changes in the client's occupational performance and performance components.

3. Occupational therapists shall periodically re-evaluate and document the client's occupational performance and performance components.

4. Occupational therapists shall document the occupational therapy services provided and the frequency of the services within time frames established by facilities, government agencies, and accreditation programs.

STANDARD VI: DISCONTINUATION OF SERVICES

1. Occupational therapists shall discontinue services when the client has achieved the goals or has achieved maximum benefit from occupational therapy.

2. Occupational therapists shall document the comparison of the initial and current state of functional abilities and deficits in occupational performance and performance components.

3. Occupational therapists shall prepare a discharge plan that is consistent with the occupational therapy, client, interdisciplinary team, family and goals, and the expected prognosis. Consideration should be given to appropriate community resources for referral and environmental factors or barriers that may need modification.

4. Occupational therapists shall allow sufficient time for the coordination of and the effective implementation of the discharge plan.

5. Occupational therapists shall document recommendations for follow-up or re-evaluation.

STANDARD VII: QUALITY ASSURANCE

1. The occupational therapist shall periodically and systematically review all aspects of individual occupational therapy programs for effectiveness and efficiency.

2. Occupational therapists shall periodically and systematically review the quality and appropriateness of total services delivered, using predetermined criteria that reflect professional consensus and recent development in research and theory.

STANDARD VIII: INDIRECT SERVICES

1. Occupational therapists shall provide supervision of other personnel as assigned in accordance with the AOTA Guide for Supervision (AOTA-Adopted, 1981).

2. Occupational therapists shall maintain records to meet facility, government agency, and accreditation program requirements.

3. Occupational therapists shall maintain a level of professional knowledge and skills to assure continued competency.

4. Occupational therapists shall facilitate research as it applies to the active practice of occupational therapy.

5. Occupational therapists shall provide administration and management services that ensure the use of AOTA standards.

6. Occupational therapists shall provide consultation services in order to develop or coordinate occupational therapy services, provide in-service education, adapt environments, and promote preventive health care in the home, client care facility, or community.

STANDARD IX: LEGAL/ETHICAL COMPONENTS

1. Occupational therapists shall maintain current AOTA certification or licensure where required by the state.
2. Occupational therapists shall practice and manage occupational therapy programs as defined by federal and state laws and regulations.
3. Occupational therapists shall be familiar with and abide by the ethical practices of the specific facility or system in which the service is provided.
4. Occupational therapists shall observe the ethical practices as defined by The American Occupational Therapy Association, Inc., *Principles of Ethics* (AOTA, Revised 1980).
5. Occupational therapists shall provide all aspects of direct and indirect services according to Standards and Policies of The American Occupational Therapy Association, Inc.

GLOSSARY*

Occupational Therapy Assessment: the process of determining the need for, nature of, and estimated time of treatment, determining the needed coordination with other persons involved, and documenting these activities.

EVALUATION: the process of obtaining and interpreting data necessary for treatment. This includes planning for and documenting the evaluation process and results. These data may be gathered through record review, specific observation, interview, and the administration of data collection procedures. Such procedures include, but are not limited to, the use of standardized tests, performance checklists, and activities and tasks designed to evaluate specific performance abilities.

MAINTENANCE OF FUNCTION: the process of preserving and supporting an individual's current abilities to engage in interpersonal relationships and to manipulate the non-human environment.

OCCUPATIONAL PERFORMANCE: life tasks (self-care, work, play/leisure) that are all those activities that individuals must perform to meet their own needs and to be contributing members of the community.

PERFORMANCE COMPONENTS: the skill areas (sensorimotor, cognitive, psychosocial) a person develops to facilitate carrying out self-care, work and play/leisure.

PROGRAM PLANNING: the development of an individual client's treatment plan.

SCREENING: the review of the potential client's case to determine the need for evaluation and treatment.

THERAPEUTIC ADAPTATIONS: the design and restructuring of the physical environment to assist self-care, work, and play/leisure performance. This includes selecting, obtaining, fitting, and fabricating equipment, and instructing the client, family, and staff in proper use and care of equipment. It also includes minor repair and modification for correct fit, position, or use. Categories of therapeutic adaptations consist of: orthotics, prosthetics, and assistive and adaptive equipment.

compiled by:

Doris J. Shriver, OTR
Mary Foto, OTR
Members, AOTA Commission on Practice

for

AOTA Commission on Practice
John Farace, OTR, Chair

Approved by the Representative Assembly, April 1983

*Uniform Terminology for Reporting Occupational Therapy Services, adopted March 1979 by The Representative Assembly, AOTA.

Reference: AOTA: Generic Standards of Practice for Occupational Therapy. *Am J Occup Ther* 37(12):802–804, 1983.

Uniform Occupational Therapy Evaluation Checklist

APPLICATION

The following Uniform Occupational Therapy Evaluation Checklist is designed as a generic occupational therapy guide for baseline data gathering. In order to use this checklist, each therapist will need to select the specific method of evaluation to be utilized. Data may be gathered through such means as suggested in the *Uniform Terminology System for Reporting Occupational Therapy Services*. For example, record, review, specific observation, interview and the administration of data collecting procedures. Such data collecting procedures include, but are not limited to, use of standardized tests, performance checklists and activities designed to evaluate specific performance abilities. The occupational therapist should use evaluation procedures that reflect the philosophical base of occupational therapy.

Occupational therapists need to thoroughly understand how to use the Uniform Occupational Therapy Evaluation Checklist. The therapist should:

1. compare/overview the client in all areas.
2. determine areas that require specific tests
3. select specific tests (for example, client may not need Activities of Daily Living, but only tests for sensory integration function; this must be stated in the report),
4. report on all major categories (I: A,B,C—II: A,B,C,D,E,F) even though all subcategories may not apply,
5. document the type of evaluation used (i.e., record, review, standard tests, etc.).

Procedure

I. *Demographic Information*
  A. Personal Information
    1. Name
    2. Address
    3. Telephone
    4. Date of Birth
    5. Age
    6. Sex
  B. Referral-Related Information
    1. Date of Referral
    2. Reason for Referral
    3. Referral Source
    4. Date client first seen by Occupational Therapist
    5. Diagnosis
    6. Presenting Problems/ Symptoms
    7. Date of Onset
    8. Medications
    9. Precautions/Complications

10. Date of Evaluation
11. Evaluator
C. Personal History
1. Developmental History
2. Educational History
3. Vocational History
4. Socio-economic History
5. Medical History

II. *Skills and Performance Areas* (1)
(See the AOTA *Uniform Terminology System for Reporting Occupational Therapy Services*, January 1979, for definition of categories. **Note:** Published as a pullout in the November 1981 issue of the *Occupational Therapy Newspaper*.

A. Independent Living/Daily Living Skills and Performance
Physical Daily Living Skills
a. Grooming and Hygiene
b. Feeding/Eating
c. Dressing
d. Functional Mobility
e. Functional Communication
f. Object Manipulation
2. Psychological/Emotional Daily Living Skills
a. Self-concept/self-identity
b. Situational Coping
c. Community Involvement
3. Work
a. Homemaking
b. Child Care/Parenting
c. Employment Preparation
4. Play/Leisure
B. Sensorimotor Skills and Performance Components
1. Neuromuscular
a. Reflex Integration
b. Range of Motion
c. Gross and Fine Coordination
d. Strength and Endurance
2. Sensory Integration
a. Sensory Awareness
b. Visual-Spatial Awareness
c. Body Integration

C. Cognitive Skill and Performance Components
1. Orientation
2. Conceptualization/Comprehension
a. Concentration
b. Attention span
c. Memory
3. Cognitive Integration
a. Generalization
b. Problem solving
D. Psychosocial Skills and Performance Components
1. Self-Management
a. Self-Expression
b. Self-Control
2. Dyadic Interaction
3. Group Interaction
E. Therapeutic Adaptation
1. Orthotics
2. Prosthetics
3. Assistive/Adaptive Equipment
F. Prevention
1. Energy Conservation
2. Joint Protection/Body Mechanics
3. Positioning
4. Coordination of Daily Living Skills
1. This Outline was taken and adapted from the AOTA *Uniform Terminology System for Reporting Occupational Therapy Services*, prepared by AOTA Commission on Uniform Reporting System Task Force, Rockville, MD, AOTA, January 17, 1979.

By Doris Shriver, OTR, Task Force Chair; Maralynne Mitcham, M.H.E., OTR; Sharon Schwartzberg, Ph.D., OTR; Mary-Helen Ranucci, OTR.

In collaboration with:
Barbara Bath, OTR
Mari Lynn Werner, OTR
Susan Hydle, OTR
Julia Zanon, OTR

For the AOTA Commission on Practice, John Farace, OTR, Chair

Adopted March 1981 by the Representative Assembly, AOTA

REFERENCE

AOTA: Uniform Occupational Therapy Evaluation
Checklist, Rm. J. Occup. Ther. 35(12): 817–
818, 1981.

Index

Grandview

Penny Petro

453-4000